AF787920

The Intertrochanteric Osteotomy

Edited by J. Schatzker

Contributors

J. Aronson R. Bombelli R. Feinstein J. Holder
E. Morscher M.E. Müller F. Pauwels J. Schatzker
R. Schneider H. Wagner

With 204 Figures

Springer-Verlag
Berlin Heidelberg New York Tokyo 1984

JOSEPH SCHATZKER, M.D., F.R.C.S. (C)
Professor of Orthopaedic Surgery
110 Crescent Road
Toronto, Ontario, M4W 1T5/Canada

ISBN 978-3-642-68054-0 ISBN 978-3-642-68052-6 (eBook)
DOI 10.1007/978-3-642-68052-6

Library of Congress Cataloging in Publication Data. Main entry under title: The intertrochanteric osteotomy. Includes index. 1. Femur neck – Surgery. 2. Osteotomy. 3. Osteoarthritis – Surgery. 4. Hip joint – Surgery. I. Schatzker, J. (Joseph), 1934-. [DNLM: 1. Osteoarthritis – surgery. 2. Osteotomy – methods. 3. Hip joint – surgery. 4. Femur Head Necrosis – surgery. WE 860 I61] RD549.I58 1984 617'.582 84-13836. ISBN-13:978-3-642-68054-0 (U.S.)

This work is subject to copyright. All rights are reserved, whether the whole or part of the material is concerned, specifically those of translation, reprinting, re-use of illustrations, broadcasting, reproduction by photocopying machine or similar means, and storage in data banks.

Under § 54 of the German Copyright Law, where copies are made for other than private use, a fee is payable to "Verwertungsgesellschaft Wort", Munich.

© by Springer-Verlag Berlin · Heidelberg 1984

Softcover reprint of the hardcover 1st edition 1984

The use of registered names, trademarks, etc. in this publication does not imply, even in the absence of a specific statement, that such names are exempt from the relevant protective laws and regulations and therefore free for general use.

Product Liability: The publisher can give no guarantee for information about drug dosage and application thereof contained in this book. In every individual case the respective user must check its accuracy by consulting other pharmaceutical literature.

2124/3130-543210

Contents

Contents

Contributors

Prof. J. Aronson
University Arkansas Hospitals
Little Rock, Ark., U.S.A.

Proff. Dott. R. Bombelli
L.D. Clinica Ortopedica
Primario Ortopedico Ospedale Di Circolo
I-21052 Busto Arsizio

Dr. R. Feinstein
Orthopädische Universitätsklinik
Felix-Platter-Spital
Burgfelderstr. 101
CH-4055 Basel

Dr. J. Holder
Orthopädische Klinik Wichernhaus, Krankenhaus Rummelsberg
D-8501 Schwarzenbruck/Nürnberg

Prof. Dr. E. Morscher
Orthopädische Universitätsklinik
Felix-Platter-Spital
Burgfelderstr. 101
CH-4055 Basel

Prof. Dr. M.E. Müller
Stiftung M.E. Müller
Murtenstr. 35
CH-3001 Bern

Prof. Dr. F. Pauwels †
Zweiweiherweg 3
D-5100 Aachen

J. Schatzker, M.D., F.R.C.S. (C)
Professor of Orthopaedic Surgery
University of Toronto
110 Crescent Road
Toronto, Ontario, M4W 1T5, Canada

Prof. Dr. R. Schneider
Alpenstr. 15
CH-2502 Biel

Prof. Dr. H. Wagner
Orthopädische Klinik Wichernhaus, Krankenhaus Rummelsberg
D-8501 Schwarzenbruck/Nürnberg

Introduction

J. Schatzker

Friedrich Pauwels first postulated that excessive joint pressure could cause the destruction of articular cartilage and lead to osteoarthritis, and that the reduction of this pressure would bring about regeneration of articular cartilage and regression of the disease. The first chapter of this book is a synthesis of Pauwels' lifelong devotion to the biomechanics of the hip. It presents the reader with a clear exposition of the intertrochanteric osteotomy as a procedure based on clear biomechanical principles, and illustrates how biomechanical regeneration of the joint can be influenced by a reversal of the mechanical causes. Although some of the views expressed by Pauwels are no longer valid, the chapter has great historic significance.

Renato Bombelli has expanded Pauwels' two-dimensional concept to a three-dimensional one. His text is lucid and beautifully illustrated. Drawing on his wide range of experience and profound grasp of pathomechanics of deformity and disease process, he not only defines for us precisely the indications for both varus and valgus osteotomy, but also provides us with a biomechanical classification of arthritis which will be most helpful in treatment.

Robert Schneider discusses the preoperative selection of patients and describes the evaluation of the arthritic joint through functional X-rays, as well as the techniques of the various intertrochanteric osteotomies using the fixed angle plates of Maurice E. Müller and following the principles of stable internal fixation as practised by the AO/ASIF group. His conclusions are based on a series of 786 intertrochanteric osteotomies and in particular on a group of 109 osteotomies followed up for 13–15 years after surgery.

Erwin Morscher supports the long-term results of Bombelli and Schneider in his analysis of a study of over 2,000 osteotomies performed in several Swiss centers.

He also presents a careful analysis of his own smaller series. Based on all these data, he defines for us the ideal parameters which should be present in order to make the patient an ideal candidate for an intertrochanteric osteotomy.

Heinz Wagner and J. Holder address the problem of the insertion of the abductors in the greater trochanter and evaluate the role it plays in the pathogenesis and treatment of osteoarthritis. The clarity of their presentation is marred somewhat by the combination of the trochanteric osteotomy with other reconstructive procedures which makes it impossible in a number of their cases to define clearly the advantages of the procedure.

In a brilliant chapter, Maurice E. Müller focuses on the success of intertrochanteric osteotomy in the treatment of conditions which would inevitably progress to osteoarthritis if left untreated.

This volume will prove invaluable to the surgeon concerned with the preservation of the hip joint and seeking alternatives to total hip arthroplasty. He will find it detailed and complete in its discussion of preoperative selection and planning, surgical technique, postoperative care, and prognosis.

Biomechanical Principles of Varus/Valgus Intertrochanteric Osteotomy (Pauwels I and II) in the Treatment of Osteoarthitis of the Hip

F. PAUWELS

In treating mechanically induced disorders and deformities of the hip joint we must have a clear conception of:

1. The normal (physiological) stress on the hip joint and how it is influenced by a change in the neck-shaft angle.
2. The manner in which living supporting tissue reacts to the magnitude and quality of mechanical stress.

The following statements are, therefore, based both on recent addition to the knowledge of functional anatomy and on some elementary rules of the theory of statics and elasticity, which are indispensable for an understanding of the reciprocal effects between living tissue and mechanical influences.

Load and Stress

The concepts of load and stress are fundamentally different. They should, therefore, under no circumstance be confused with each other, something which unfortunately still occurs in modern literature. Load refers exclusively to the *external forces* which influence the body. In contrast, the term *stress* is reserved for all effects of the forces within the material itself. The magnitude and distribution of the stresses in the material characterize the stress condition.

Influence of Mechanical Stress on Mature Bony Tissue

According to our concept, the reaction of mature bony tissue is determined solely by the *magnitude* of the stress and not by its quality. Thus, it is irrelevant whether the stress consists of compression, tension, or shear. The physiological *magnitude* of stress constitutes the driving force for the permanent bone remodelling in which apposition and resorption of bony tissue balance each other. Within certain limits, an increase in stress leads to predominant bone apposition, depending on the extent by which normal stress has been exceeded.

The form of the subchondral bony sclerosis in the acetabular roof, so aptly termed "sourcil" (eyebrow) in the French literature, reflects very clearly this relationship between bone formation and magnitude of stress.

The articular pressure in a normally developed hip joint under normal stress is distributed evenly over the weight-bearing surface (Fig. 1a). The sclerotic zone in the acetabular roof is even throughout (Fig. 1b).

A primary or secondary subluxation of the head of the femur leads to a concentration of the articular pressure at the edge of the acetabulum. Frequently, the articular pressure is increased to several times its normal magnitude (Fig. 2a). In these cases, the subchondral bony sclerosis assumes the form of a laterally ascending triangle (Fig. 2b), which corresponds well to the form of the appropriate stress diagram.

Thus, the form of the subchondral bony sclerosis in the acetabular roof allows one to deduce the distribution of the compressive stresses in the joint. This observation is of great practical significance for diagnosis.

If the stress exceeds the upper limit of tissue tolerance, the bony tissue is resorbed instead of being laid down. In certain forms of osteoarthritis of the hip, the limit of tolerance is apparently lowered. Thus, levels of stress which in normal bony tissue would lead to an increase in the sclerosis (Figs. 14, 15, 17) result in a complete breakdown of normal bone remodelling and lead to rapid proliferative and degenerative changes.

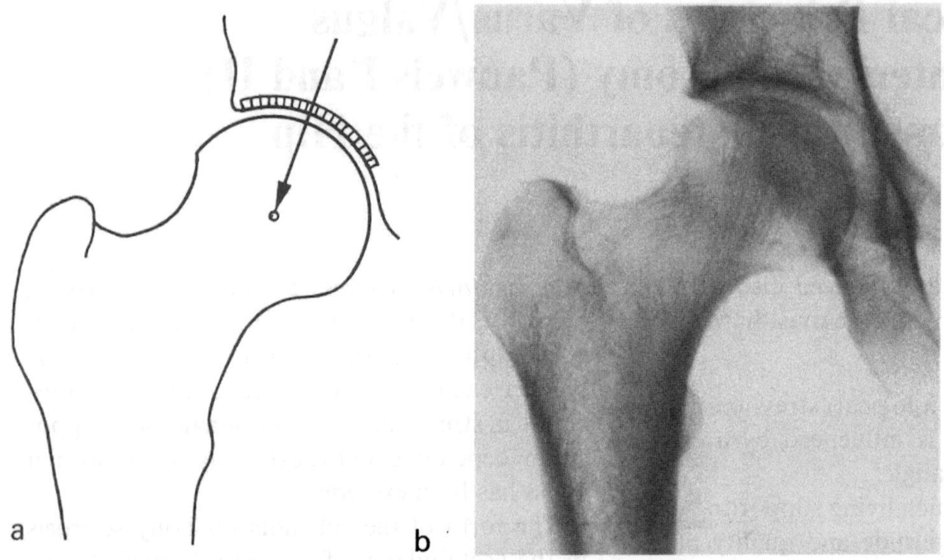

Fig. 1a, b. The distribution of stress in a normal hip joint is embodied in the subchondral bony sclerosis in the acetabular roof. **a** Diagram of the compressive stresses in the acetabulum. **b** Sclerosis of even width in the acetabular roof (sourcil)

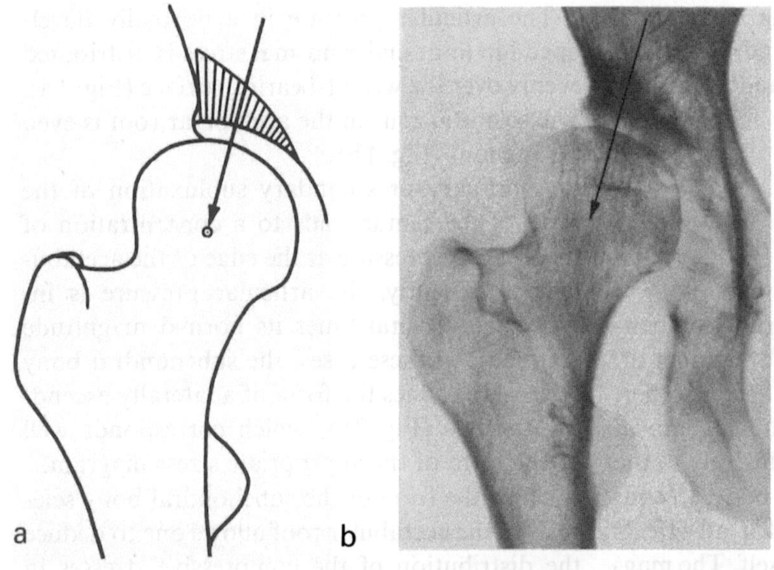

Fig. 2a, b. If the resultant compressive force moves toward the edge of the acetabulum, the distribution of stress and sclerosis in the acetabular roof assumes a triangular shape. **a** Diagram of the compressive stresses in the acetabulum. **b** Sclerosis in the acetabular roof in the form of a laterally ascending triangle

Load on the Upper End of the Femur Under Normal Conditions

During normal gait, the upper end of the femur of the supporting leg is loaded by the resultant force R, which is composed of all the forces acting on the hip joint. The direction of this compressive force *R* is a straight line connecting the center of rotation of the hip joint with the intersection of the lines of action of the muscle force *M* and the partial body weight *K* (Fig. 3). It runs from above downward and laterally and is inclined at 16° to the vertical.

The load exerted on the upper end of the femur is, therefore, the resultant force *R*. Al-

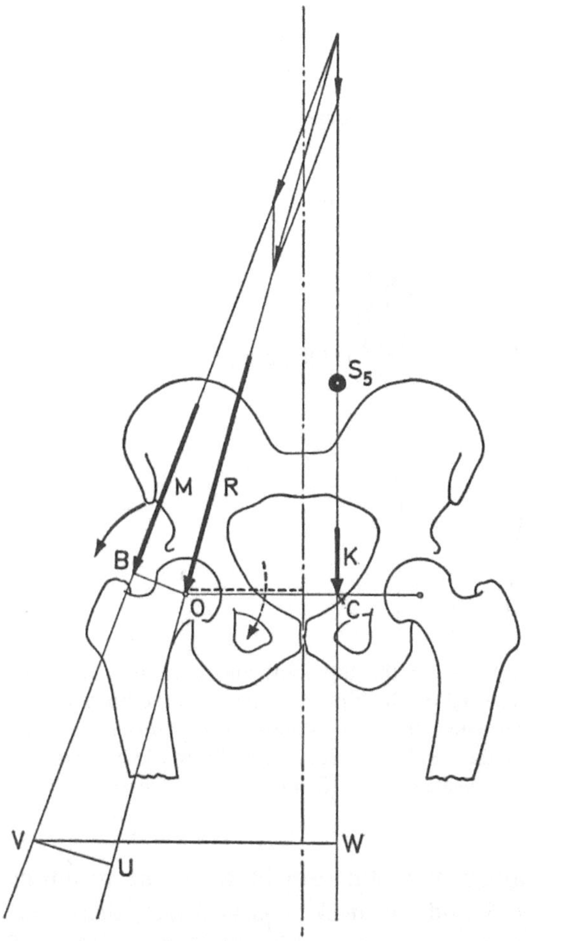

Fig. 3. The resultant compressive force R evokes stresses in the hip joint during the single support period of gait. $0B$, lever arm of the muscle force M; $0C$, lever arm of the load K; K, body weight to be borne by the weight-bearing leg; M, force of the abductor muscles; 0, center of the hip joint; R, hip joint compressive force resulting from the forces K and M; S_5, center of gravity of the body weight to be borne by the hip joint of the weight-bearing leg; U, V, W, auxiliary points

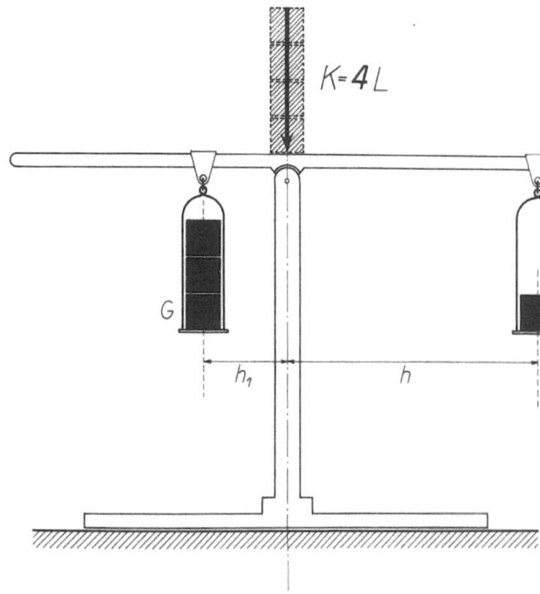

Fig. 4. Comparison of the hip joint of the weight-bearing leg with a balance. L, load (comparable to body weight); G, counterweight to be compared with the hip joint abductor muscles; h, lever arm of the load L; h_1, lever arm of the counterweight G; K, total load on the balance's joint

though R is the geometric sum of K and M, it is determined largely by the magnitude of the muscle force M, which in turn depends on the relative length of the lever arms of the body weight K and the abductor muscles M acting on the joint. The lever arm of the body weight K corresponds in Fig. 3 to the line $0C$. It is almost three times as long as the lever arm of the muscle force M (line $0B$). To maintain equilibrium at the joint, the muscular force must, therefore, be about three times greater than the weight to be supported. This relationship can be easily understood with the aid of a model of a balance (Fig. 4). Since in the hip joint the forces K and M meet at an angle, the geometric sum of K and M is somewhat smaller than a simple addition of the two forces (see the parallelogram of forces in Fig. 3). This means that, during gait, a compressive force R more than three and a half times greater than the partial body weight K acts on the upper end of the femur of the supporting leg.

If the size and weight of the man on whom Fischer (1899) carried out his classic investigations on human gait are used (total body weight 58.7 kg), then we expect a partial weight of 47.76 kg to act on the hip joint of the supporting leg. If we assume that the neck-shaft angle is 127°, we can, based on these figures, calculate the resultant force to be about 175 kp for the *static* loading. We can assume, therefore, a kinetic force of about 200 kp for slow walking. This figure will be used for further calculations.

According to the definition, the resultant force R passes through the center of rotation of the femoral head and is, therefore, directed

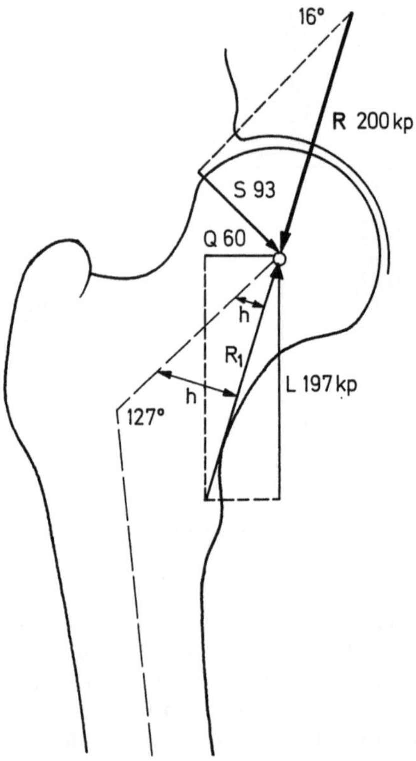

Fig. 5. The resultant force R runs obliquely to the axis of the neck and can be resolved into separate components to clarify its various effects. R, force, acting on the hip, resulting from the body weight and muscular force; $R_1 = -R$, counterforce to R; h, h, lever arm of the compressive force R in relation to the neck at various cross-sectional levels; L, (vertical) longitudinal component of the force R_1; Q, transverse component of R_1; S, shear component of the resultant force R

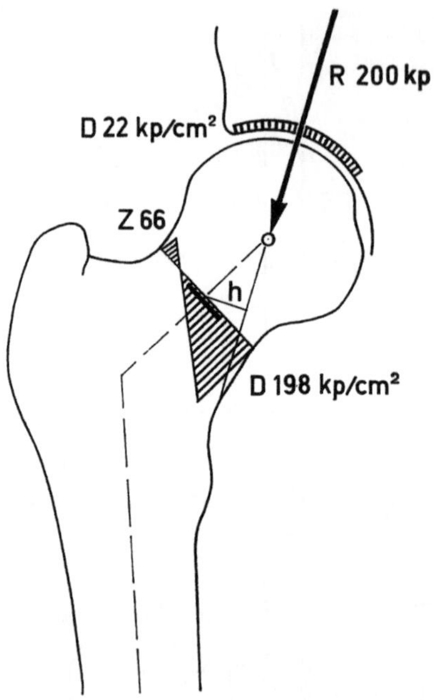

Fig. 6. Stress in the hip joint and neck (see text). R, force exerted on the hip, resulting from the body weight and muscular force; D, compressive stresses; h, lever arm of the resultant force R for the marked cross section; Z, tensile stresses (from Pauwels 1976b)

perpendicular to its surface and acts entirely on the femoral head and acetabulum as a *pure compressive force*.

The line of action of R does not, however, coincide with the axis of the neck, but diverges slightly from it medially and distally (Fig. 5). As a result, because of the lever arm h, the length of which increases distally, the neck is subjected to bending. The bending moment, i.e., the product of the force and the lever arm, is greatest at the level of the greater trochanter because there the lever arm is longest.

The compressive force R can be resolved into two components, one of which runs in the direction of the axis of the neck and the other perpendicular to it. The latter component acts on the neck as a shearing force S; it is determined by the angle of inclination between the resultant force R and the neck axis and has, therefore, at every cross section the same magnitude of 93 kp (see Fig. 5).

Stress in the Upper End of the Femur Under Normal Conditions

The compressive force R acting on the hip joint is distributed over the weight-bearing surface of the hip joint in the form of compressive stresses (D) (see Fig. 6). The articular pressure is determined by the magnitude of the resultant force R but even more by the size of the area which transmits R. Under normal conditions, the compressive stresses are distributed almost evenly over the weight-bearing surface. Their average magnitude can be readily determined if the force R is divided by an area which corresponds to a projection of the curved weight-bearing surface on a plane perpendicular to the direction of R. When the diameter of the head

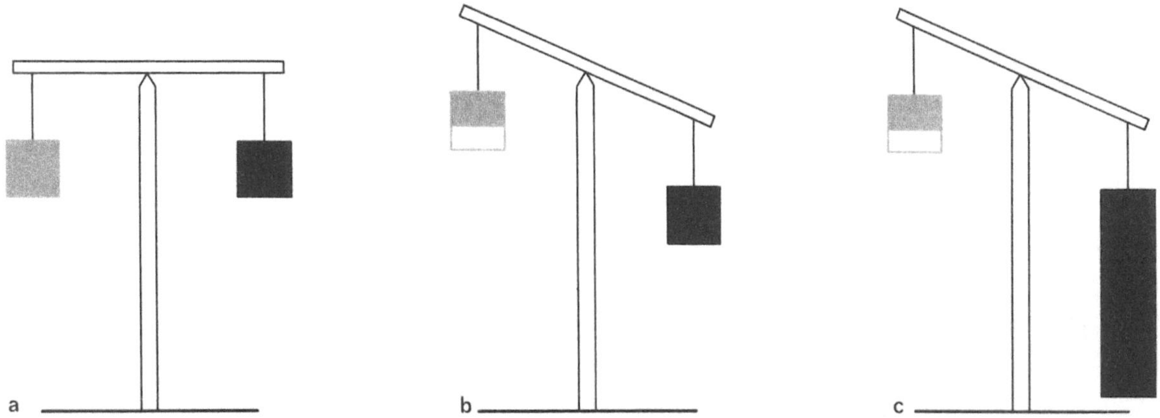

Fig. 7 a–c. The biomechanical equilibrium between stress and the mechanical resistance of a joint can be illustrated using a balance as a model. The tissue resistance is represented by the *light-colored* weight and the stress by the *dark-colored* weight. **a** In a normal joint, resistance and stress counterbalance each other. **b** The equilibrium is disturbed by a reduction in resistance. **c** The equilibrium is disturbed by an increase in stress and reduction in resistance

is 5 cm, the projection of the weight-bearing surface is approximately 9 cm^2 (Kummer 1969). Based on these figures, it was calculated that a resultant force of 200 kp provokes an average articular pressure of about 22 kp/cm^2.

The bending effect of the resultant compressive force R causes compressive stresses (D) in the medial border of the neck and tensile stresses (Z) in the lateral border where the line of action of R lies outside the "core" (see Fig. 6). If one assumes the weight-bearing surface of the neck at the level of the cross section shown in Fig. 6 to be approximately 3 cm^2, then the maximum compressive stress is 198 kp/cm^2 on the medial side, and on the lateral side the maximum stress is 66 kp/cm^2. Shear stresses (shear force S divided by the area affected by the force) are approximately 31 kp/cm^2.

Clinical Picture of Osteoarthritis of the Hip and Its Relationship to Mechanics

In a normal hip joint, the resistance of the cartilaginous and bony tissue to mechanical stress, and the magnitude of the articular pressure are in equilibrium (Fig. 7a). In osteoarthritis, this equilibrium is disturbed. The cause for this can be either biological or mechanical or both (Fig. 7b, c).

The resistance of cartilage and bone can be so severely diminished by a congenital or acquired insufficiency that even normal articular pressure can cause the pathologic tissue alterations typical of osteoarthritis (Fig. 7b).

The initial stage of primary osteoarthritis affecting a joint of normal articular configuration is characteristic of the sequelae of this type of disturbance of the equilibrium.

The equilibrium can also be disturbed by an increase in the articular pressure, possibly to several times the physiological level. A good example of this is provided by primary and secondary subluxations of the femoral head (see Fig. 7c), where the load is carried only by a small area because of the incongruence of the articular surfaces. In the majority of cases of osteoarthritis, both components are responsible in varying degrees for the disturbance of the equilibrium and for the development and inexorable progression of the disorder. In any case, the level of articular pressure undoubtedly plays a decisive role. The biological component of this biomechanical equilibrium, the tissue tolerance of stress, can be disturbed in a variety of ways. At present we are unable to evaluate the tissue resistance either qualitatively or quantitatively,

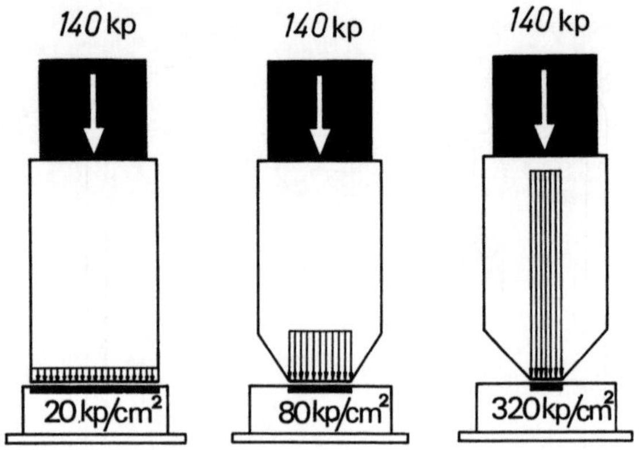

Fig. 8. The articular pressure is force per unit area. At constant loading, the pressure (i.e., the compressive stresses!) increases as the surface decreases

nor can we affect it therapeutically with any degree of certainty.

In contrast, the way the mechanical components disturb the equilibrium can be determined fairly accurately, because the biomechanics of the hip is now well understood (Pauwels 1976) and because the bony sclerosis in the acetabular roof, which can be identified by X-rays very precisely, reflects the distribution and the magnitude of articular pressure (Fig. 13a–g).

Osteoarthritis can be treated surgically. Suitable surgical measures can reduce excessive and concentrated articular pressure to normal or even below normal. This is due to the fact that the magnitude of the stress depends not only on the magnitude of the compressive force, but also on the area of the surface subjected to stress (Fig. 8).

The significance of the weight-bearing area on the magnitude of the compressive stress is clearly demonstrated in everyday life by the devastating effect of the stiletto heel of the 1950s, on floors (Fig. 9).

The pressure exerted on the floor by a normal flat heel is approximately 6 kp/cm², in comparison to the 160 kp/cm² exerted by a stiletto heel. This example makes it clear why a reduction in the weight-bearing surface of the hip joint, as in the case of a subluxation of the femoral head, greatly increases the articular pressure (Fig. 10a, b).

The above mentioned observations illustrate how important it is to determine the magnitude and distribution of the articular pressure if one is to arrive at the correct treatment and prognosis.

The radius of the bony head of the femur is significantly smaller than the radius of the bony acetabulum. The space between the two contours, which can be observed in the X-ray, is filled by two layers of articular cartilage which exercise considerable influence on the magnitude and distribution of the articular pressure. If both cartilaginous coverings were absent, so that the bony acetabulum would rest directly on the bony head, the articular pressure could affect only a small area of the head and would be concentrated to a high degree (Fig. 11a).

If only *one* layer of cartilage were present (either on the acetabular side or on the femoral head), the pressure would be significantly smaller than if both cartilaginous coverings were missing because it would be distributed over nearly the entire articular surface, although unevenly. The stress diagram would be delineated by a convex line as shown in Fig. 11b.

For a uniform distribution of articular pressure, it is necessary that both the head and acetabular cartilage be present (Fig. 11c). This is

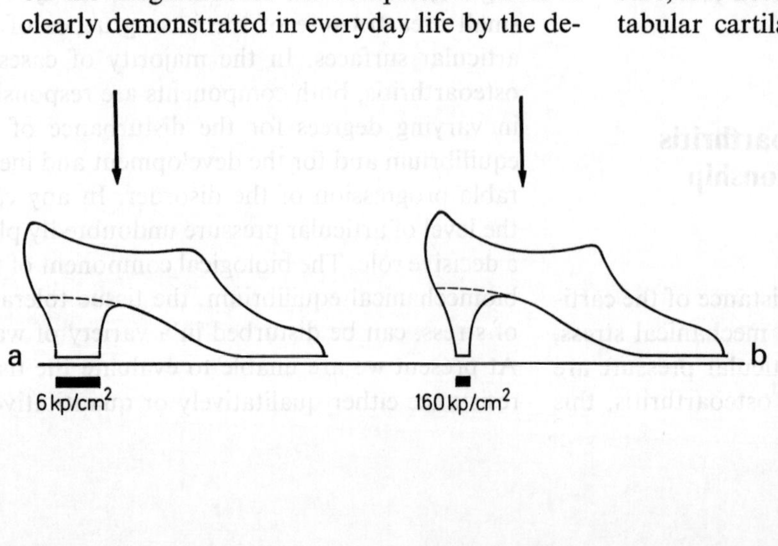

Fig. 9a, b. Comparison of the pressures exerted on a floor by flat-heeled and stiletto-heeled shoes. The pressure in subluxation of the hip joint can be compared to the pressure exerted by the stiletto-heeled shoe

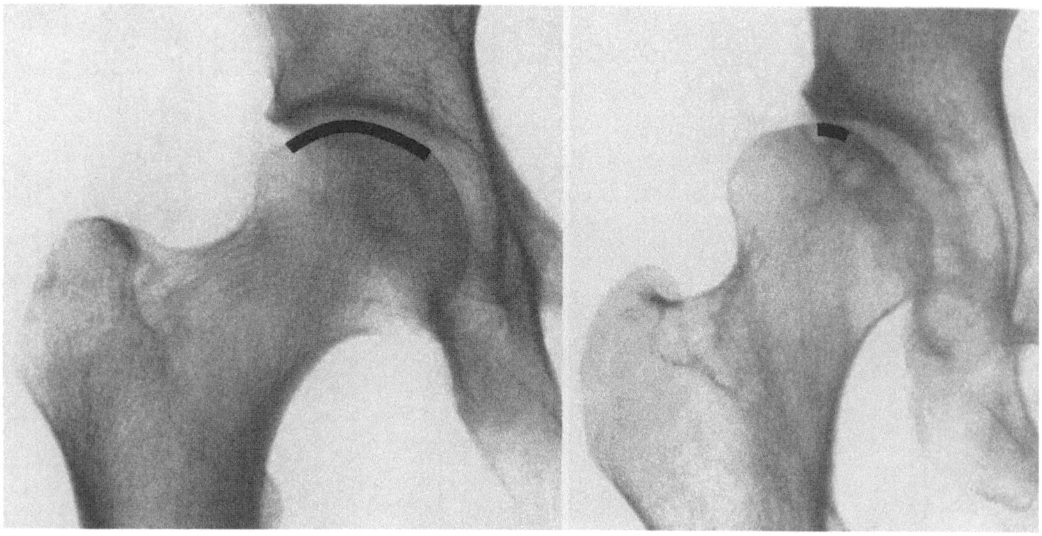

Fig. 10a, b. Surface subjected to pressure in the hip joint. **a** Normal hip joint. **b** Severely reduced weight-bearing surface in subluxation of the hip joint

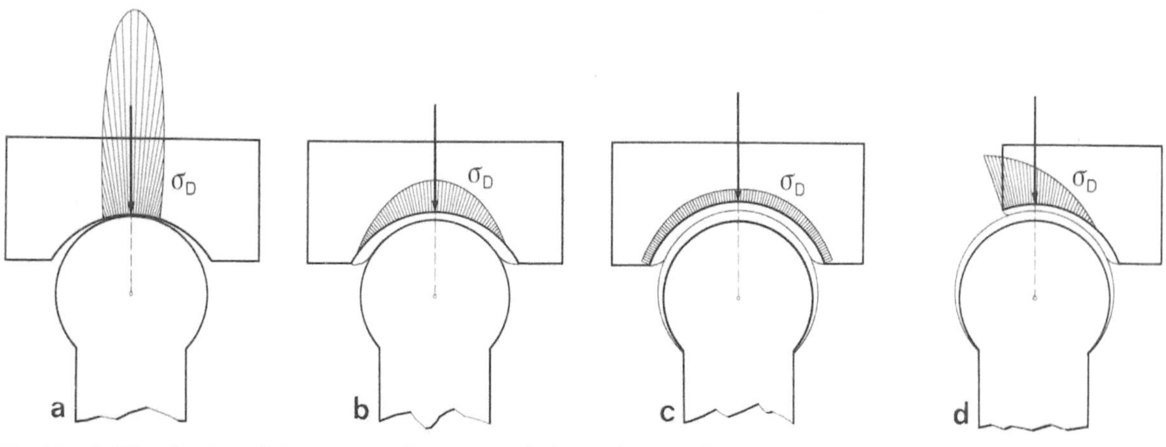

Fig. 11a–d. Distribution of the compressive stresses (σ_D) in a ball-and-socket joint depends on the effectiveness of the articular cartilage and the position of the resultant force. **a** Both articular cartilages are missing: excessive stresses on the small weight-bearing surface. **b** Cartilage on the femoral head missing: convexly limited symmetrical stress diagramm. **c** Effect of both articular cartilages: overall a uniform diagram with relatively small compressive stresses (sourcil). **d** Eccentric position of the resultant force (corresponding to a subluxation): triangular increase of the stress diagram toward the edge of the acetabulum

probably related to a difference in structure of the two articular cartilages, as was described to be the case in the gleno-humeral joint (Pauwels 1959). In any case, in order to attain uniform distribution, the resultant force must be situated in the middle of the weight-bearing surface of the joint.

If the compressive force is exerted eccentrically, for example, when it is displaced toward the edge of the acetabulum in the case of subluxation of the femoral head (see Fig. 11d), the articular pressure is distributed *unevenly* over the weight-bearing surface even if functionally normal articular cartilage is present. The compressive stresses increase from a value of zero at the inner edge of the weight-bearing surface to a maximum at the outer margin (edge of the acetabulum). This asymmetrical distribution

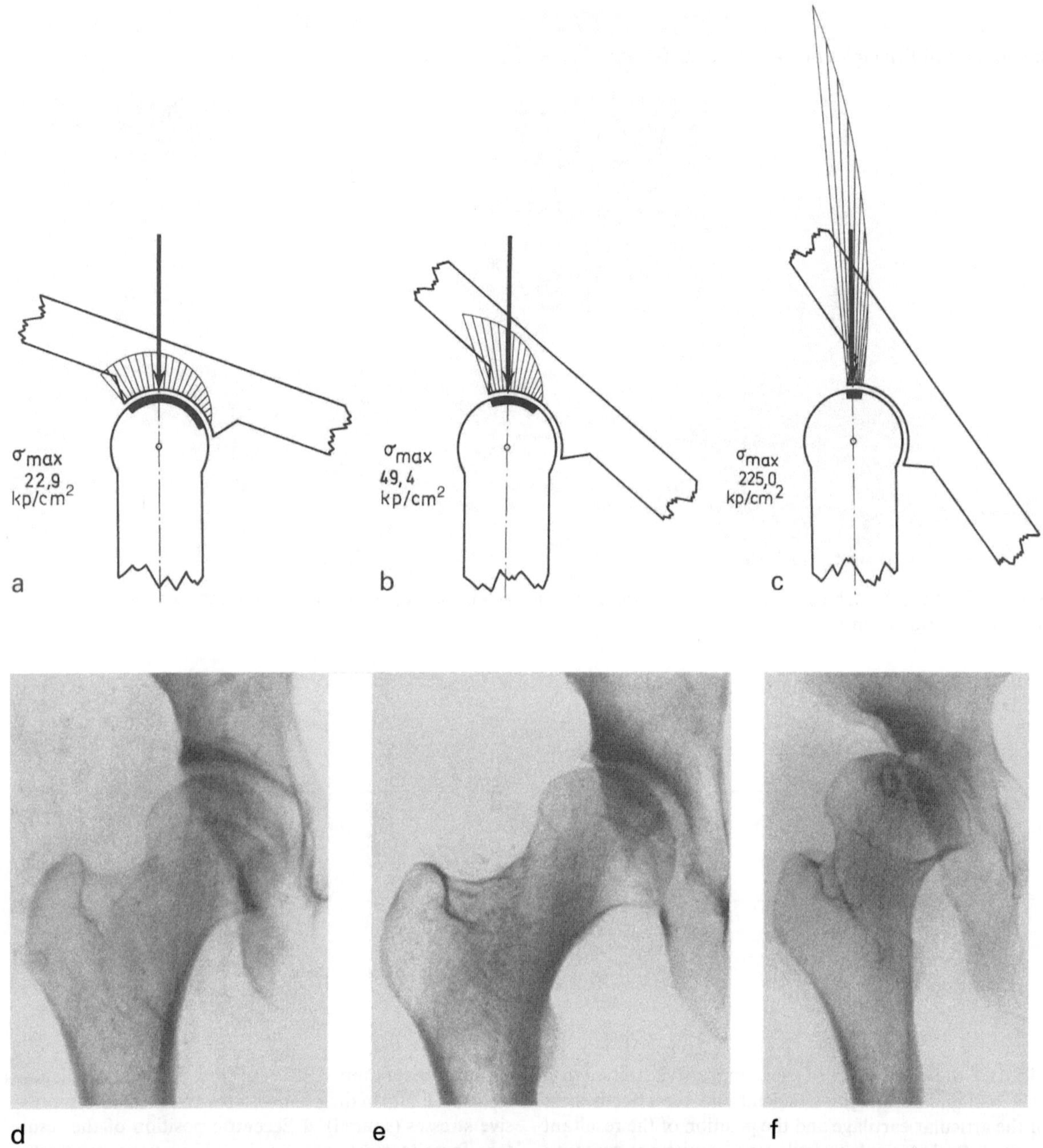

Fig. 12a–f. The shape of the sclerotic zone in the acetabular roof represents the diagram of the compressive stresses. **a–c** Distribution of the stresses in a model joint with increasing eccentricity of the load. **d–f** X-rays of hip joints with increasing subluxation of the femoral head. Initially, the dense triangle increases toward the edge of the acetabulum (**d**), then the width of the articular cartilage also decreases (narrowing of the "joint space" in **e**), and finally a deformation of the femoral head ensues and degenerative cysts appear, indicating an overstressing of the bony tissue (**f**)

causes the maximum stress to be considerably greater than one would expect solely from a reduction in the weight-bearing surface.

The influence of a progressive subluxation of the femoral head on the magnitude and distribution of the compressive stresses in the joint is illustrated in Fig. 12a–f. One can see that the shorter the distance of the resultant force from the edge of the acetabulum, the more quickly the weight-bearing surface of the joint dimin-

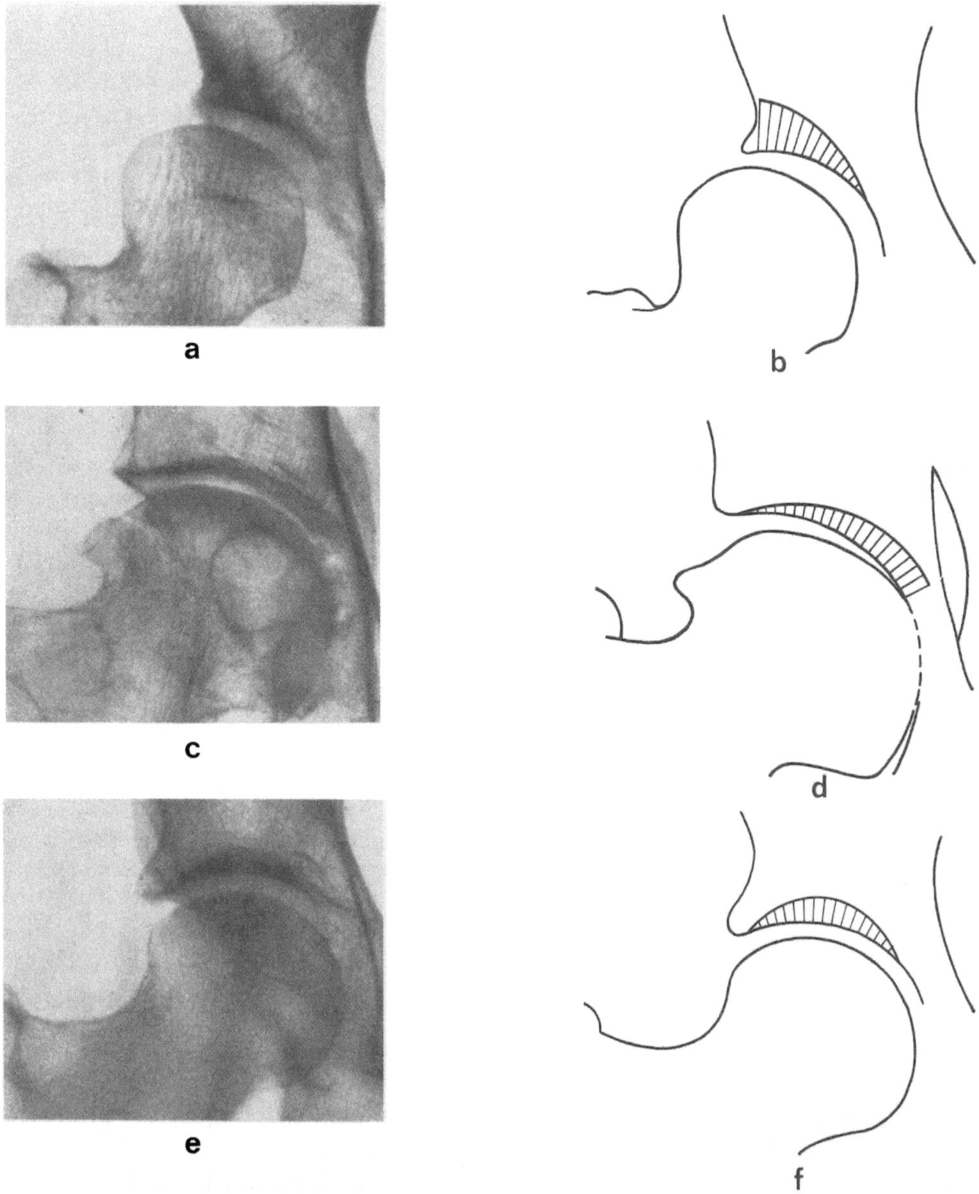

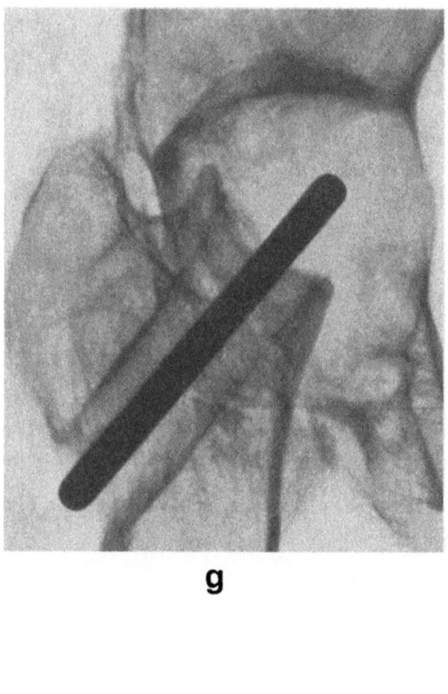

Fig. 13a–g. Different forms of subchondral sclerosis in the acetabular roof representing various degrees of stress. **a, b** Increase in the compressive stresses at the edge of the acetabulum in a case of subluxation of the femoral head. **c, d** Increase in the compressive stresses in the depths of the acetabulum in a case of protrusio acetabuli. **e, f** Central increase in the compressive stresses in a case of deficient distribution of the articular pressure caused by cartilage insufficiency. **g** Crescent-shaped sclerosis in the acetabular roof – similar to that in **e** – after replacement of the femoral head by a Judet prosthesis

ishes and in consequence the more the articular pressure increases. This is related to the general rule that the width of the weight-bearing surface can be at most only three times the distance of the resultant force from the edge of the acetabulum, even when ideal articular contact is present (see Pauwels 1963).

At the beginning of this discussion, it was shown that the subchondral bony sclerosis in the acetabular roof accurately reflects the magnitude and distribution of the articular pressure (Figs. 1, 13). This observation is of great practical significance for both the treatment of prearthrosis and of osteoarthritis.

As shown in Fig. 12d, the sclerotic zone in the acetabular roof becomes increasingly more wedge-shaped with progressive subluxation of the femoral head. Compare this with the stress diagrams in the joint models under similar stress illustrated in Fig. 12a, b. In the case of extreme subluxation with the resultant enormous stresses at the edge of the acetabulum, the bony sclerosis can no longer follow the steeply inclined stress diagram; signs of destruction become visible (see Fig. 12c and f). The destruction must be considered as a sign that the tolerance of the bony tissue to the stress has been exceeded in this case. Because of this, the bone begins to degenerate.

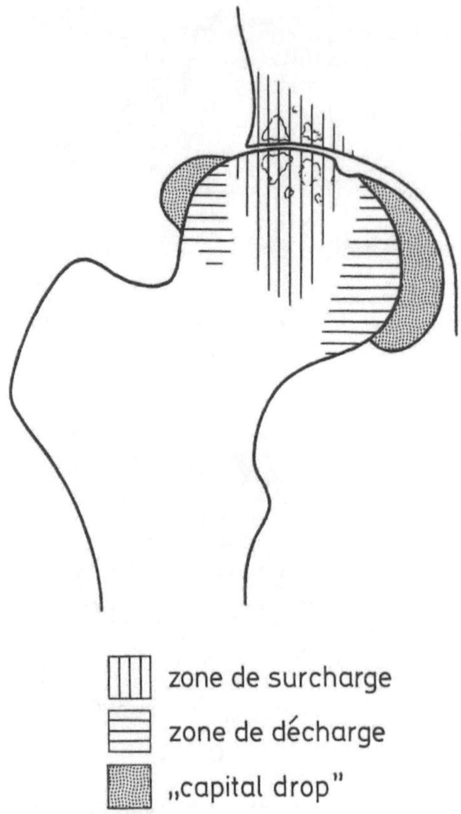

Fig. 14. Diagram of the areas of degeneration (*vertical bars*) and proliferation (*dotted*) in an osteoarthritic hip joint (adapted from Grasset 1960)

The pathologic bony sclerosis in the acetabular roof appears in three different forms (see Fig. 13a–g). The above-described subluxation of the head leads to the laterally based sclerotic wedge (Fig. 13a, b). In the case of protusio acetabuli, the articular pressure increases towards the depths of the acetabulum and results in a medial triangle of sclerosis (Fig. 13c, d).

The normal zone of sclerosis (sourcil) is dependent among other things on the pressure-distributing effect of *both* layers of articular cartilage. This is very clearly illustrated by the cases in which only one layer of cartilage is present, as for exemple when the femoral head has been replaced by a Judet prosthesis (Fig. 13g). In this instance, the zone of sclerosis has the shape of a crescent. Such a convex subchondral bony sclerosis in a hip joint, which otherwise appears to be normal, indicates a mechanical insufficiency of the articular cartilage. Such cartilage has apparently lost the ability to distribute the articular pressure uniformly. It has not been appreciated until now that such a convex sclerosis is an early sign of primary osteoarthritis (Fig. 13e, f).

A characteristic feature of osteoarthritis of the hip is the fact that a relative or absolute increase in articular pressure which becomes excessive causes tissue alterations which are totally different in the overloaded zone and in the zone of low pressure (cf. Grasset 1960).

The *overloaded zone* is characterized by rapid bony proliferation. In addition to sclerosis of the bony tissue (which is only a functional adaptation at the beginning of the disease), alterations such as fibrocartilaginous and fibrous degeneration, atrophy of the articular cartilage and pseudocysts of various sizes in the bone (Fig. 14) become apparent in the femoral head and acetabulum.

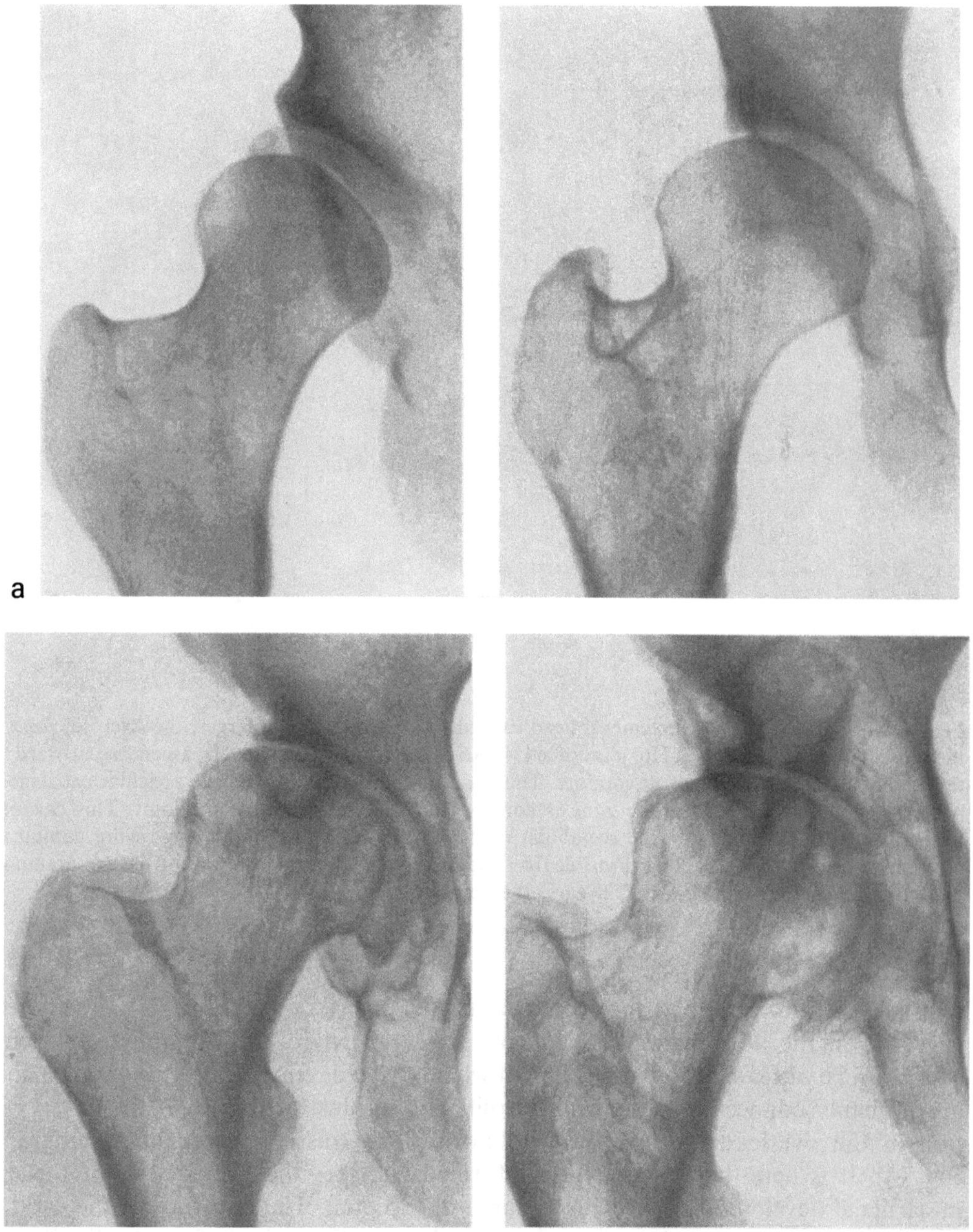

Fig. 15a–d. Chronological survey of the most important alterations in X-rays of osteoarthritic hips. **a** Triangular compression zone in the acetabular roof ascending laterally in a case of a subluxation of the femoral head. **b** Upon further overloading, the sclerotic triangle ascends further in the acetabular roof and the joint space becomes narrower (atrophy of the articular cartilage). **c** The sclerotic triangle in the acetabulum is accentuated, a degenerative cyst appears in the head on the opposite side, the articular cartilage is further thinned, and a medial osteophyte ("capital drop") becomes visible over the contour of the head. **d** In an advanced case, the cystic deformation in the femoral head has increased and a large cyst has also developed in the acetabulum. A capital drop is also evident

a 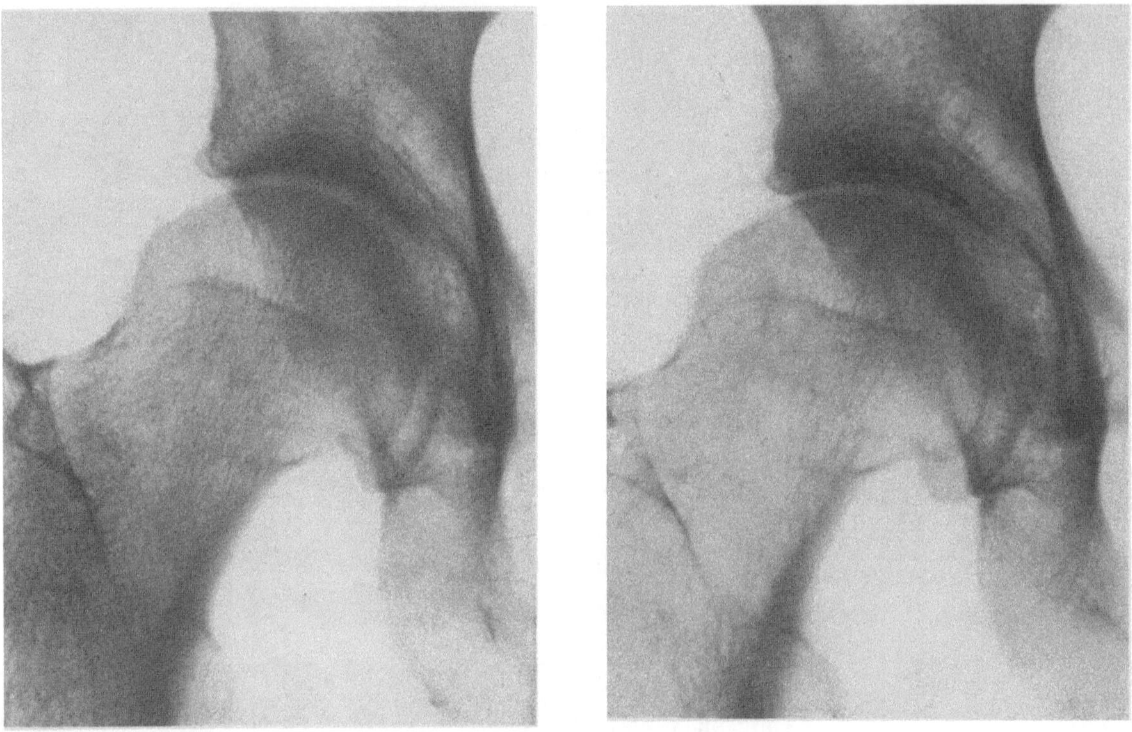 b

Fig. 16a, b. Subluxation of the femoral head caused by the growth of a capital drop. **a** Hip joint of a 45-year-old female patient at the onset of discomfort. The head is partially subluxated. The sclerotic zone is convex. Its top is located in the middle of the acetabular roof. An osteophyte (capital drop) is already visible over the medial contour of the head. **b** After 2 years, the capital drop is much larger, the sclerotic zone has assumed the form of a triangle ascending toward the edge of the acetabulum, and the articular cartilage is thinner in the lateral aspect of the joint. This can only be explained by the fact that the growing capital drop has forced the femoral head out of the acetabulum

In the *zone* of low load (horizontal bars in Fig. 14), on the other hand, proliferative processes can be observed (dotted in Fig. 14) which are probably connected to the rapid proliferation in the overloaded zone (vertical bars in Fig. 14). It is here that osteophytes preformed in cartilage develop. One particularly large osteophyte, which appears drop-shaped in the X-ray, is of special significance for the further development of the disease and for treatment. It extends over the medial contour of the femoral head from the fovea capitis to, in some instances, well past the former medial border of the articular cartilage. It is termed the "capital drop" because of its shape as observed in the X-ray. This same osteophyte is also at the origin of the development of the tête coulée (Grasset 1970) described in the French literature. The frequently observed progressive subluxation of the femoral head is directly related to the growth of this osteophyte. The characteristic X-ray development of this osteoarthritic alteration is illustrated in Fig. 15a–d.

Grasset's excellent monograph (1960) describes the histogenesis of the capital drop in detail. The influence of the capital drop on the configuration of stress distribution in the hip joint is less well known. As Fig. 16a–b shows, the growing capital drop eventually forces the femoral head out of the acetabulum. The progressive subluxation leads to overloading of the lateral articular margin which results in sclerosis of the bone and atrophy of the articular cartilage.

A more rapid development is illustrated in Fig. 17a–d, where the degeneration progressed to loss of cartilage and formation of large pseudocysts in the head and acetabulum.

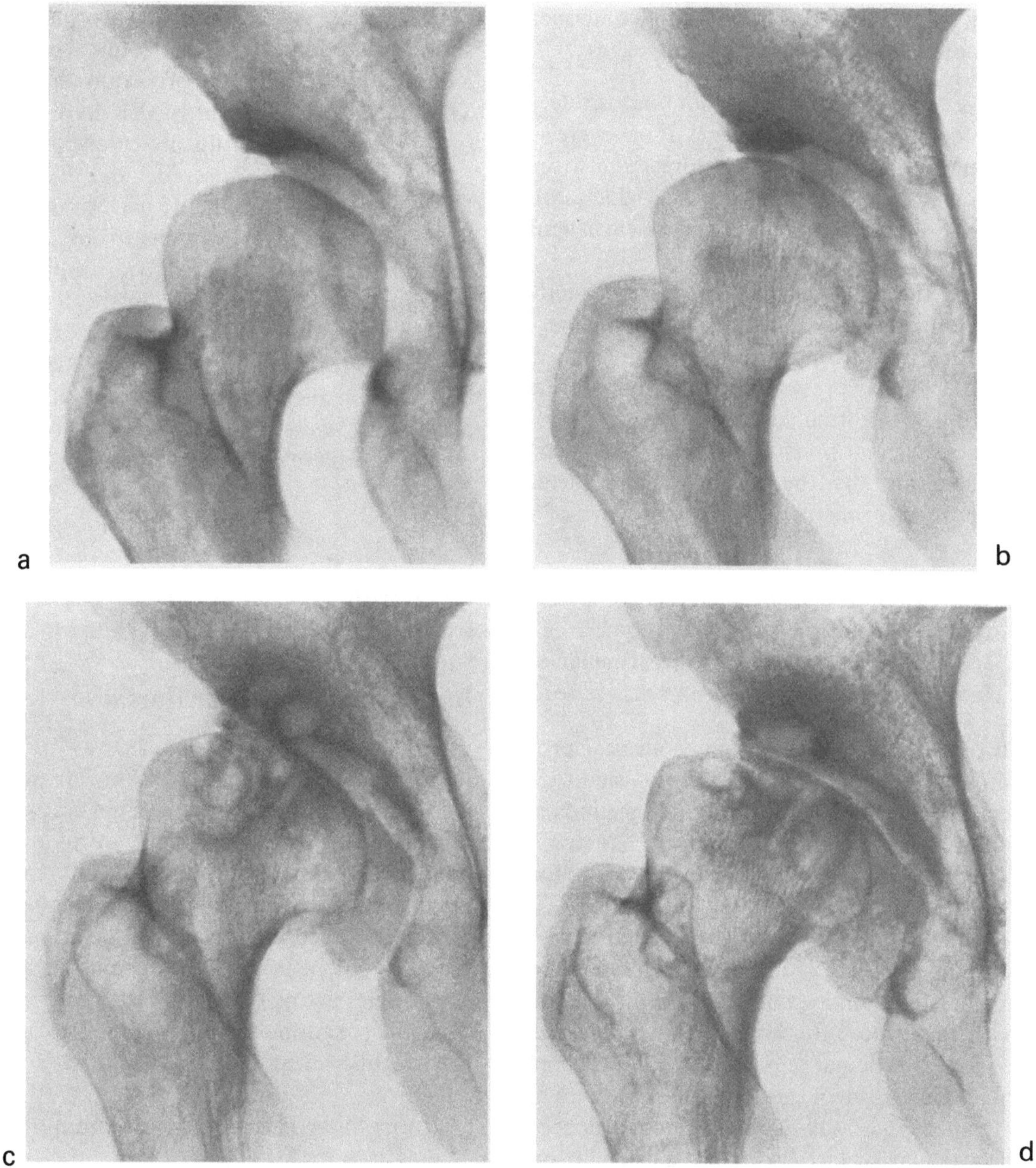

Fig. 17 a–d. Secondary osteoarthritis after a congenital subluxation. **a, b** Increasing accentuation of the sclerotic triangle and atrophy of the articular cartilage at the edge of the acetabulum. **c, d** Cystic degeneration in the femoral head and acetabulum as well as extreme enlargement of the capital drop. The contour of the acetabulum adapts by becoming flatter

Rationale of Treatment of Osteoarthritis of the Hip

Once we appreciate the pathogenesis of osteoarthritis, it becomes apparent that the treatment must be aimed at restoring the disturbed biomechanical equilibrium between the resistance of the tissue and the magnitude of the articular pressure.

Basically, this could be achieved in two ways:

1. By altering the biological components, i.e. improving the tissue resistance to stress.

2. By influencing the mechanical components in order to decrease articular pressure.

It is extremely difficult, if not impossible, to alter the biological components. If one were successful, one could at best restore them to normal. This would still leave tissue which could never adapt to pathologically excessive articular pressure.

Thus, the only feasible therapeutic maneuver is to influence the mechanical components. In fact, this is quite possible. Surgically one can reduce articular pressure which far exceeds normal to below normal levels.

Since articular pressure is determined both by the load and by the weight-bearing surface, there are in principle two possible ways of reducing it:

1. Decreasing the load, i.e., the compressive force acting on the joint.
2. Increasing that portion of the articular surface which transmits this compressive force.

To date, there have been many surgical procedures designed to attain the first possibility, i.e, decrease the loading. Two such operations will be discussed briefly; the temporary hanging hip (Voss) and the displacement osteotomy (McMurray 1935, 1939).

In the Voss's operation, the reduction in the compressive force is achieved by reducing the force of the muscles which act on the hip joint. With this procedure, however, one can at best reduce the articular pressure to half of the initial magnitude. Prerequisite for the success of this operation is a well-maintained congruence of the articular surfaces, so that the articular pressure is not pathologically increased by a decrease in the weight-transmitting surface. Incongruence of the articular surfaces, therefore, makes this operation inadvisable.

The rationale of McMurray's osteotomy lies in reducing the load on the hip joint by supporting the pelvis on the femur at the lower edge of the acetabulum. This is achieved after an intertrochanteric osteotomy by displacing the shaft fragment upward and medially until the medial edge abuts on the lower edge of the acetabulum.

Experience has shown, however, that such support was achieved at best only accidentally, and as a rule, that the procedure has failed. The medial displacement of the shaft fragment by itself exercises no influence on the magnitude of the articular pressure. Beneficial effects of McMurray's displacement osteotomy, therefore, can only result from either a reduction of the muscular forces or from an unintentional rotation of the femoral head in the acetabulum which accidentally eliminated the existing incongruence of the joint. However, the elimination of joint incongruence was not claimed by McMurray and may not, therefore, be considered as a principle of his method.

Decreasing the Articular Pressure by Increasing the Weight-Bearing Surface in the Case of Incongruent Articular Surfaces

In the case of incongruent articular surfaces, increasing the area of the weight-transmitting surface is the only practical way of restoring biomechanical equilibrium. It leads to a far greater reduction in the articular pressure than can be achieved by decreasing the compressive force, as for instance by reducing the force of the muscles acting on the joint (Voss).

Two operations were developed to increase the weight-bearing area of the joint:

1. Varus intertrochanteric osteotomy (Pauwels I; see Fig. 18a, b);
2. Valgus intertrochanteric osteotomy (Pauwels II; Fig. 18c, d).

These two operations which I have performed since 1931 (P I) and 1956 (P II) are *joint-preserving procedures* (Pauwels 1950, 1960).

If properly selected, either one of these two procedures will result in the largest decrease in articular pressure. In addition to the increase in the surface of the weight-bearing area, the concomitant muscle release results in a decrease of the compressive force acting on the joint.

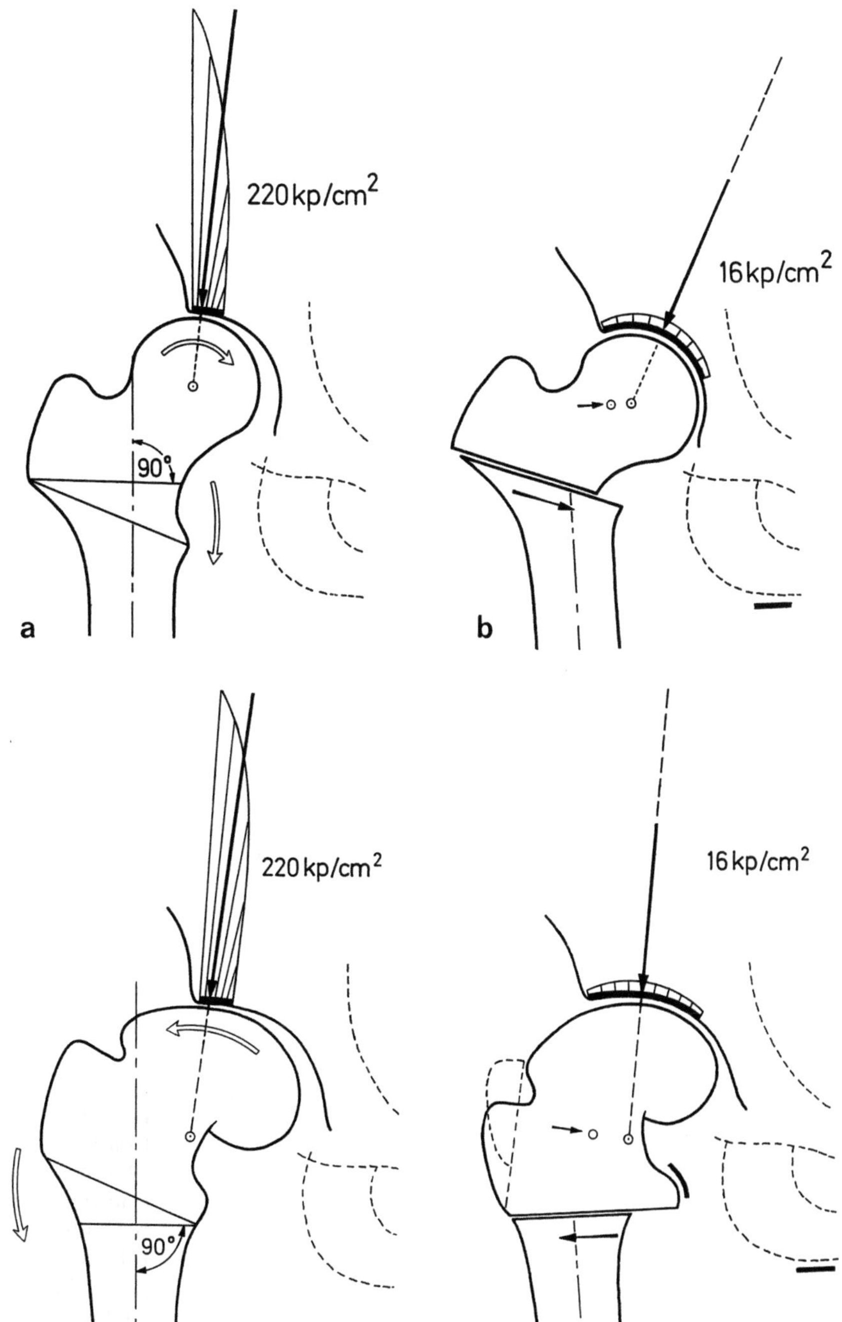

Fig. 18a–d. Rationale of the osteotomies aimed at enlarging the weight-bearing surface. *Varus osteotomy* (*P I*): **a** Subluxation of the femoral head; the large compressive force acts near the edge of the acetabulum and therefore evokes extremely high stresses. The bony wedge to be removed, is shown with a medial base. **b** After osteotomy. The resultant force has become smaller and has moved to the middle of the weight-bearing surface; the stresses are low and even (sourcil). The shaft fragment has been moved somewhat proximally; the adductor muscles are relaxed by tenotomy. *Valgus osteotomy* (*P II*): **c** A large, deformed femoral head with a huge capital drop is subluxated. The large resultant force acts near the edge of the acetabulum, resulting in very high stresses on the reduced weight-bearing surface. Note that the bony wedge to be resected has a lateral base. **d** After osteotomy, the weight-bearing surface of the joint is considerably increased, the resultant force has moved medially, the stresses have been greatly reduced and are evenly distributed. The shaft fragment is displaced laterally, a tenotomy of the adductor and iliopsoas muscles is performed, and the greater trochanter, after being chiseled off, is moved upward reducing the power of the abductor muscles

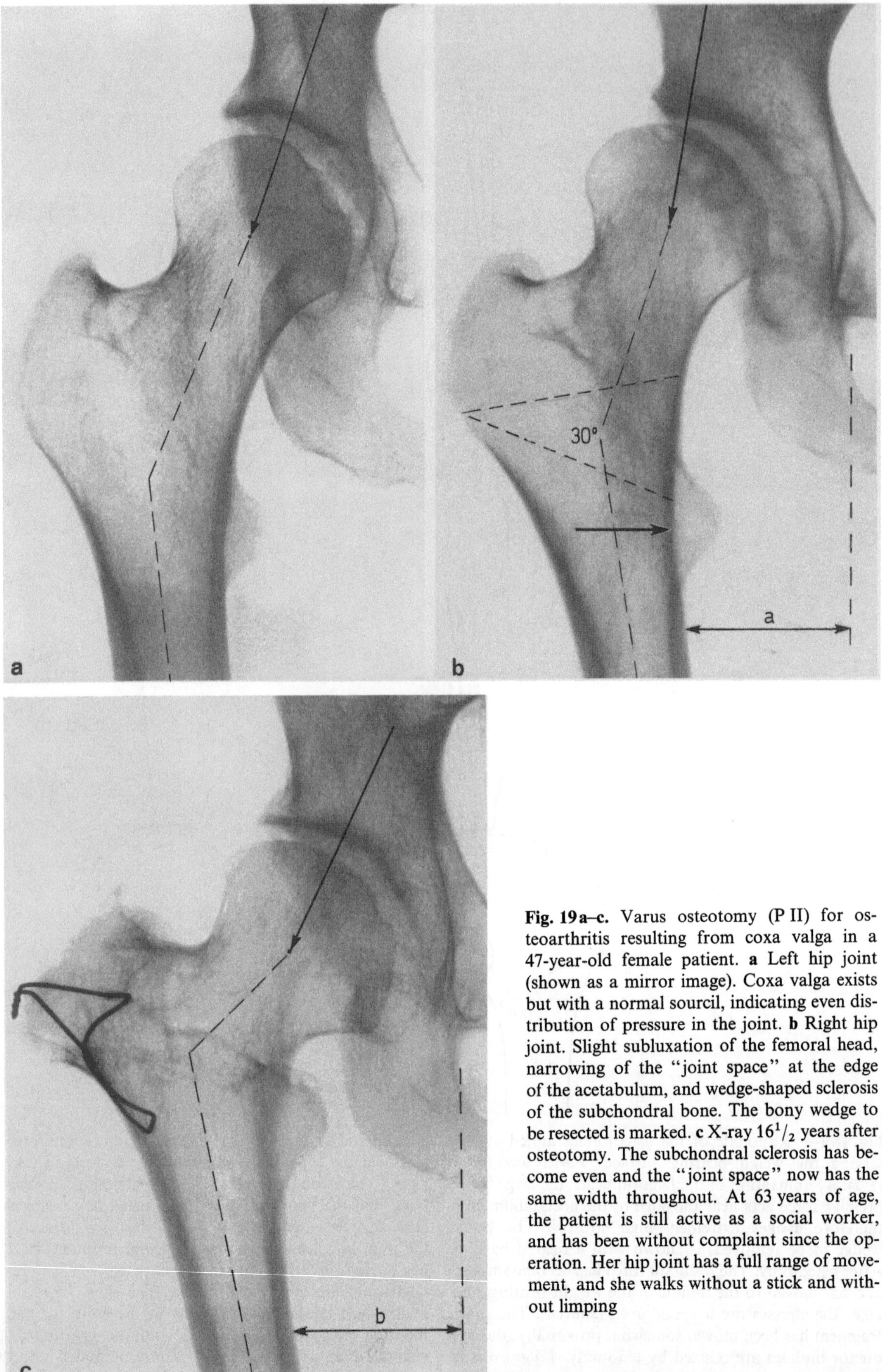

Fig. 19a–c. Varus osteotomy (P II) for osteoarthritis resulting from coxa valga in a 47-year-old female patient. **a** Left hip joint (shown as a mirror image). Coxa valga exists but with a normal sourcil, indicating even distribution of pressure in the joint. **b** Right hip joint. Slight subluxation of the femoral head, narrowing of the "joint space" at the edge of the acetabulum, and wedge-shaped sclerosis of the subchondral bone. The bony wedge to be resected is marked. **c** X-ray $16^1/_2$ years after osteotomy. The subchondral sclerosis has become even and the "joint space" now has the same width throughout. At 63 years of age, the patient is still active as a social worker, and has been without complaint since the operation. Her hip joint has a full range of movement, and she walks without a stick and without limping

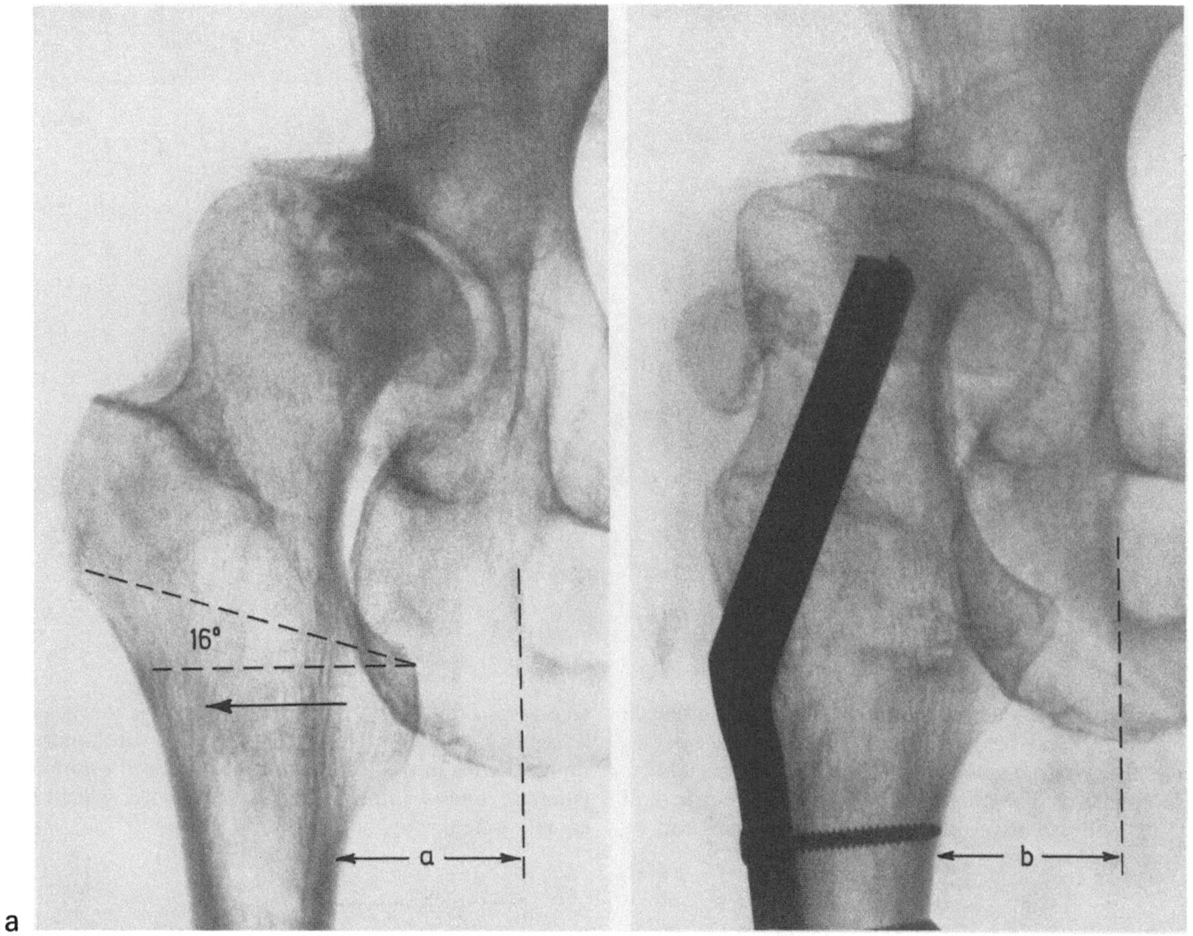

Fig. 20 a, b. Advanced case of osteoarthritis in a 54-year-old female patient with subluxation of the right hip joint. **a** X-ray shortly before operation. The articular cartilage at the edge of the acetabulum has disappeared, the sclerotic zone in the acetabular roof is triangular, and several cysts are present in the head. The bony wedge to be removed is marked. **b** X-ray 5 years and 1 month after a valgus osteotomy; the greater trochanter has been chiseled off. The sclerosis in the acetabular roof has become normal, the cysts in the femoral head have disappeared, and the articular cartilage once again exhibits normal and even width. The hip joint is mobile except for some limitation of rotation and the patient walks without a stick and without limping

When the amount of varus or valgus correction necessary has been precisely determined for each individual case (most reliably by careful preoperative drawings), then both of these operations achieve the same therapeutic effect.

The decision of whether to perform a varus or a valgus osteotomy depends on whether the femoral head has to be turned inward or outward in order to enlarge the weight-bearing surface of the joint.

In the *varus osteotomy,* by resecting a precisely planned medially based wedge, the femoral head is turned inward as far as possible and displaced medially until the articular contours are congruent. This provides the maximal surface area for weight-transmission. Depending on the case, a varus angle of 15–40° may be necessary. The adductor muscles are divided subcutaneously or by open tenotomy; the tension of the abductor and iliopsoas muscles is automatically reduced by the upward movement of the greater and lesser trochanters. Finally, the shaft fragment is displaced medially about 1 cm, i.e., returned to its physiological position. A typical example (Fig. 19 b, c) illustrates how, in a case of osteoarthritis due to coxa valga

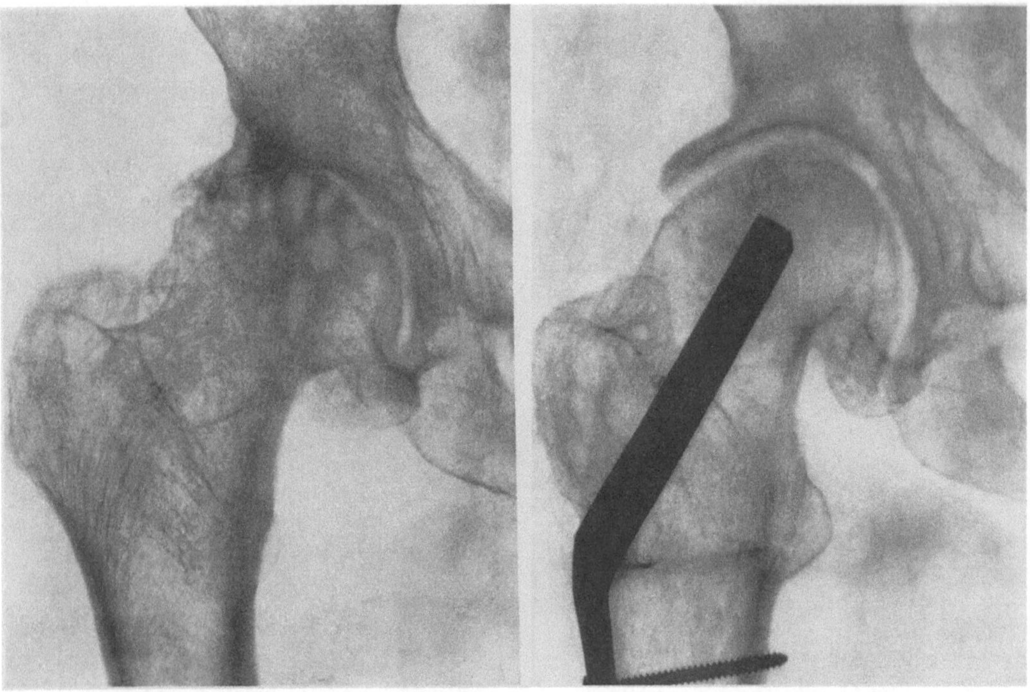
a b

Fig. 21 a, b. Severe osteoarthritis in a 63-year-old female patient. **a** X-ray before operation. No joint space is visible, there is triangular bony sclerosis in the acetabular roof, sclerotic bony tissue in the head containing several cysts, and extensive osteophytes (capital drop) can be seen, especially over the medial contour of the head. **b** Eight years after valgus osteotomy. The subchondral bony sclerosis in the acetabular roof has become normal (sourcil), and a joint space has developed which is equally wide throughout

subluxans, a varus osteotomy achieved an excellent result which was maintained at the time of the follow-up examination $16^1/_2$ years postoperatively. It is, therefore, justifiable to claim that this procedure results in long-term recovery.

The left hip joint (Fig. 19a) of the same woman, with the same degree of coxa valga (150°), shows that the size of the neck shaft angle alone is not reason enough to operate since the normal sourcil proves that the articular pressure on this side is not excessive. In support of this contention were the facts that no pathologic alterations were observed and that the patient had no subjective complaints.

If the congruence of the articular surfaces which results in an increase of the weight-bearing surface can be achieved only by turning the femoral head outward in the acetabulum, then a *valgus osteotomy* is indicated. As in the varus osteotomy, it is extremely important to determine precisely the size of the laterally based wedge which has to be removed. Its lower border is at right angles to the femoral shaft at the level of the lesser trochanter (Fig. 20a). This procedure (P II) also decreases the compressive force acting on the joint, since the muscles are slackened, the adductor and iliopsoas muscles by a tenotomy and the abductor muscles by an osteotomy and upward displacement of the greater trochanter by about 3 cm or by division of the muscles. The shaft fragment is displaced laterally in order to avoid a genu valgum.

A preexisting coxa valga does not by itself contraindicate a valgus osteotomy, as can be seen in Fig. 20a, b. Only the restoration of congruence of the joint is decisive. The medial capital drop plays an important role because it becomes incorporated into the weight-bearing surface.

Figure 21a shows very advanced osteoarthritis of the hip in a 63-year-old female patient. The head of the femur contains several cysts,

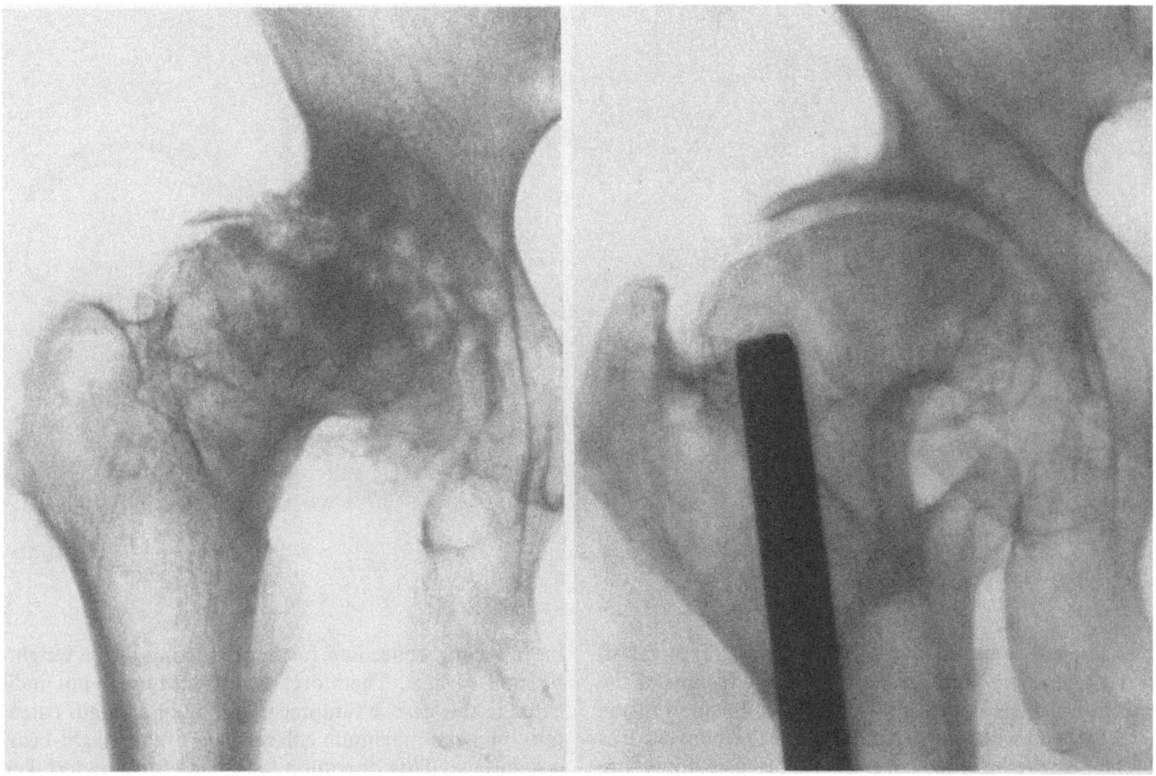

a b

Fig. 22 a, b. Extremely severe osteoarthritis in a 56-year-old female patient. **a** Shortly before operation, the joint is severely disturbed, the joint space has practically disappeared, there is a large triangular subchondral bony sclerosis in the acetabular roof, numerous cysts are present in the acetabulum and head, and a large capital drop is clearly visible. **b** 11 years postoperatively after a valgus osteotomy (with an oblique cut), the joint is completely regenerated and free from abnormality. The sclerosis in the acetabular roof looks like a normal sourcil and the articular cartilage is again of normal width. The patient, a housewife, has been fully active

indicating excessive stress. The joint space has disappeared, and an extensive capital drop is present. The result of a valgus osteotomy remains excellent after more than 8 years. Note specifically the width of the joint space shown in the X-ray. This suggests regeneration of the articular cartilage (Fig. 21 b).

Initially I carried out the valgus osteotomy by making the cut obliquely in order to relax the adductor and iliopsoas muscles by an upward displacement of the shaft fragment. This is in no way identical to McMurray's osteotomy in which the femur is supported by the pelvis in order to reduce the load on the joint. In my operation the importance was placed on enlargement of the weight-bearing surface through restoration of congruence of the hip joint by removal of a bony wedge with a precisely predetermined angle.

However, several disadvantages were observed with the oblique osteotomy:

1. Shortening of the leg,
2. Accentuation of the physiological genu valgum due to medial displacement of the upper fragment,
3. Insufficient contact of the osteotomy surfaces due to possible derotation.

For these reasons, the oblique osteotomy was abandoned in favor of the previously described horizontal cut at the level of the lesser trochanter with the wedge taken out of the proximal fragment. As far as long-term success is concerned, results were the same with the oblique and transverse sections; in the example in Fig. 22, nearly 11 years after the valgus osteotomy the joint still has a smooth contour with

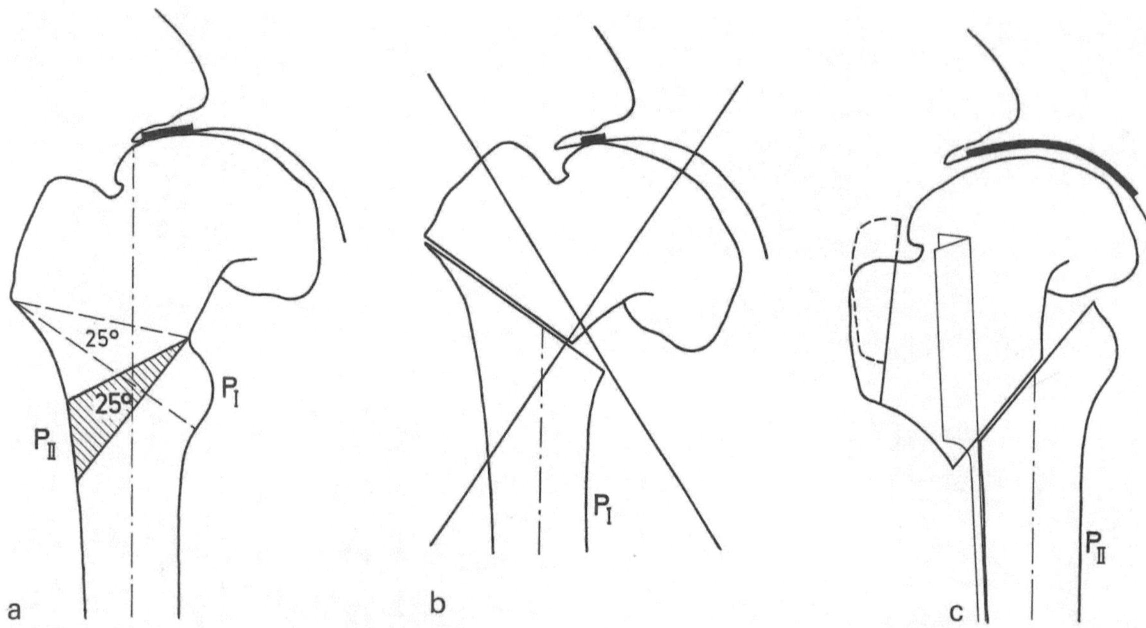

Fig. 23a–c. Examination of whether varus (P I) or valgus (P II) osteotomy is indicated. **a** Severe reduction of the weight-bearing surface in the case of subluxation of the femoral head with a large capital drop. The bony wedges to be removed for a varus or valgus osteotomy are marked. **b** Graphic planning of a varus osteotomy shows more incongruence and further reduction in the weight-bearing surface. Therefore, this procedure is not indicated in this case. **c** Graphic planning of a valgus osteotomy shows a maximum enlargement of the weight-bearing surface. This operation was, therefore, undertaken (see Fig. 22b)

a distinct joint space in the X-ray and a uniform, narrow sourcil, which would indicate much reduced and evenly distributed articular pressure.

Indications for Varus (P I) and Valgus (P II) Osteotomy

In certain cases, the decision can be extremely difficult as to whether a varus or valgus osteotomy is indicated to enlarge the weight-bearing surface of the joint. It is not the form of the deformity or its etiology which are decisive, but rather the magnitude and distribution of the articular pressure. It is, therefore, as Fig. 20 shows, erroneous to assume that a varus osteotomy is always indicated in the case of subluxation of the femoral head. This fallacy has often led to failures which were then unfairly ascribed to the method itself.

Suitable X-rays and preoperative diagrams should serve as an empirical basis for determining which of the two procedures will achieve the maximum enlargement of the weight-bearing surface of the joint (see Pauwels 1976a, pp. 159ff.). Often X-rays with the leg in abduction and adduction clearly show whether a varus or valgus osteotomy is indicated. However, the type of osteotomy to be performed can only be reliably determined by graphic planning of the operation. This is especially important for determining the degree, i.e., choosing the size and position of the bony wedge to be resected. In case of doubt, preoperative diagrams must be drawn for both varus and valgus osteotomies (Fig. 23).

Should either procedure be executed with erroneous indication, then failure is inevitable. Then a further operation can and should be undertaken. According to our experience, when correctly indicated, such a reoperation can be expected to give good long-term results. This topic has been discussed in greater detail elsewhere (Pauwels 1976a, p. 225ff.).

Summary

Osteoarthritis of the hip is caused and maintained by articular pressure of pathologic magnitude and distribution. Logical therapy of this disease must, therefore, affect the mechanical stress and aim at reducing the articular pressure. When the articular contours are incongruent, this is only possible by enlarging the weight-bearing surface. The necessary alteration in magnitude and distribution of the articular stress is achieved solely by changing the neck-shaft angle. The indication for opening or closing this angle depends on whether the increase of the weight-bearing surface of the joint can be achieved by rotating the femoral head inward or outward. The success of the operation depends on the precise determination of the amount by which the neck-shaft angle is to be reduced or increased. For this reason, the operation cannot be a standard procedure. It must be carried out according to a correctly executed drawing adapted to the individual case and based on a definite biomechanical rationale. Only in this manner can satisfactory long-term results be reliably achieved and that even in older patients (Pauwels 1976a, pp. 200–209).

References

Fischer O (1899) Der Gang des Menschen. II. Teil: Die Bewegung des Gesamtschwerpunktes und die äußeren Kräfte. Abh Kgl sächs Ges Wiss math-phys Kl, 25:1–163

Grasset EJ (1960) La coxarthrose. Etude anatomique et histologique. Georg, Genève; Masson, Paris

Kummer B (1969) Die Beanspruchung des Gelenkes, dargestellt am Beispiel des menschlichen Hüftgelenks. 55. Kongreß Verh Dtsch Orthop Ges Kassel, 1968, pp 301–311

McMurray TP (1935) Br J Surg 22:716–227

McMurray TP (1939) J Bone Joint Surg 21:1–11

Pauwels F (1950) Über eine kausale Behandlung der Coxa valga luxans. Z Orthop 79:305–315

Pauwels F (1961) Neue Richtlinien für die Behandlung der Coxarthrose. 48. Kongreß Verh Dtsch Orthop Ges Berlin, 1960, pp 332–366

Pauwels F (1976a) Biomechanics of the normal and diseased hip. Theoretical foundation, technique and results of treatment. Springer, Berlin Heidelberg New York

Pauwels F (1976b) Über die gestaltende Wirkung der funktionellen Anpassung des Knochens. Anat Anz 139:213–220

Intertrochanteric Osteotomy: Indication, Preoperative Planning, Technique

M.E. Müller

Introduction

Pauwels showed many years ago that an intertrochanteric osteotomy can change the loading of a hip, and demonstrated the profound effects that such a change in loading can bring about. A full discussion of this subject can be found in the chapters here by Pauwels, Bombelli, and Schneider. These biomechanical principles form a basis for the understanding of the effects of an intertrochanteric osteotomy in the treatment of pseudarthrosis of the femoral neck, coxa valga with subluxation, and osteoarthritis.

I have organized my discussion of the intertrochanteric osteotomy under indications, grouping them into very good, good, and questionable.

The *preoperative planning and drawing* of each intertrochanteric osteotomy is most important, and is therefore discussed in detail for each operation. Prerequisites for planning are knowledge of the normal axial relationships, performance of the necessary clinical and radiological examinations, and familiarity with the technical details of an intertrochanteric osteotomy and the principles of stable fixation. The surgeon must also know the causes and treatment of the two chief complications of the procedure, avascular necrosis of the femoral head and loss of fixation and position.

In the special section of this chapter I shall discuss only very briefly the *technical details* of repositioning osteotomy, varus and valgus osteotomies, and derotation osteotomy and the use of the special seating chisel, as these have already been published in the English literature [5, 7, 9]. On the other hand, the technical details of the complex intertrochanteric osteotomy necessary in the treatment of coxa valga with subluxation or of slipped capital epiphysis have so far been published only in the German literature [4, 6]. These I shall discuss therefore at length. I shall also discuss some extremely important but poorly appreciated technical details of a cervical osteotomy used in the treatment of a slipped capital epiphysis of over 50°, as these profoundly affect the likelihood of success.

General Section

Aims and Indications

Intertrochanteric osteotomies are successful in the treatment of many disease processes in the region of the proximal femur. This is particularly true in those diseases which have a *clearly demonstrable cause*. In these, the success of an intertrochanteric osteotomy can be predicted almost with mathematical certainty as long as a careful preoperative plan is made and no mishap occurs during surgery.

Very Good Indications. The following conditions are very good indications for an intertrochanteric osteotomy, as with proper preoperative planning and proper execution an excellent result is almost a certainty.

1. All *malunions* of fractures in the trochanteric region, as long as normal anatomical relationships can be reconstructed (Figs. 10, 11).
2. All *pseudarthroses of the neck with a viable head,* as long as the repositioning osteotomy will convert the forces of shearing and displacement into forces of compression (Figs. 14, 15).
3. *Congenital coxa vara,* as long as the hip is freely mobile (Fig. 17).
4. *Avascular necrosis* involving a small well-circumscribed area, as long as it is possible by means of intertrochanteric osteotomy to ro-

tate this segment out of the weight-bearing area. Such cases of avascular necrosis usually occur as complications of a fracture of the neck or traumatic dislocation (Fig. 18). Osteochondritis dissecans falls into this category [7].

5. An *arthrodesis* which has healed in malposition or one in which the shaft was excessively medialized is relatively easy to correct (Fig. 19).
6. *Shortening and lengthening osteotomies* up to 2.5 cm are simple and sure in the intertrochanteric area (Figs. 21, 22).

Good Indications. Under good indications, I have grouped the cases whose prognosis can be profoundly changed by means of an intertrochanteric osteotomy despite the fact that complete healing or disappearance of the causative problem cannot be anticipated. These are the cases in which normal anatomy and biomechanics of the hip cannot be reestablished or those in which the underlying disease process remains unaffected.

1. *Coxa valga and subluxation* in patients of 10 years or older with retained abduction, a broad cartilage space, and in whom an adduction (varus) osteotomy significantly improves the congruence of the joint (Figs. 24, 26). Occasionally, one has to combine the procedure with osteotomy of the greater trochanter (Figs. 7, 27), curettage and bone grafting of acetabular cysts [7], or shelfplasty of the acetabular roof (Fig. 28).
2. *Oval femoral head with a medial capital drop osteophyte* which by means of an abduction or a valgus osteotomy can be brought into the weight-bearing zone (Fig. 29).
3. Chronic *slipped capital epiphysis* with a slip of 25°–50° and rotational deformity of the limb (Figs. 34, 35). In cases of a slip of over 50°, we must consider cervical osteotomy rather than intertrochanteric osteotomy (Figs. 37, 38).
4. *Excessive anteversion in a child.* Intertrochanteric osteotomy may be combined with a pelvic osteotomy of Salter or Chiari (Figs. 40, 41).
5. *Legg-Perthes disease,* in order to bring the lateral portion of the head into the weight-bearing zone. This will result in the development of a concentric femoral head (Figs. 43, 44).
6. *Abduction deformity* after a *healed acetabular fracture* (Fig. 45) or after a healed *posttraumatic avascular necrosis* which has resulted in a deformity of the femoral head but where there is well-preserved articular cartilage space (Fig. 46).
7. *Spastic cerebral palsy* in those children who are able to walk, but who walk in marked equinus. Through the correction of the marked anteversion, it is frequently possible to correct permanently the equinus and scissoring (Fig. 47).
8. Fresh *femoral neck fractures* in patients with severe osteoporosis or intertrochanteric fractures with severe comminution of the medial buttress. In an intertrochanteric fracture with comminution, the osteotomy makes it possible to secure a stable medial buttress (Fig. 49).

Questionable Indications. In patients with *advanced osteoarthritis*, particularly in those with so-called primary idiopathic osteoarthritis, it is much more difficult to delineate indications and goals of treatment. In patients over 60 with severe pain and disability, it is difficult to conceive of anything but total hip replacement. In the younger individual, one can at times achieve a symptom-free interval of 10 years or more (Figs. 50, 51). The intertrochanteric osteotomy alone results in local hyperemia, improved venous drainage, and remodeling of the internal architecture. In addition, the varus or valgus should result in an increase in the surface area of contact with a resultant decrease in stress, an increase in the length of the muscle effort arm, and a relaxation of the periarticular musculature [7, 10].

Since the indications for intertrochanteric osteotomy and treatment of advanced osteoarthritis in patients over 60 are rather rare [12], and as they are discussed at length by others in this book, I shall confine myself chiefly to a discussion of those conditions which present very good or good indications for an intertrochanteric osteotomy.

Normal Anatomical Axial Relationships

The intricate relationships between the mechanical axis and the body axis and between the anatomical axis of the femoral shaft and the knee joint axis in the frontal plane (Fig. 1) are responsible for genu varum and genu valgum and thus for the degree of loading of the medial and lateral halves of the knee joint. The mechanics of a congruous hip joint is determined by the angle of femoral neck inclination (CCD angle), by the angle denoting femoral head coverage (CE angle of Wiberg), and by the angle of inclination of the acetabular roof (AC angle). The angle between the knee joint axis and the femoral neck axis is called the angle of anteversion (AT angle).

It is extremely important to remember when one inserts implants into or about the greater trochanter that the axis of the greater trochanter subtends an angle of 25°–30° with the axis of the femoral neck (Figs. 1.4, 8). Thus malinsertion of the seating chisel could result in injury to the retinacular vessels and lead to subsequent avascular necrosis, and malinsertion of the hook plate could result in failure to achieve stable fixation.

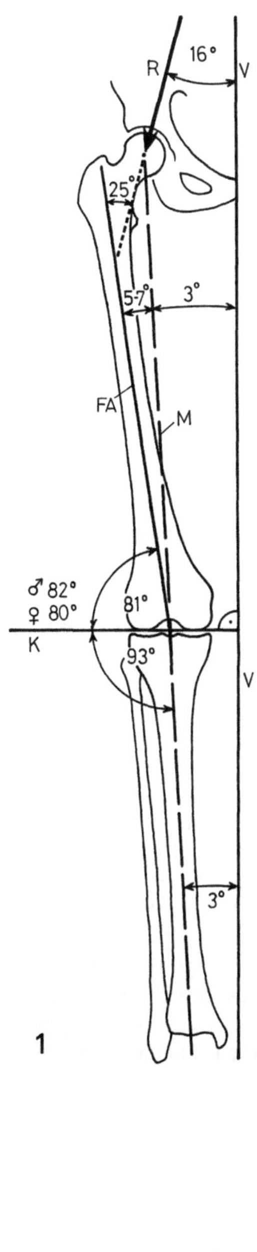

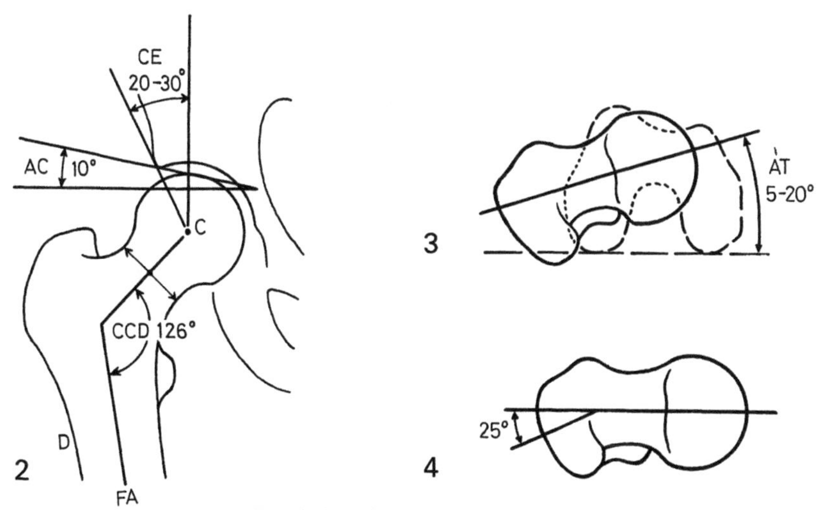

Fig. 1. Physiological axial and angular correlationships of lower extremity. **1** Frontal plane. The mechanical axis *M* goes through the center of the femoral head, the center of the knee, and the center of the ankle. It subtends an angle of 3° with the vertical *V* and 5°–7°, depending on the sex of the patient, with the anatomical axis of the femoral shaft *FA*. The axis of the knee joint *K* is perpendicular to the body axis or the vertical, and the angle which the resultant *R* of the compressive forces on the hip subtends with the vertical is 16°. **2** The axis of the femoral neck corresponds to the line which joints the center of the femoral head *C* with the center of the neck. The CCD angle is the angle subtended between the neck and shaft axis and averages 124°–130°. The CE angle should be at least 20° and the AC angle 10° or less. **3** In the transverse plane we have the AT angle, which varies from 5° to 25° (average 12°). It is the angle between the neck axis and the condylar axis. **4** The angle subtended between the axis of the greater trochanter and the neck axis is somewhere between 25° and 30°

Clinical Examination

The important findings whose presence or absence must be determined are the Duchenne-Trendelenburg limp and the Trendelenburg sign, genu varum or valgum, hip joint contracture, and a fixed pelvic tilt due to lumbosacral deformity. The passive range of movement of the hip without anesthesia must also be investigated. The degree of extension is best determined with the patient lying on the opposite side with the opposite limb in maximum flexion (the Thomas test performed with the patient on his side), and the degree of flexion is similarly determined with the opposite limb in maximum extension. Abduction and adduction are best determined with the patient supine. The opposite limb should fix the pelvis by being held in abduction or adduction respectively. Internal and external rotation are best determined with the patient prone. One must determine the true and apparent leg length discrepancy with the patient lying and standing. The true leg length is measured from the anterior superior iliac spine to the tip of the lateral malleolus while both legs are held in exactly the same alignment and flexion.

Radiological Examination

An AP view of the pelvis taken with the patient supine and with the beam centered one finger breadth above the pubic symphysis is usually all that one needs to establish the diagnosis (Fig. 2). In order to display abduction and adduction contractures on the same X-ray, one should bind both legs together at the knees. If the affliction is only unilateral, the X-ray should also be taken with the normal leg in internal rotation (Fig. 2.2). The AP view of the hip in internal rotation provides one with a real view of the femoral neck, which is usually all that one needs for preoperative planning in a post-traumatic malalignment (Fig. 11). The cross-table lateral view is taken with the healthy leg crossed over the involved leg. The latter should be held in slight adduction (Fig. 2.3). In order to determine the degree of abduction and adduction, and, if one is contemplating an osteotomy, the congruence in varus or valgus, the so-called functional X-rays should be obtained. These are taken either with the patient supine and the involved hip in maximum abduction and adduction or with the patient prone and the hip in maximum abduction and internal rotation (Fig. 2.4–2.6).

In the preoperative planning of an intertrochanteric osteotomy for the treatment of a subluxed hip or chronic epiphyseal slip, one requires specific X-ray projections in order to be able to determine the mechanics of the involved hip. These special projections are discussed in detail in the section of this chapter which deals with these particular conditions (Figs. 23, 30). Anteversion is most accurately and most easily evaluated with the CT scan. However, this is still a very expensive procedure and one which is not universally available.

General Operative Technique

Construction of an intertrochanteric osteotomy (Fig. 3) begins for me principally with a transverse osteotomy of the femur just proximal to the lesser trochanter. This allows rotational correction and displacement. Once this is accomplished, angular corrections can be obtained and wedges removed from the proximal fragment in both the frontal and sagittal plane. For the fixation of adduction or varus osteotomies, we use 90° osteotomy plates. For the fixation

Fig. 3. General operative technique of intertrochanteric osteotomy. Always begin with an osteotomy at right angles to the femoral shaft axis. **1** Adduction or varus osteotomy in the adult: transverse osteotomy with a medial wedge. **2** Adduction or varus osteotomy in a child: transverse osteotomy with an opening wedge laterally. Internal fixation in children over 5 is carried out with the special 90° plate and under 5 with the special children's plate which is bent to the desired angle. **3** Valgus osteotomy up to 25° is fixed with a condylar plate. The wedge is taken from the proximal fragment. **4** Abduction or valgus osteotomy of 30°. Use the 120° blade plate for fixation and remove the 30° wedge from the distal fragment. **5** Abduction or valgus osteotomy of more than 30°. Remove a 30° wedge from the distal fragment and the remaining wedge from the proximal fragment ▷

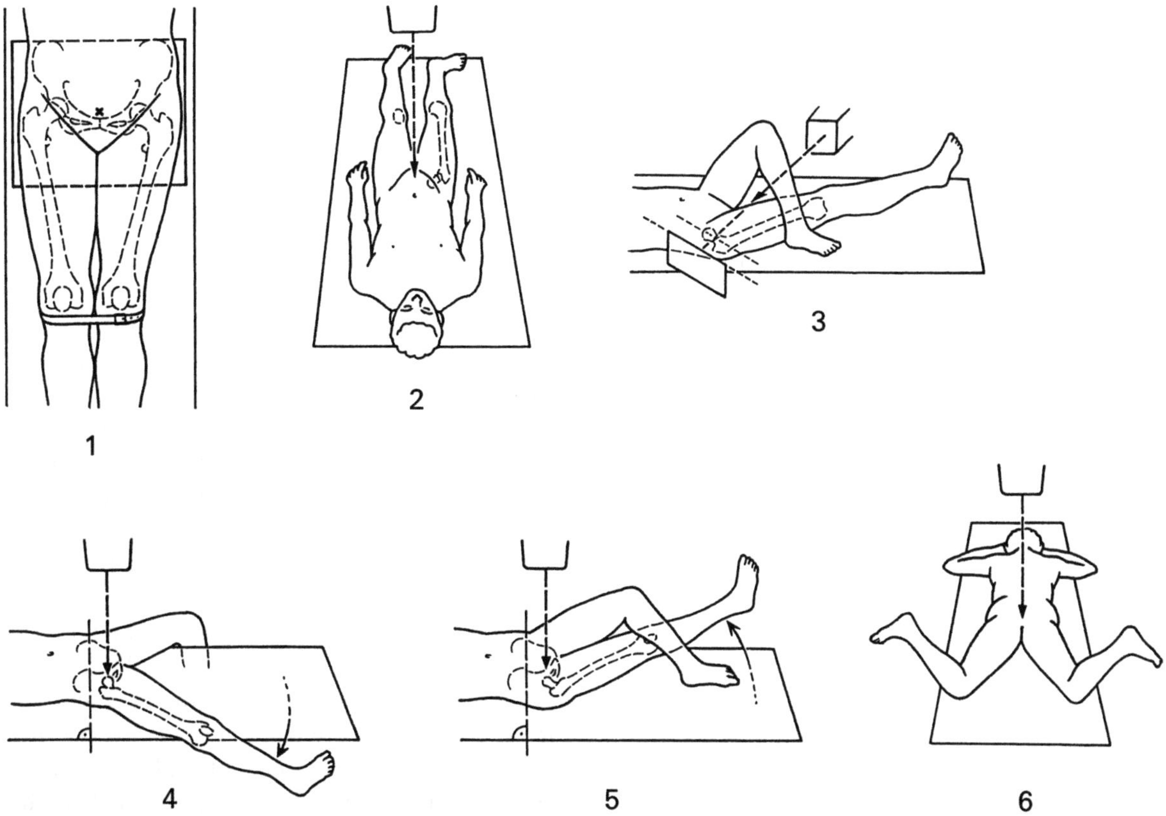

Fig. 2. Common X-rays of hip necessary for planning. **1** The AP survey film of the pelvis in the adult is taken with the beam centered one finger above the pubic symphysis. The patellae should be pointing forward and the knees should be touching. **2** In unilateral disease, the normal hip should be in internal rotation when the AP of the pelvis is taken. This gives one the orthogonal projection of the femoral neck (see also Fig. 30.1). **3** In order to obtain the cross-table lateral of the femoral neck and trochanter area, the normal leg should be crossed over the involved leg. **4–6** Functional X-rays of the hip consist of AP projections in maximal abduction and maximal adduction and a PA projection with the patient prone with both hips in maximal internal rotation and abduction

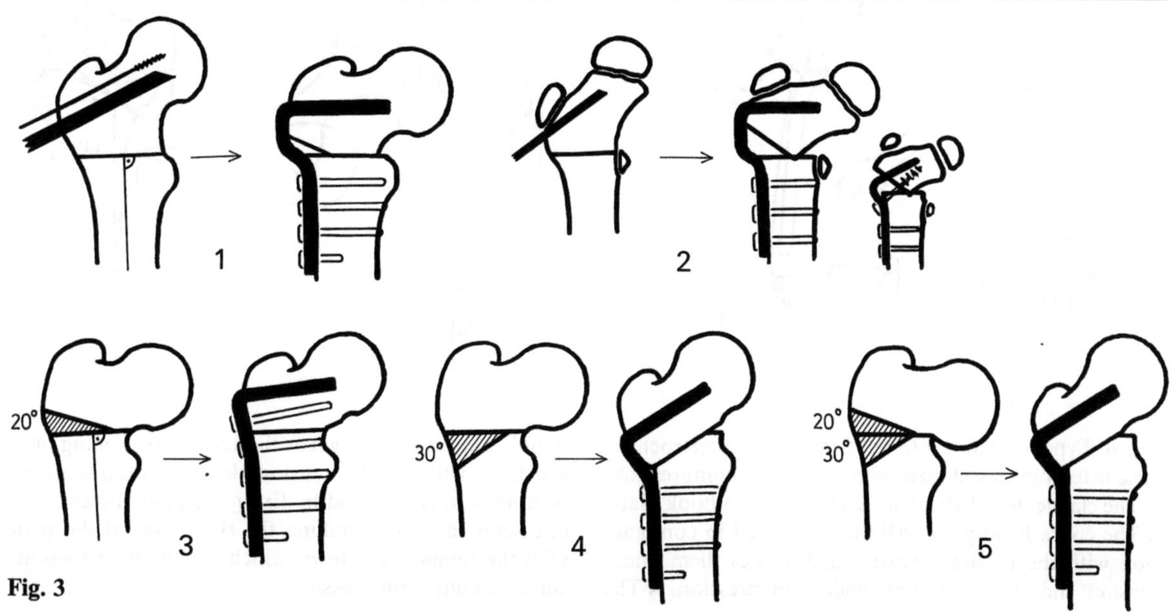

Fig. 3

of abduction or valgus intertrochanteric osteotomies of 30° or more which are necessary to correct corresponding adduction contractures, we most commonly use the double-angled plates which permit the resection of wedges not only from the distal but also from the proximal fragment. In children under 15, resection of wedges is unnecessary, particularly if the involvement is unilateral. We simply tip the fragments and leave them as opening wedge osteotomies, because in children, despite the gaps which one creates in this manner, union occurs rapidly.

Fixation of the Intertrochanteric Osteotomy (Fig. 4)

Hip spicas, if ever used, should be applied only in children under 6 or 7 years of age. This is possible because the degree of stability of internal fixation which can be achieved today, usually by means of interfragmental compression, prevents any change of position of the fragment. This degree of stability also allows early postoperative mobilization without the fear of loss of position. Furthermore, union can be anticipated in 5–8 weeks. The 90° osteotomy plate, the condylar plate, and the cobra head plate are placed under tension with the tension device, which results in axial compression. When the double-angled 120° plate is used, interfragmental compression is achieved in a special way, involving first screwing the plate to the femoral shaft distally (Fig. 4.4). Because the blade plates have a fixed angle, the blade of the plate chosen for a particular intertrochanteric osteotomy must be inserted into the femoral neck at an inclination to the shaft axis determined in the

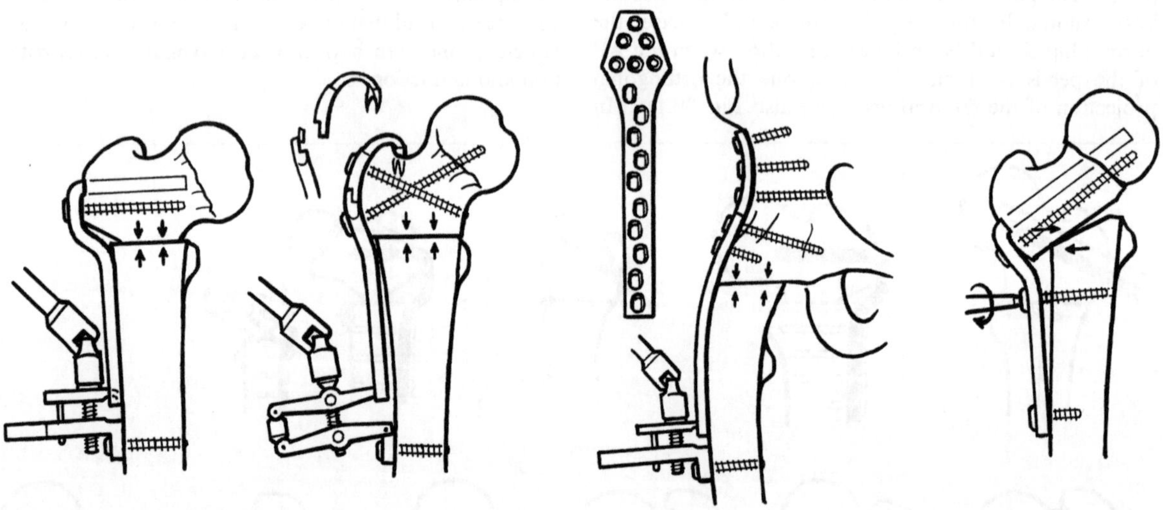

Fig. 4. Types of stable internal fixations of intertrochanteric osteotomies stabilized with the aid of compression. **1** The classic 90° blade plate. **2** The bipartite hook plate. **3** The cobra head plate. All three are used in combination with the tension device, which places them under tension and the osteotomy under compression. **4** The double-angled plates such as the 120° repositioning plate are used without the tension device. Interfragmental compression is achieved by fixing the plate distally with one screw and then pulling the shaft toward the plate with the remaining screws, which brings the osteotomy surfaces under compression

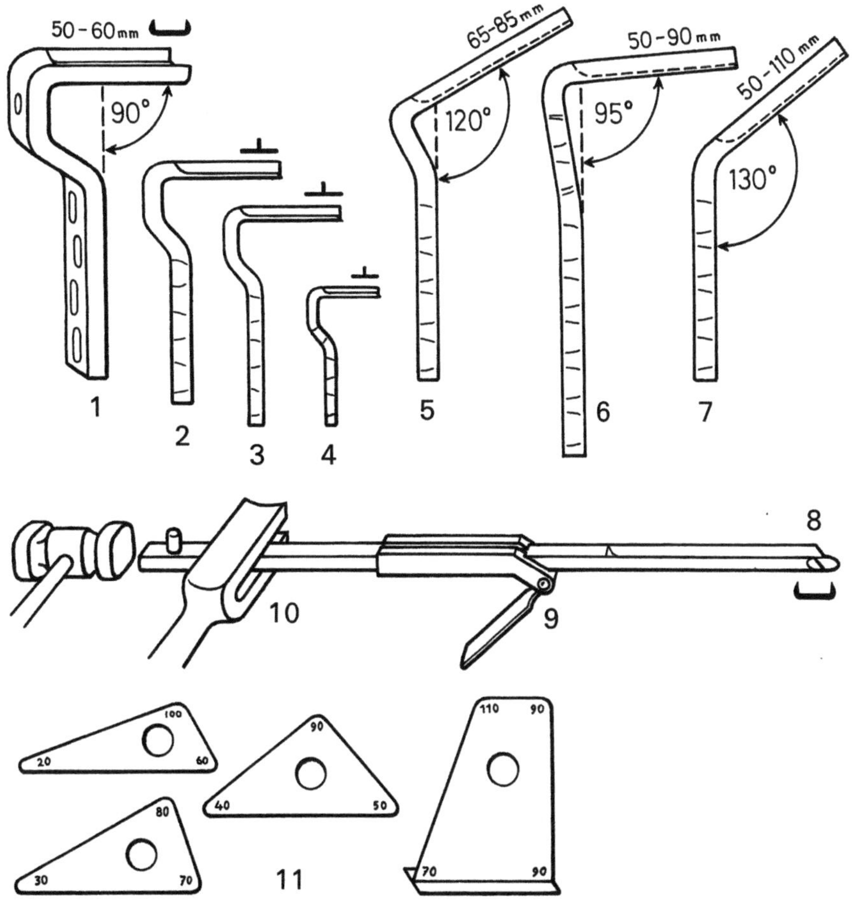

Fig. 5. Most common plates, seating chisel, and triangles used in carrying out an intertrochanteric osteotomy. **1–4** The 90° plate for adults, adolescents, children, and small children. **5** The double-angled 120° plate. **6** The condylar blade plate. **7** The 130° blade plate. **8** The U-shaped seating chisel. **9** The seating chisel guide. **10** The slotted hammer. **11** The triangles used in the determination of angles

preoperative plan. At the time of surgery, the correct insertion is accomplished with the help of the seating chisel and the various osteotomy aiming devices (Fig. 5).

Interrelated Phenomena

Any corrective osteotomy carried out on a tubular bone results not only in a change of angle but also in a transposition of the fragments. Thus, an intertrochanteric osteotomy allows not only angular corrections in three planes (abduction/adduction, flexion/extension, and internal/external rotation), but also transposition of the fragment in three planes: medialization/lateralization, anterior/posterior transposition, and axial transposition, i.e., shortening or lengthening. Furthermore, one must recognize that with each angular correction, the trochanters move either proximally or distally. Each angular correction and each transposition must be carefully calculated preoperatively and compensated for if necessary. The most common interrelated changes are portrayed in Fig. 6. The only change which we have not discussed is that in the inclination of the neck which comes about with changes in the sagittal plane; for instance, an extension osteotomy results in a certain degree of varus. Furthermore, each medialization of the shaft results in genu valgum and each lateralization in

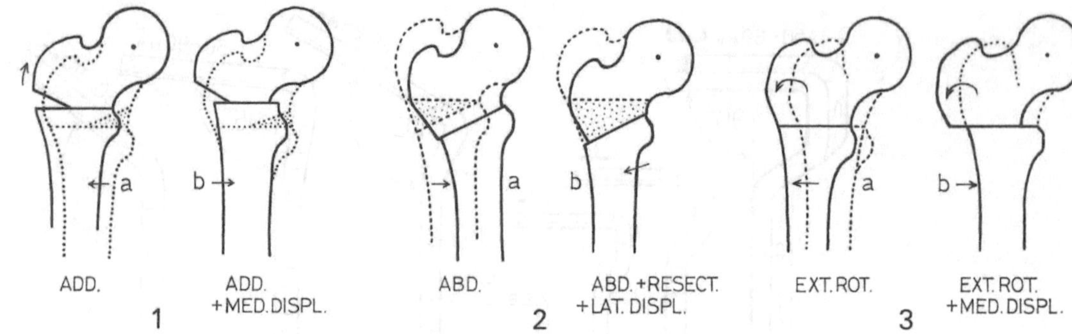

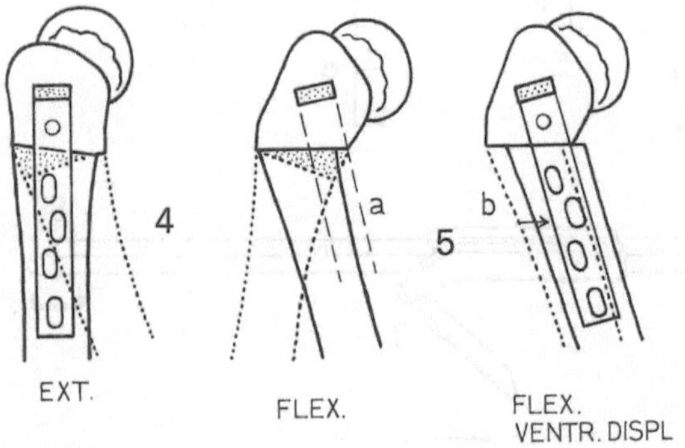

Fig. 6. Interrelationship between angular correction and shaft transposition. **1 a** In an adduction or varus osteotomy the shaft is lateralized and a genu varum results; **b** medialization is necessary in order to bring the femoral shaft axis to its correct preoperative position. **2 a** Abduction or valgus results in lengthening and medialization of the shaft; **b** the situation is normalized by resection of bone to equalize length and by lateralization of the shaft. **3** External rotation causes medialization, at least as long as the joint is freely mobile. **4** In an extension osteotomy, the shaft fragment must be transposed dorsally so that the plate will come to lie along the shaft. The extension results always in varization of 5°–10° or more. **5** In a flexion osteotomy, the shaft must be transposed ventrally or the plate would not make contact with it

---

Fig. 7. 1–6 Preoperative planning and drawing of a complex adduction (varus) osteotomy. **1** The preoperative X-ray. **2, 3** On separate sheets of tracing paper, draw first the outline of the proximal femur (**A**) and then the acetabulum (**B**). On **A** mark in the femoral shaft axis and at right angles to it just proximal to the lesser trochanter, the projected osteotomy line (*IO*), as well as the projected osteotomy of the greater trochanter (*TO*). On **B** mark similarly the shaft axis corresponding to **A**. **4** Place **B** over **A** and turn **B** until the head becomes covered by the acetabulum. Take a different-colored pencil and draw in the proximal femur without the trochanter and draw in the femoral axis which will now subtend with the previous axis *FA* an angle of 25°. This will become the subsequent angle of varization or adduction. **5** Position the two sheets of tracing paper so that the two femoral shaft axes *FA* are superimposed. Move **B** distally until the medial edge of the proximal femur touches the intertrochanteric osteotomy line. Draw in the distal femur and the greater trochanter. The triangular wedge *a* which has to be resected can now be clearly outlined. This corresponds to the angle of correction, that is, to an angle of 25°. **6** On a third sheet of tracing paper (**C**) draw in the projected final result with the suitable 90° blade plate. **7, 8** Tactical drawings and steps. On a fourth sheet of tracing paper (**D**) draw in the contours of the proximal femur (**A**) together with the *IO*, the *TO*, the triangular segment *a*, and the blade plate. On a fifth sheet of tracing paper (**E**) draw in the contours of the projected final result **C**. On these two drawings, mark in the steps of the procedure in numerical order. Thus on tracing paper **D**: *1* First Kirschner wire (K1) along femoral neck as guide to anteversion. *2* Second Kirschner wire (K2) at right angles to shaft at level of lesser trochanter. *3* IO. *4* Seating chisel parallel to K2 inserted partway into greater trochanter. *5* TO. *6* IO to middle of shaft. *7* At right angles to IO, excision of the triangular wedge *a*. *8* Third Kirschner wire (K3) with a threaded end is inserted into cranial portion of proximal femur. *9* Resection of K2 2 cm from shaft. *10* Point of entry of seating chisel. *11* Insertion of seating chisel to a depth of 60 mm. Immediately thereafter, backing out of seating chisel by 20 mm. *12, 13* Insertion of two Kirschner wires at right angles to shaft on each side of IO line for rotational control. *14* IO now complete and proximal fragment tilted into varus. *15* Any projecting piece of bone now resected. *16* Withdrawal of seating chisel. On tracing paper **E**: *17* Blade of chosen *90°* blade plate is first pushed through slot cut in greater trochanter and then inserted into previously prepared channel in femoral neck. *18* Insertion of proximal screw. *19* With a Verbrugge, plate is held to femoral shaft. *20* Tension device fixed to femur. *21* Resected triangular wedge *a* inserted between osteotomy surfaces. With tension device, triangular fragment *a* and osteotomy surfaces are brought under compression. *22* Plate fixed to shaft with four screws. **9** X-ray 1 year after surgery

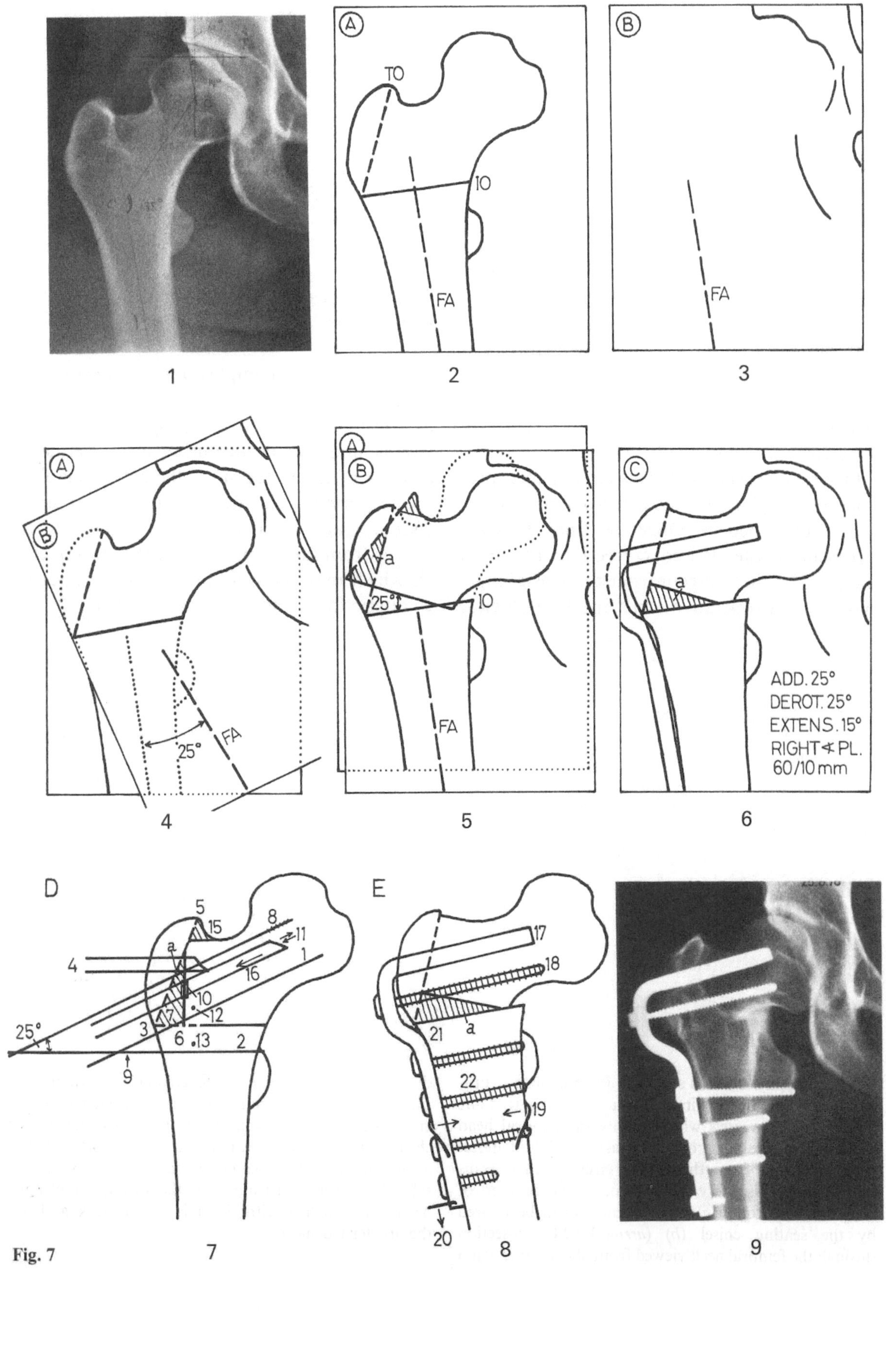
1
A
TO
IO
FA
2
B
FA
3
A
B
25°
FA
4
A
B
a
25°
IO
FA
5
C
a
ADD. 25°
DEROT. 25°
EXTENS. 15°
RIGHT∢PL.
60/10 mm
6
D
5
15
8
11
1
4
a
16
10
12
25°
3
17
6
13
2
9
7
E
17
18
21
a
22
19
20
8
9

Fig. 7

genu varum. This is discussed extensively in my respective articles [5, 7]. All these interrelated changes must be taken into account during preoperative planning.

Preoperative Planning and Drawing

The planning of a simple adduction or varus or of an abduction or valgus osteotomy has been carefully described on more than one occasion by Pauwels, Blount, and Müller [1, 4, 5, 7, 10]. We shall concern ourselves therefore only with difficult examples, such as the planning of a complex osteotomy of 25° varus with derotation to correct excessive anteversion of 25° and extension of 15° plus a distal transposition of the greater trochanter (Fig. 7.1).

One requires sheets of transparent paper, protractors, templates for the corresponding plates, and colored pencils. Once the final drawing, representing the desired correction, has been completed, the surgeon must painstakingly mark all the operative steps in chronological order on the preoperative and postoperative drawings (Fig. 7.2). Such careful planning results in a much faster operative procedure; X-rays during the procedure become unnecessary, all the necessary instruments can be prepared prior to surgery, and if complications arise, the surgeon can deal with them more quickly and definitively. For a description of the technique of the procedure see p. 49.

Complications of Intertrochanteric Osteotomies

The most feared complication of intertrochanteric osteotomy is avascular necrosis. It arises as a result of injury to the posterior retinacular vessels, and may occur during surgery either as a result of the reflexion of the soft tissue from the posterior or dorsal aspect of the intertrochanteric area or as a result of damage to the vessels from faulty insertion of the seating chisel, which may inadvertently enter the intertrochanteric fossa and cut the vessels (Fig. 8).

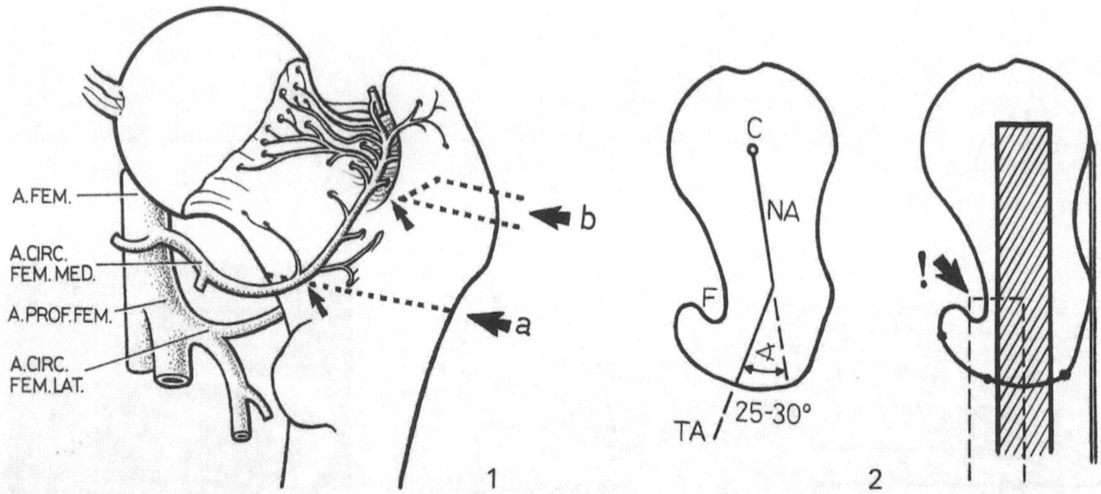

Fig. 8. Anatomy of blood supply to femoral head. **1** Posterior view of the proximal femur according to Lanz [3]. The blood vessels which supply the femoral head are found on the posterosuperior aspect of the femoral neck and arise from the arteria circumflexa dorsalis (after Lanz). This artery can be damaged by the intertrochanteric osteotomy (*a*) or its branches can be injured by the seating chisel (*b*) (*arrows*). **2** Cross-section through the femoral neck viewed from above: note again the 25°–30° angulation of the greater trochanter axis. The arrow shows where the posterior retinacular vessels are to be found and what would happen if the seating chisel were to be inserted not ventrally or anteriorly but in the middle of the greater trochanter, i.e. too far dorsally. It also demonstrates that the seating chisel must be inserted in line with the axis of the neck and not the greater trochanter

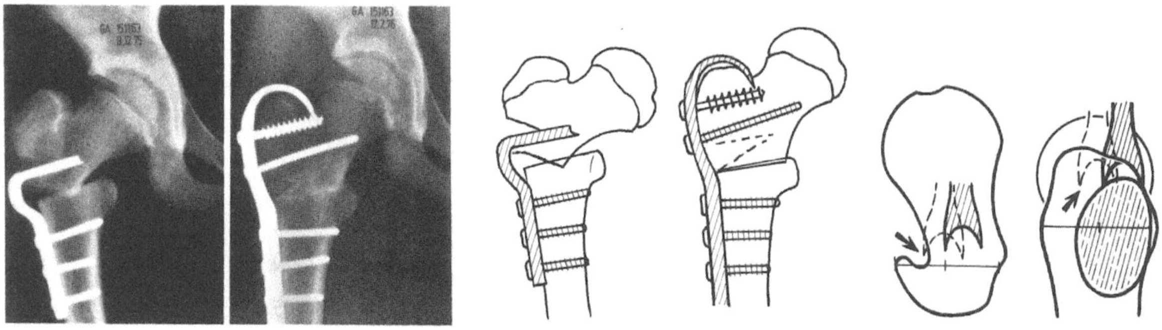

Fig. 9. Fracture of bony bridge between plate and intertrochanteric osteotomy and correction of this complication. **1** X-ray of a 12-year-old girl 12 days after intertrochanteric osteotomy. Note that the bridge between the point of entry of the blade and the intertrochanteric osteotomy was too narrow, and broke. **2** One month after revision and fixation with a hook plate. **3, 4** Preoperative planning. **5** The two hooks of the hook plate must be hammered in so that they straddle the highest point of the neck, i.e., they must be anterior and *not* in the middle of the greater trochanter. If the plate is in the middle of the trochanter, the posterior hook will be in space, the plate will engage the neck with only one prong, and the fixation will be unstable (*arrow*). On the *right*, the proximal femur in a longitudinal cross-section

In the treatment of massive avascular necrosis of the femoral head, total hip replacement arthroplasty is pretty well the procedure of choice. In the treatment of more localized areas of avascular necrosis, one must consider rotational osteotomies such as the Sugioka osteotomy [13]. These complex operations, which are carried out in the intertrochanteric area, may endanger the vessels. One must pay therefore great attention to the anatomy of the retinacular vessels supplying the femoral head and be aware of the different ways in which they can be injured.

Loss of position of the fragment, the second most important complication, can occur when the fixation is not sufficiently stable. This can happen if the blade cuts out of the proximal fragment or if there is insufficient contact of bone medially, giving rise to a deficient medial buttress. Similarly, if the ridge of bone between the osteotomy and the blade of the plate is too thin, the blade may loosen or the bridge may actually break, with loss of fixation (Fig. 9). If displacement occurs due to any of the above factors, all is not lost, as revision can be successfully carried out with the hook plate. When one uses the hook plate, it is important to remember that the hooks must be inserted on the neck as far anteriorly as possible, in order to achieve good purchase and prevent any possible damage to the retinacular vessels, which lie posteriorly.

Special Section

Posttraumatic Malalignment

Malalignment of fragments in the intertrochanteric area following fracture may result either from inadequate reduction or from unstable fixation because of a deficient medial buttress [8]. Malalignment following subcapital fractures is almost always combined with either avascular necrosis or pseudarthrosis and is discussed at length on p. 37.

The aim of the intertrochanteric osteotomy in the treatment of these malalignments is to recreate normal anatomical relationships as they exist on the normal side. Thus, when one comes to treat these cases, it is most important to obtain, in addition to the axial X-ray projection of the involved side, an AP view of the pelvis with the normal side in slight abduction and internal rotation in order to obtain an exact view of the femoral neck (Fig. 2.2). The outline of the involved as well as of the normal side is then traced on a separate piece of tracing

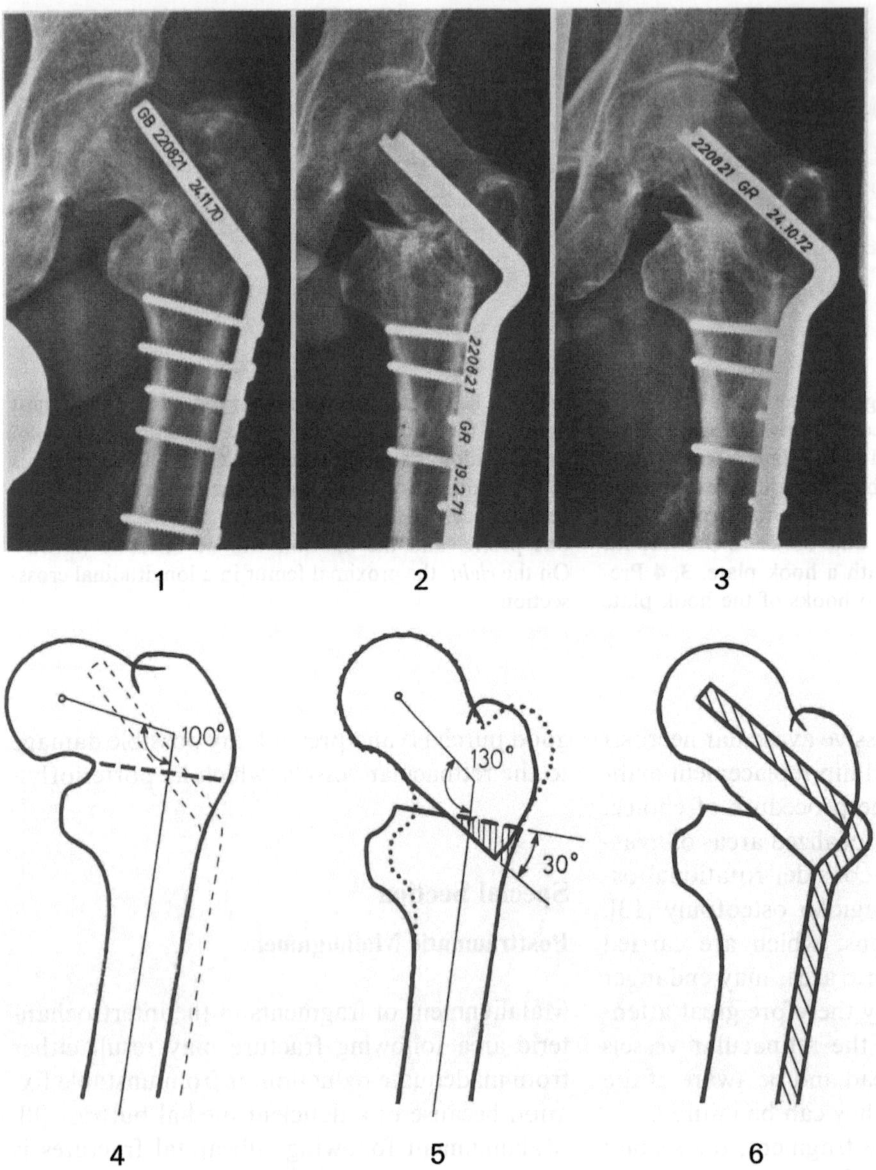

Fig. 10. Posttraumatic malalignment. G.R., 49-year-old man. **1** Note the varus malunion, which resulted from unstable fixation (the plate protruded through the back of the neck). **2** The 130° plate was used because a mistake was made in introducing the seating chisel and it was driven in too steeply. At $2^1/_2$ months after an abduction osteotomy of 30° and an extension of 20°. The shaft was medialized too much. **3** At 2 years: the patient is symptom-free but has developed a slight genu valgum. **4** The outline of the preoperative state with a neck-shaft angle of 100°. **5** The outline of the normal side has been dotted in and the outline of the proximal femur and of the distal femur of the previous drawing drawn in. This indicated a necessary resection of 30°. **6** The planned lateralization of the plate with a bone wedge was not carried out because it would have resulted in too small a contact area for the intertrochanteric osteotomy

paper. On the normal side, draw in the anatomical shaft axis of the femur as well as an osteotomy line just above the lesser trochanter at right angles to the long axis. The tracing paper is now turned over. On the tracing of the involved side mark in the femoral shaft axis as well as the osteotomy line. The latter must be drawn at the same distance from the lesser trochanter as it was on the normal side. The tracing of the abnormal femur is now placed under the tracing of the normal side so that the outlines of the proximal femur overlap. On the tracing of the normal side, the osteotomy line of the abnormal side is now drawn in. The angle subtended between the two osteotomy lines is the angle of the wedge which must be resected in the frontal plane (Fig. 10.4–10.6). Frequently, one must combine this wedge resection with an extension as well as with a derotation. The plate to be used for the fixation of the osteotomy is chosen with the help of the AO (ASIF) templates [7, 9]. The preoperative X-ray, the postoperative result, and the scheme of the planning of two typical osteotomies, one with a 130° plate and one with a 90° plate, are illustrated in Figs. 11 and 12 respectively. These illustrations also demonstrate the resection of the different wedges, whose size is determined by the plate used.

Pseudarthrosis of the Femoral Neck

Pauwels recognized as early as 1927 that a pseudarthrosis of the femoral neck would unite within a few months if one changed the inclination of the pseudarthrosis in such a way that the resultant of forces ceased to exert a shearing force on the pseudarthrosis and was converted into forces of compression. Such a repositioning osteotomy results in stability. Once the micromotion between fragments ceases, the interposed fibrocartilage mineralizes, is invaded then by vessels, and gradually undergoes endochondral ossification [10, 11]. Pauwels' principle of placing the pseudarthrosis at right angles to the resultant of forces by resecting a laterally based wedge has stood the test of time and continues to be used most successfully to this day (Fig. 12).

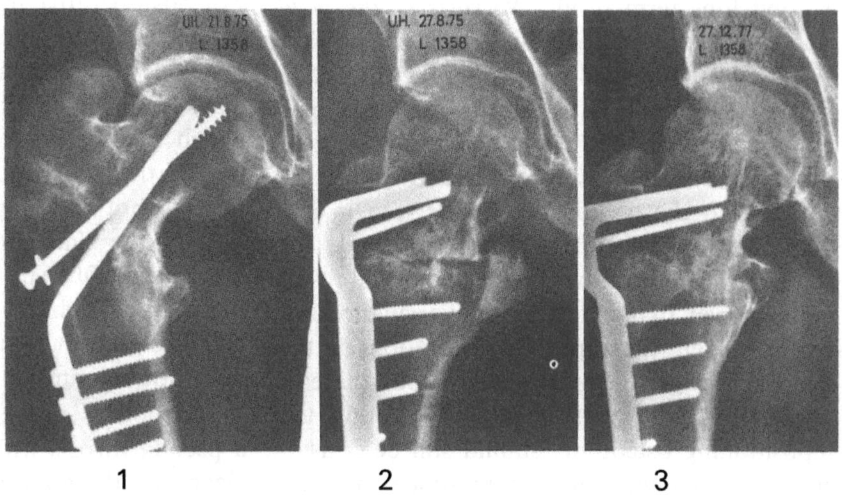

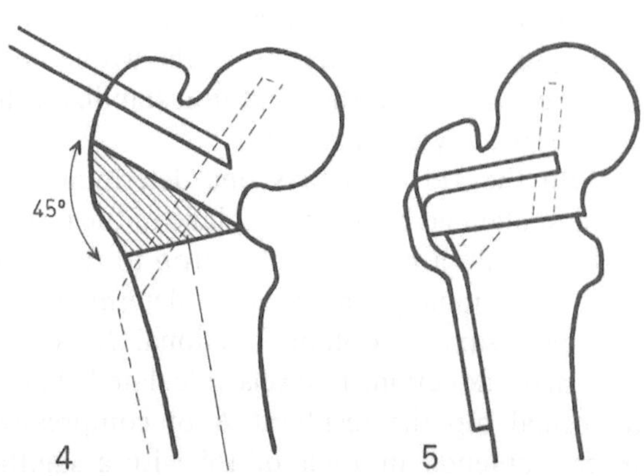

Fig. 11. Posttraumatic malunion. U.H., 47-year-old man. The use of the 90° plate for such a correction is an exception to the rule. Because the 90° plate was used, the osteotomy had to be made at right angles to the shaft. **1** Varus malunion as a result of instability (the plate was protruding posteriorly through the neck). **2** Use of the 90° plate: the situation right after the intertrochanteric osteotomy. **3** The result after 2 years was clinically and radiologically perfect. **4, 5** The preoperative drawing shows the resection of a 45° wedge entirely from the proximal fragment, which is a departure from the usual procedure. Because the 90° plate was used for fixation, the osteotomy was planned at right angles to the shaft

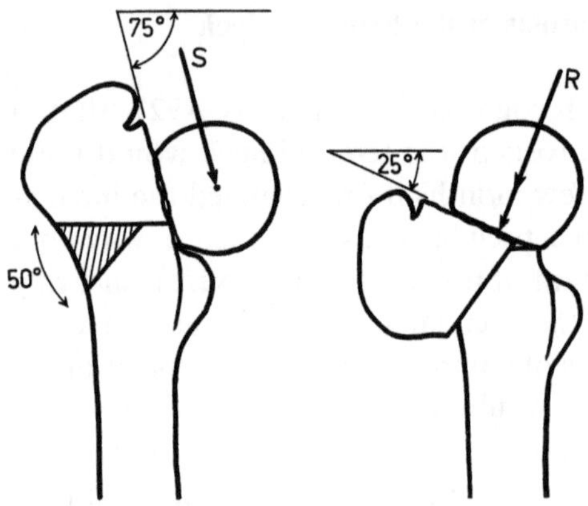

Fig. 12. Pauwels' Y repositioning osteotomy. This scheme illustrates how the resection of a lateral wedge results in the conversion of the shearing forces into forces of compression. In order to support the head, inferiorly the shaft is excessively medialized. This results in considerable shortening and in genu valgum

A living femoral head is the prerequisite for a good long-term result. *Necrosis of the head* is likely if there is a generalized relative increase in density of the head with rounding off of the fracture fragment. On the other hand, similar bone density of the greater trochanter and of the femoral head, as well as a reactive sclerosis adjacent to the pseudarthrosis, as seen in elephant foot pseudarthrosis, speaks strongly for *viability*. The repositioning osteotomy will result in union even in the presence of avascular necrosis. However, the rapid fragmentation of the femoral head which usually occurs soon thereafter destroys the hip. If the patient is young, the repositioning osteotomy should still be considered as a possible form of treatment as long as the avascular segment is strong (Fig. 16). A certain degree of collapse is to be anticipated. If progressive fragmentation of the whole head does not occur, and the condition stabilizes, the hip can usually be salvaged.

With the aid of X-rays one determines the angle subtended between the plane of the pseudarthrosis and a perpendicular drop to the shaft axis. Occasionally, in order to determine this it is necessary to obtain functional X-rays in maximal adduction. Pauwels calculated that in a normal hip the resultant *R* of compressive forces subtends an angle of 16° with a sagittal or body axis (Fig. 1.1). The angle between the sagittal body axis and the anatomical axis of the femoral shaft is 8°–10°. Thus, a pseudarthrosis which subtends an angle of 25° with the perpendicular to the femoral shaft axis is placed under pure compression. The angle of correction is determined by subtracting 25° from the angle which the pseudarthrosis plane subtends with a perpendicular drop to the femoral shaft axis. The angle of correction in the frontal plane corresponds to the wedge which must be resected. The rotational malalignment measured with the patient in the prone position determines the necessary correction in the horizontal plane and the fixed flexion deformity determines the degree of extension necessary.

Pauwels usually carried out a simple wedge osteotomy, but if the head had slipped down, he then carried out the so-called Y osteotomy (Fig. 12), which allowed him to medialize the shaft and in this way prop up the femoral head. For postoperative immobilization patients were placed in a hip spica. This type of osteotomy resulted not only in shortening, but also in marked medialization of the femoral shaft, which usually led to severe genu valgum. The use of the 120° double-angled plate makes it possible not only to prevent excessive medialization of the shaft, but also to maintain equal leg length. Of even greater importance is the fact that with this type of fixation, patients can begin to recover function at an early stage, and need not be immobilized in plaster.

As soon as one establishes the diagnosis of a pseudarthrosis with a viable head it becomes clear that the goal of treatment is to carry out a Y-shaped repositioning osteotomy which will convert the shearing forces to compression. The implant to be used is the 120° plate. The next information necessary is the desired rotational correction in the frontal plane and extension in the sagittal plane. Once the information is available, one can proceed straight on to the preoperative planning and drawing (Fig. 13).

On a sheet of tracing paper mark in the outlines of the proximal femur and the pseudarthrosis, the anatomical axis of the femoral shaft, and the osteotomy line at right angles to the femoral shaft axis. Determine now the angle

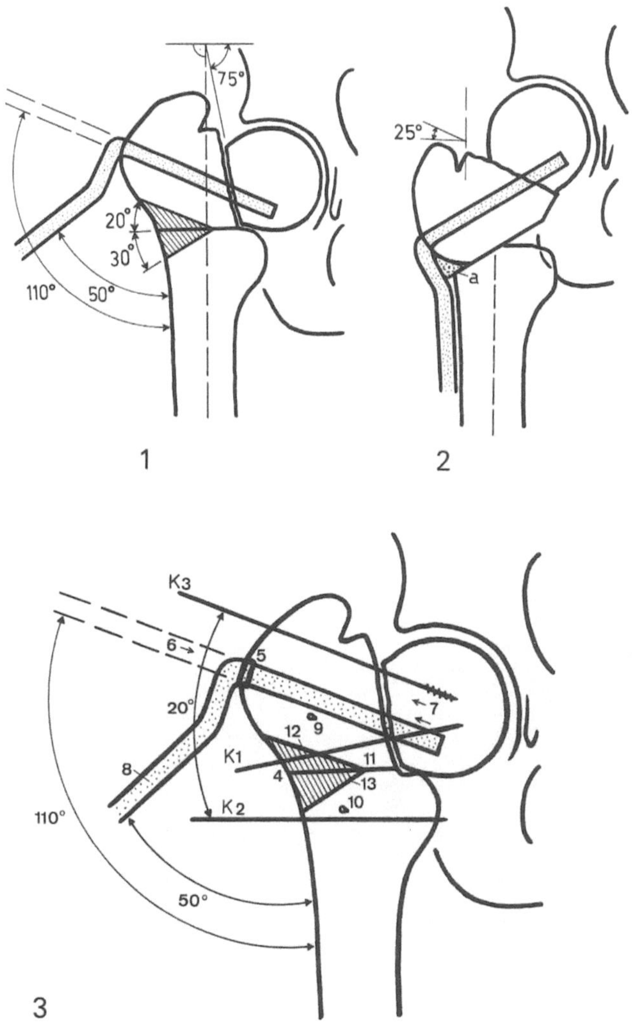

Fig. 13. 1, 2 Principle of a repositioning osteotomy of 50° with a 120° double-angled plate. **1** Note that the tip of the blade is inserted into the inferior segment of the head. A 30° wedge is cut from the proximal fragment and a 20° wedge from the distal fragment adjacent to the intertrochanteric osteotomy (IO) line. Note that the angle between seating chisel and shaft is 110° and that between plate and shaft 50°. **2** In lateralizing the shaft, one must remember that the minimal permissible contact area between the osteotomy surfaces is one-third of the diameter of the shaft. Some times a bone graft (*a*) is inserted between neck and plate. **3** Tactical steps of repositioning osteotomy. *1* A 2-mm Kirschner wire (*K1*) is placed over the femoral neck. *2* A second 2-mm Kirschner wire (*K2*) is inserted at right angles to shaft axis at level of lesser trochanter. *3* A 2.5-mm threaded Kirschner wire (*K3*) is inserted through tip of greater trochanter at 20° angle to K2 in frontal plane and parallel to K1 in transverse plane. K1 is removed. *4* Level of osteotomy is marked with a saw. *5* Portal of entry for seating chisel is prepared. *6* Seating chisel is inserted parallel to K3. Its guide is tilted 10° dorsally in order to subsequently carry out a 10° extension osteotomy. Note that seating chisel is inserted into inferior half of femoral head. *7* Seating chisel is removed. *8* Chosen blade plate is inserted. *9, 10* Two parallel Kirschner wires are inserted, one on each side of the IO, for rotational control. *11* Transverse IO. Once completed, any rotational correction necessary (transverse plane) is executed. *12* Resection of 20° cranial wedge parallel to seating chisel in both frontal and sagittal planes. *13* Resection of distal wedge of 30°. Once this wedge is resected, shaft is abducted and plate is fixed to shaft with a short screw. Osteotomy is then placed under compression by insertion of remaining screws (see Fig. 4.4), which pull shaft towards plate

subtended between the pseudarthrosis and the perpendicular to the shaft axis. This angle, less 25° (Fig. 13.1), is the angle of correction, and determines also the size of the wedge to be resected. The blade of the 120° plate, and of course the seating chisel, must come to lie parallel to the proximal osteotomy line. With the help of the plate templates, now mark in the position of the plate in such a way that the tip of the blade comes to lie in the inferior half of the femoral head. Take a second sheet of tracing paper and mark in first the distal fragment, and subsequently the proximal fragment in such a way that at least one-third of the osteotomy surfaces will be in contact. The plate of the 120° blade plate should now lie along the femoral shaft. The final result is discernible (Fig. 13.2). All that remains is to draw in the steps of the procedure (Fig. 13.3).

The degree of extension of the distal fragment which is necessary is easily determined from the fixed flexion contracture which was established clinically. It is not drawn in on the preoperative plan, but comes into play when the seating chisel is hammered into the bone. The angle which the seating chisel guide subtends with the shaft axis in the sagittal plane should equal the desired degree of extension. Once the transverse cut is executed, one should correct any rotational malposition before the resection of any wedges. The distal wedge of 30° is the first to be resected. If the wedge based laterally is

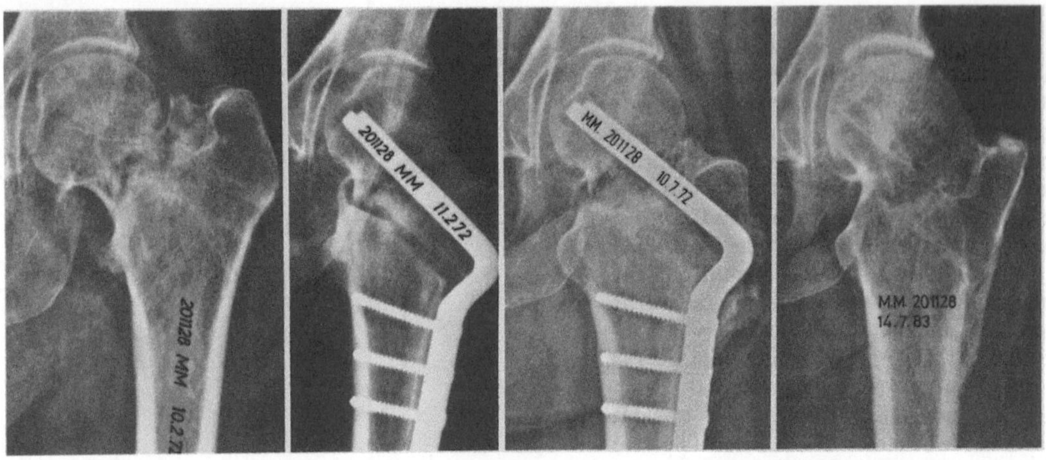

1 2 3 4

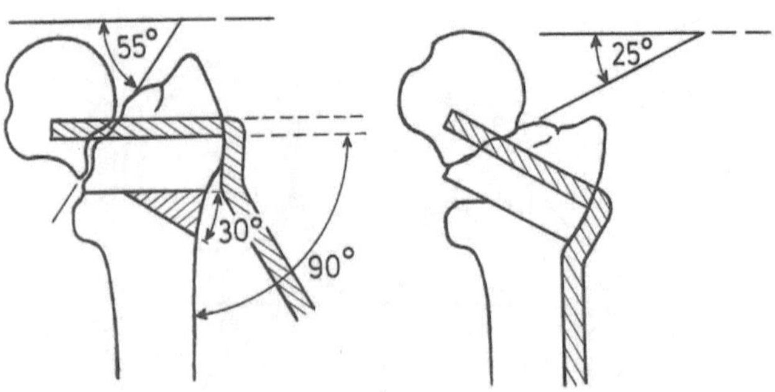

5 6

Fig. 14. Pseudarthrosis of femoral neck with viable head. M.M., 44-year-old woman. **1** Note the state prior to the corrective procedure. **2** After an abduction intertrochanteric osteotomy of 30° and its fixation with a 120° plate. **3** Five months after the intertrochanteric osteotomy. Note that the pseudarthrosis has united. **4** After 11 years. The patient is symptom-free, able to work without any disability, and even able to ski. **5, 6** Preoperative planning: From the X-ray, we see that the angle between the pseudarthrosis and a perpendicular to the shaft axis is 55°. Note the removal of a 30° wedge from the distal fragment. The fixation was carried out with a 120° plate

greater than 30°, then the remainder is resected from the proximal fragment, paying attention not only to the valgus, but also to the extension component. The examples which I have chosen are as follows: (a) a classic example (Fig. 14), (b) partial avascular necrosis of the femoral head (Fig. 15), and (c) extensive avascular necrosis in a 16-year-old boy (Fig. 16).

Coxa Vara Congenita (Fig. 17)

The basic lesion of coxa vara congenita is a pseudarthrosis in the metaphysis. A surgical procedure will be successful only if it can reverse the pathogenesis. Thus the repositioning osteotomy must be designed in such a way that it will lead to consolidation of the pseudarthrosis. The pseudarthrosis in the metaphysis will ossify as soon as the epiphyseal plate is placed at right angles to the resultant of the compressive forces. In small children, it is somewhat difficult to achieve stable internal fixation. At first, we attempted to secure the fixation with Schanz screws (Fig. 24). Today the Schanz screws have been replaced with a special 90° blade plate. The preoperative planning of the procedure is executed in exactly the same way as for pseudarthrosis of the femoral neck, the object being to convert shearing forces into pure compressive forces. In small children, when a lateral wedge is resected, there is the distinct danger of damaging the epiphyseal plate of the greater trochanter. Therefore, in children under 6 years we resect the whole wedge even if it is greater than 30° only from the distal fragment. In older children, as well as in adults, the procedure is carried out in exactly the same way as in pseudarthrosis of the femoral neck.

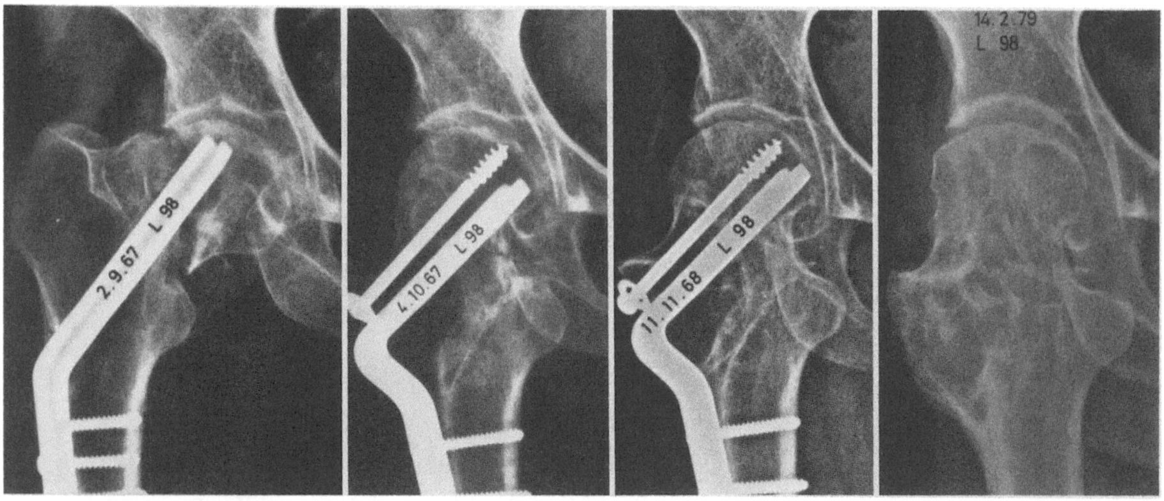

1 2 3 4

Fig. 15. Pseudarthrosis of femoral neck. G.E., 38-year-old woman. **1** Partial avascular necrosis of the femoral head with a defect in the head, the result of the blade. **2** The result after an abduction intertrochanteric osteotomy of 60° and its fixation with a 130° plate. **3** One year after the intertrochanteric osteotomy. Note the considerable improvement within the femoral head. **4** After 12 years, the hip is symptom-free despite the slight flattening of the femoral head. The shaft had to be medialized considerably, resulting in genu valgum which has become symptomatic

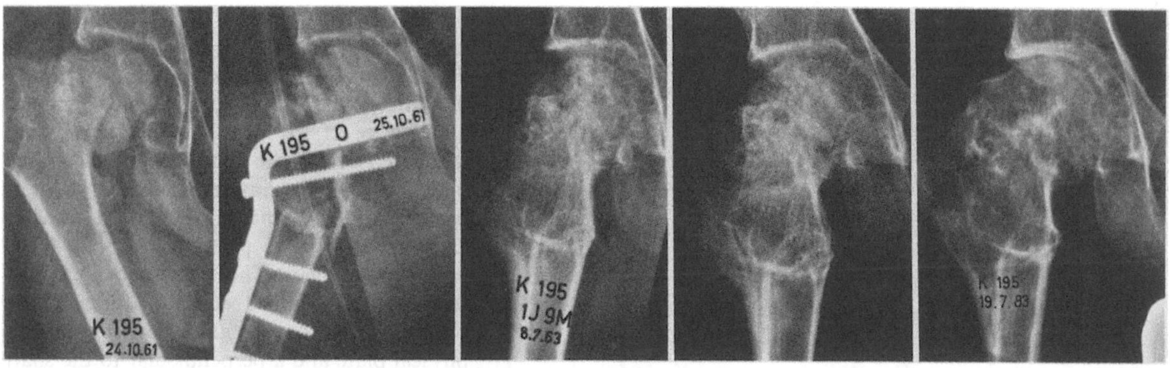

1 2 3 4 5

Fig. 16. Pseudarthrosis of femoral head. J.U., 16-year-old male. **1** Two years after fracture, the femoral head is severely necrotic without any trabecular detail. **2** Two years after a repositioning osteotomy fixed with a 120° plate. The plate was hammered into the pelvis because the head fragment was too small to give any fixation. The hip was immobilized in a spica for 3 months. **3** After $1^1/_2$ years. **4** After 8 years. Flexion is possible to 70°. **5** After 22 years. Flexion is only possible to 45°. The patient limps despite a lift in his shoe but is able to walk for 2 h. Because of the 5 cm shortening, a shortening and lengthening osteotomy was recommended

Localized Segmental Avascular Necrosis and Osteochondritis Dissecans

An intertrochanteric osteotomy can reverse the process and lead to reossification of the avascular fragment, as long as the avascular fragment can be brought out of the loading zone. Usually, at the time of osteotomy, we also perform a cancellous graft to the avascular zone [2]. In teenagers, this usually leads to a rapid reossification of the decompressed avascular zone. The same procedure is carried out in treating im-

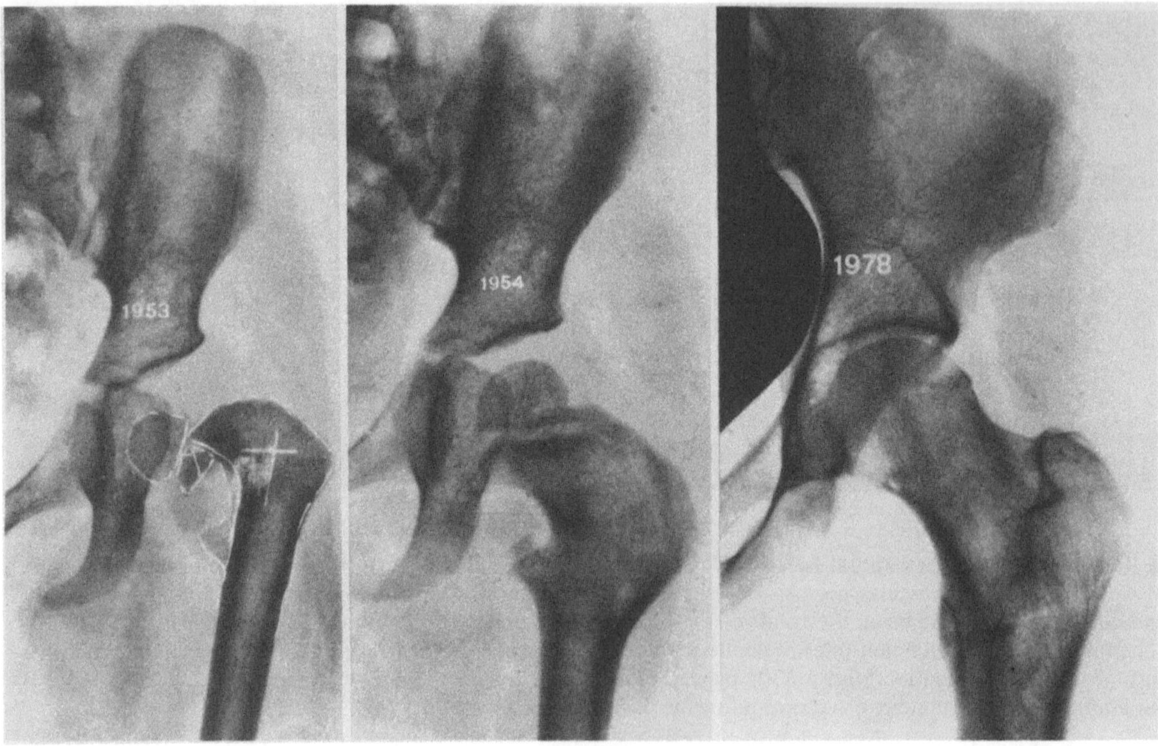

1 2 3

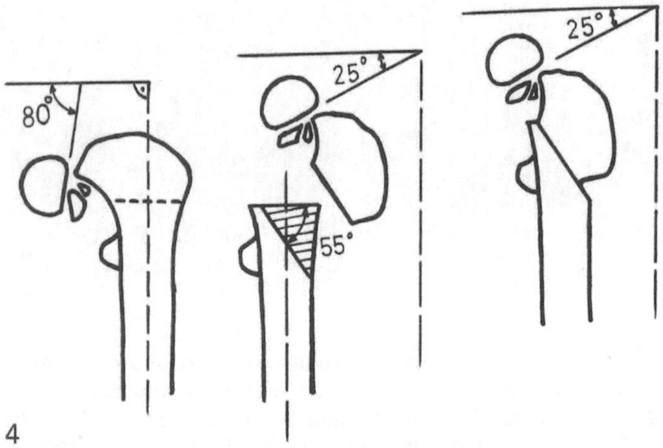

4

Fig. 17. Coxa vara congenita. K.B., 20-month-old girl. **1** Note the pathognomonic triangular appearance of the proximal metaphysis and the epiphyseal plate almost parallel to the body axis. **2** One year after an abduction intertrochanteric osteotomy of 55°. **3** After 23 years, the hip is perfectly normal. **4** The preoperative plan. The intertrochanteric osteotomy was planned at right angles to the shaft axis. Because the angle between the epiphyseal plate and a perpendicular to the shaft axis is 80°, a 55° wedge was removed entirely from the distal fragment, as otherwise the lesser trochanter would have been pushed too far distally. Fixation was with the external fixator and a hip spica (see Fig. 25)

pacted fractures of the weight-bearing portion of the femoral head, which may occur as a result of an obturator dislocation of the hip (Fig. 18).

Arthrodesis of the Hip

Many arthrodeses malunite in too much flexion or abduction or with too much medialization, which results in genu valgum. Such a malunion can be easily corrected by means of an intertrochanteric osteotomy. The example in Fig. 19 is of a Z-shaped osteotomy. This allowed for simultaneous lengthening and lateralization. The fixation was achieved with a cobra head plate. Such lateralization and lengthening can also be achieved by means of an oblique osteotomy which runs from proximal-medial to distal-lat-

1 2 3 4

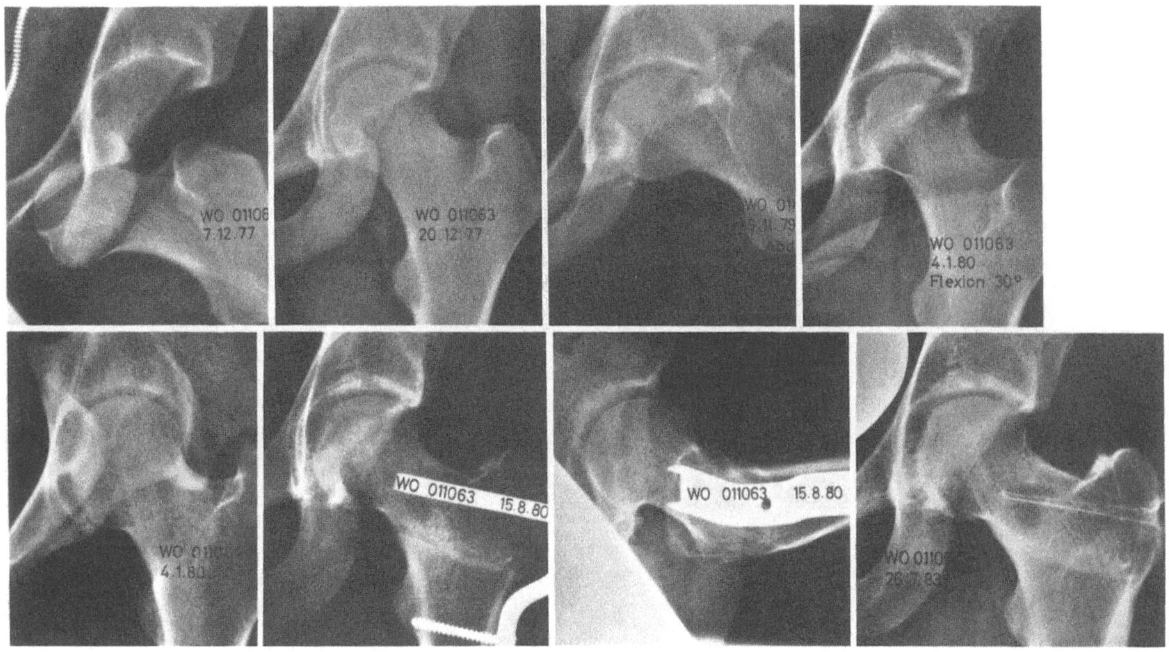

5 6 7 8

Fig. 18. Obturator dislocation of hip. W.O., 17-year-old girl. **1** Note the obturator dislocation with an impaction fracture of the femoral head. **2** After reduction, one can appreciate better the extent of the fracture and the flattening of the femoral head. **3–5** Functional X-rays 2 years later. The defect is best seen on the abduction and flexion view. Note that the tangential projection of 40° demonstrates a spherical contour of the head. **6, 7** Seven months after a 30° flexion and 15° adduction intertrochanteric osteotomy. **8** The result 3 years after surgery. The hip is fully mobile and pain-free

eral. Lengthening of 2 cm can be achieved without difficulty (Fig. 20).

Shortening

A shortening of 3 cm or more is usually carried out in the midregion of the femoral shaft [9]. If the required shortening is 2.5 cm or less, then it is best to carry out a cylindrical osteotomy in the intertrochanteric area (Fig. 21). The 90° osteotomy plate is used for fixation. The fixation achieved is usually so stable that the patient can begin full weight-bearing at 2 weeks following surgery with the help of only one cane.

If one wants to carry out a simultaneous lengthening of the other side, then with the aid of the distractor one can distract the osteotomy in the intertrochanteric area and insert the resected cylindrical fragment from the other side as a graft (Fig. 22).

Coxa Valga Luxans

If one has to deal with a residual subluxation of the hip or with a congenital subluxation with a CE angle of less than 15°, it is frequently possible to achieve much better congruence of the articular surfaces if one carries out an intertrochanteric adduction (varus) derotation osteotomy. This usually leads to better development of the acetabular roof and better coverage of the femoral head. In children under 12 years, one should anticipate a loss of the varus correction, because the epiphyseal plate, the result of the varus is no longer at 90° to the resultant. This leads to rapid remodeling of bone until the plate comes to lie once again at right angles to the resultant. Rotational correction, on the other hand, is frequently permanent, and a recurrence greater than 10°–15° is very rare. If one wishes to maintain a permanent varus, the osteotomy should not be carried out until the

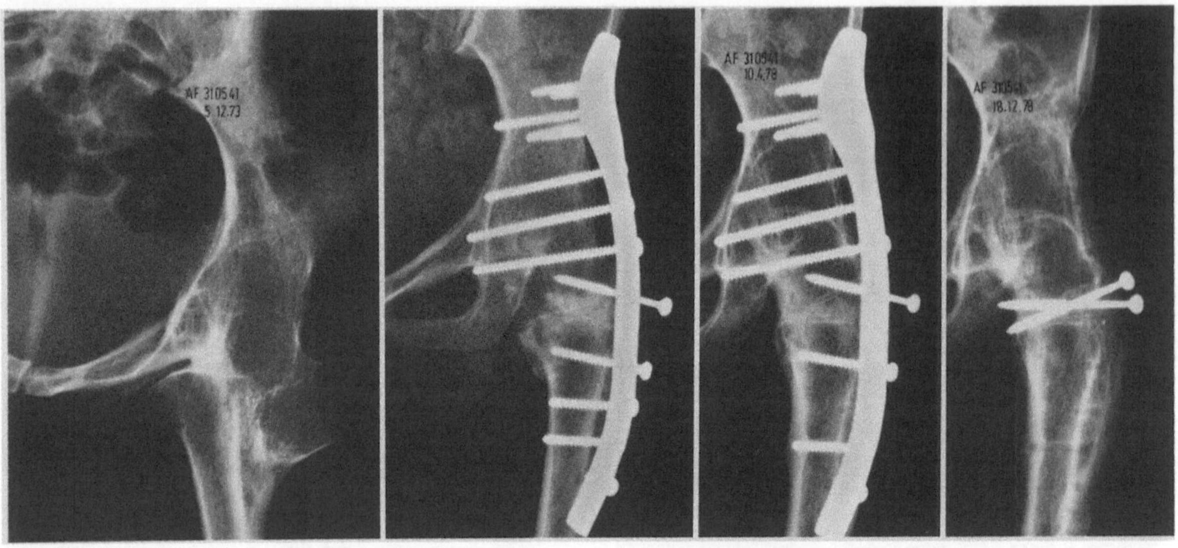

1 2 3 4

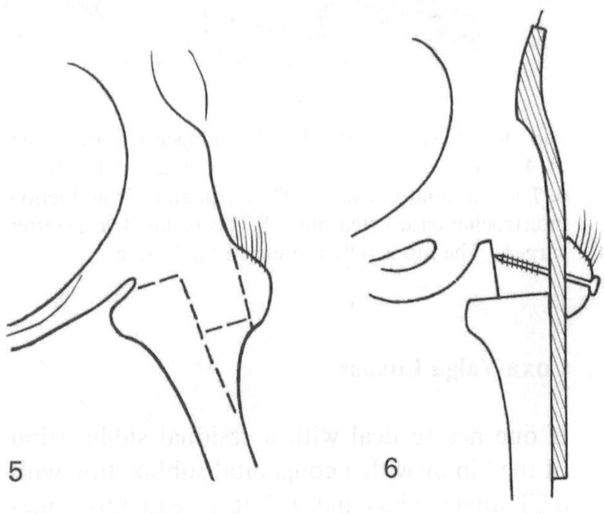

5 6

Fig. 19. Arthrodesis of hip. A.F., 34-year-old woman. **1** Twenty years after a Brittain extra-articular arthrodesis which was carried out because of tuberculous arthritis of the hip. The excessive medialization of the shaft resulted in severe genu valgum. In addition, the hip was in abduction and flexion and the leg was 5 cm short. **2** One year after an intertrochanteric osteotomy which resulted in lengthening, lateralization, adduction, and extension. Fixation was achieved with a cobra head plate. The greater trochanter was fixed on top of the plate. **3** Eight years after the intertrochanteric osteotomy. The patient is able to work and is symptom-free. **4** After removal of the plate and fixation of the greater trochanter with two screws at its proper level to facilitate a future revision to a total hip arthroplasty. **5, 6** Preoperative drawings

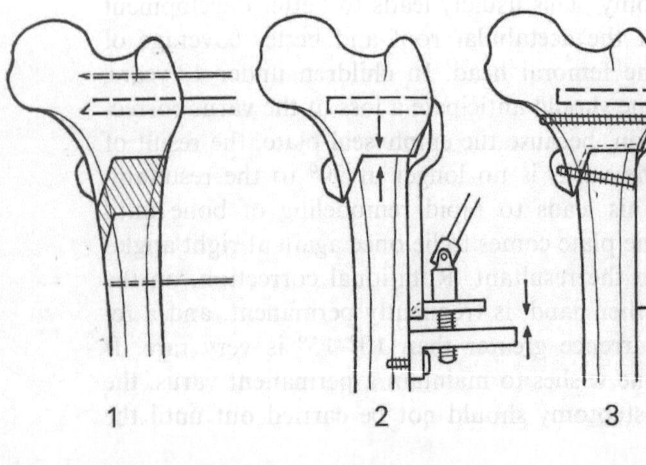

1 2 3

Fig. 20. Technique of shortening intertrochanteric osteomy of 2–3 cm. **1** Introduce the seating chisel into the greater trochanter at right angles to the shaft. Insert two Kirschner wires to mark the rotation. Resect a 2- to 3-cm-thick cylindrical segment from the femur but spare the lesser trochanter and leave it attached to the proximal fragment. **2** Replace the seating chisel with a right-angle plate with a short blade and place the osteotomy under compression with the tension device. This leads to impaction of the fragments. **3** Insert one screw through the plate in such a way that it fixes the shaft and the lesser trochanter

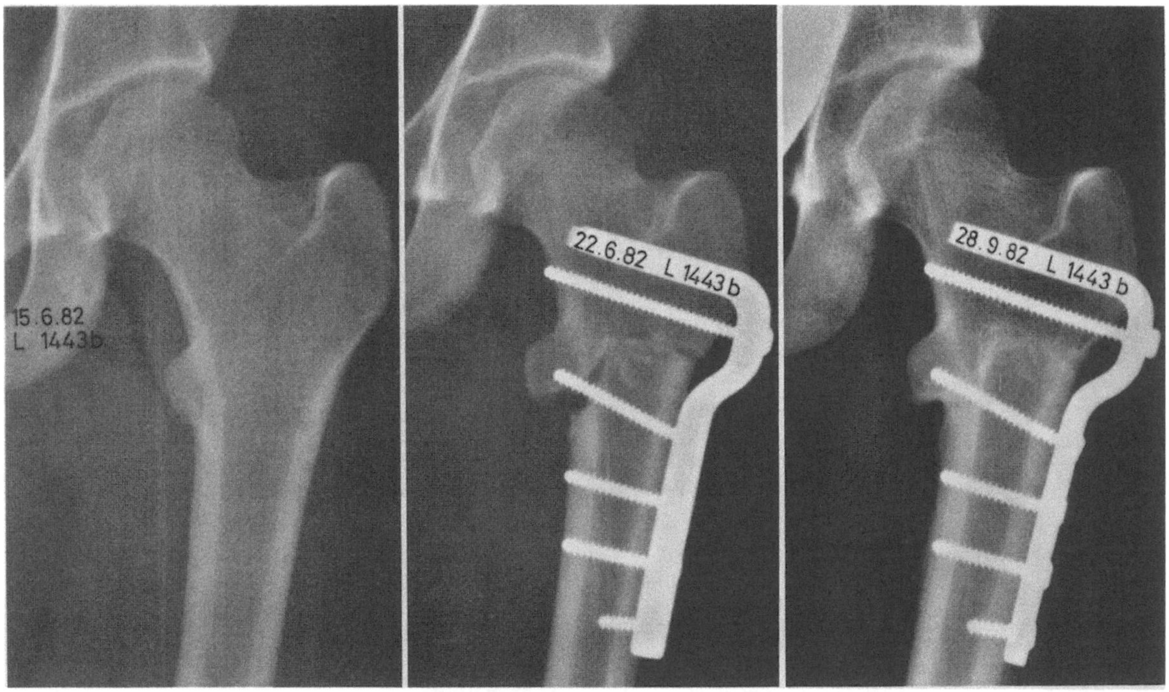

1 2 3

Fig. 21. Shortening intertrochanteric osteotomy after Legg-Perthes on right. L.A., 13-year-old girl. **1** At the age of 7 the Legg-Perthes on the right resulted in a shortening of 4 cm. **2** A 3-cm shortening was carried out on the left. **3** After 3 months, note the solid union of the intertrochanteric osteotomy with minimal callus and no osteoporosis

teens, when the epiphyseal plate has closed, which means after 12 in girls and after 15 in boys.

Prior to the procedure, it is necessary to obtain special X-rays which allow, with the aid of the special tables, determination of the true CCD and AT angles, as well as the CE and AC angles (Fig. 23). The anteversion can be measured, of course, with the help of the CT scan. To do this, one section is taken at the level of the tip of the greater trochanter and the other 3 cm proximal to the knee joint.

In children under 4 years, the fixation of the fragments under compression can be performed with Schanz screws and external clamps (Fig. 24). Postoperatively a plaster cast is applied.

An example of intertrochanteric varus and derotation osteotomy in a 12-year-old girl with 23 years follow-up is given in Fig. 25. Fig. 26 shows a varus osteotomy in a 45-year-old woman.

Varus intertrochanteric osteotomies carried out in teenagers or adults are usually combined with distal transposition of the greater trochanter (Fig. 27), shelf-plasty of the acetabular roof (Fig. 28), or cancellous bone grafting of the cysts [7].

Valgus Osteotomy in the Treatment of Coxa Valga Luxans with a Fixed Adduction Deformity. Once the head becomes deformed and oval, it is usually no longer possible to carry out a varus osteotomy. When an intertrochanteric osteotomy is considered, valgus must be chosen. A valgus osteotomy is particularly good if one can make use of the medial capital drop osteophyte and bring it into the weight-bearing zone, as shown in Fig. 29. In this case the osteotomy was combined with a shelf-plasty of the acetabular roof.

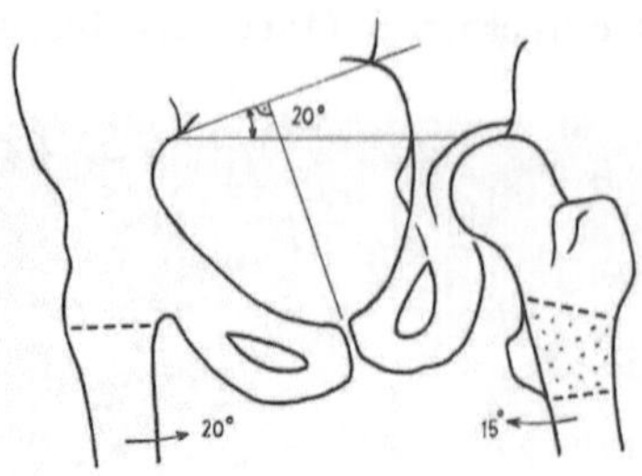
20°
20°
15°
4

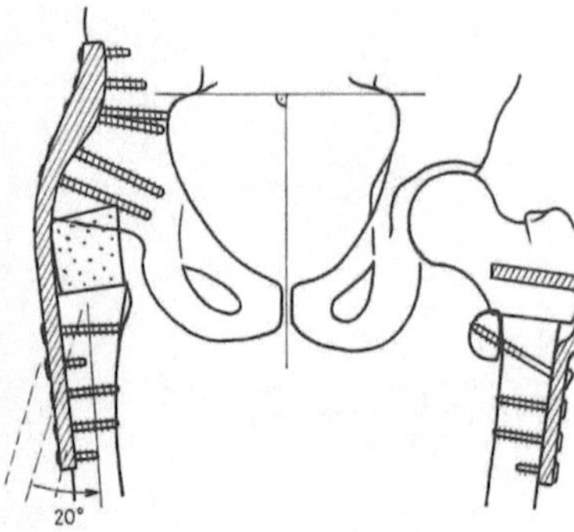
20°
5

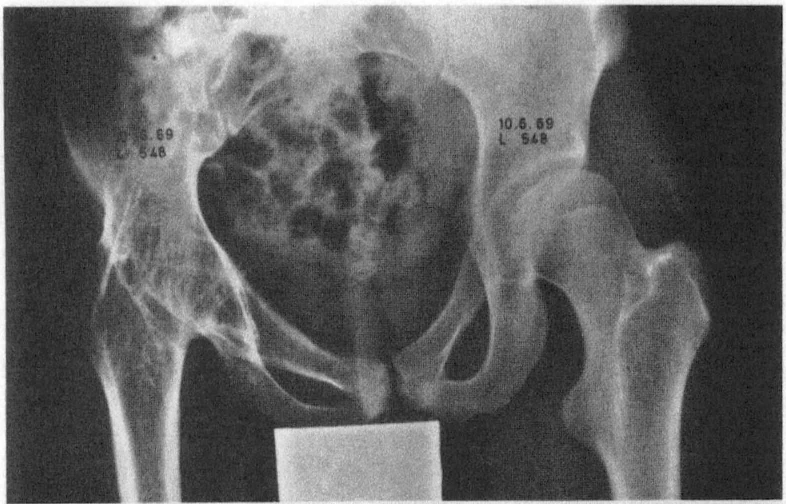
10.6.69
L 548
1

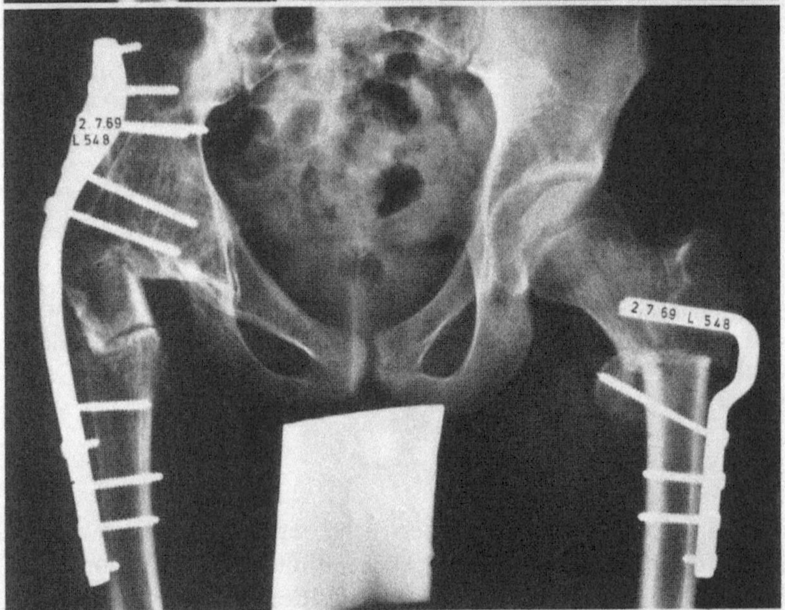
2.7.69
L 548
2.7.69 L 548
2

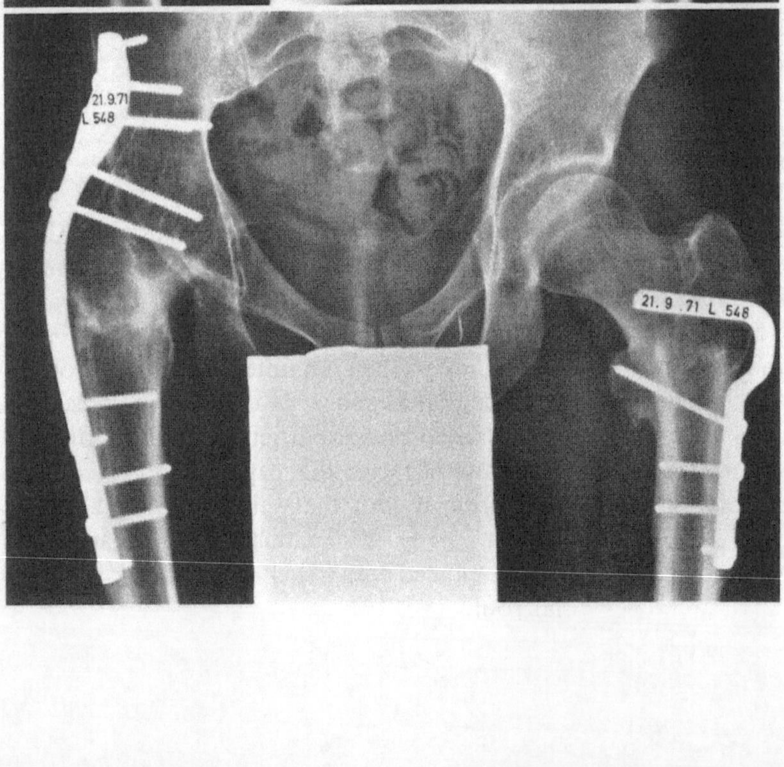
21.9.71
L 548
21.9.71 L 548
3

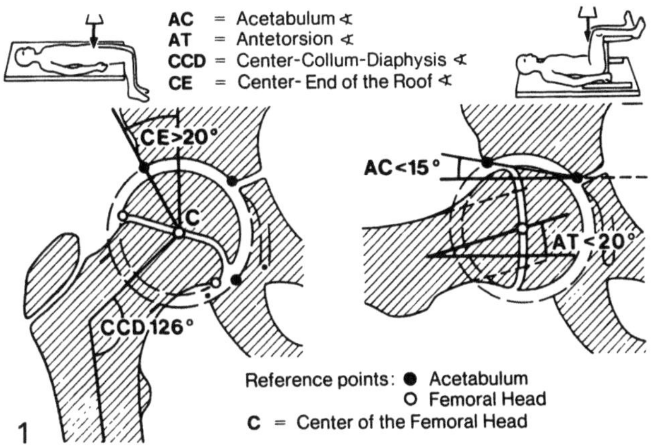

1

PROJ. AT∢

PROJ. CCD∢	30°	35°	40°	45°	50°	55°	60°	65°	70°	75°
110°	32 106	36 106	42 105	47 104	52 103	56 101	61 99	66 98	71 97	76 95
115°	32 111	37 110	43 109	48 107	52 105	57 104	62 102	67 101	71 99	76 96
120°	33 115	38 114	44 112	49 110	53 108	58 106	63 104	68 103	72 101	77 98
125°	34 119	39 118	44 116	50 114	54 112	58 109	63 107	68 105	72 103	77 100
130°	35 124	40 122	46 120	51 117	55 116	60 112	64 109	69 107	73 104	78 101
135°	36 129	42 126	47 124	52 120	56 118	61 114	65 112	70 109	74 105	78 102
140°	38 132	44 130	49 127	53 124	58 120	63 117	67 114	71 111	75 107	79 103
145°	40 136	45 134	50 131	55 128	59 124	64 120	68 117	72 114	75 110	79 104
150°	42 141	47 138	52 136	56 134	61 129	65 124	69 120	73 116	76 112	80 105
155°	44 145	50 142	54 139	58 137	63 132	67 128	71 124	74 119	77 115	81 108

REAL CCD AND AT∢

2

Fig. 23. X-ray projections of children with mobile hip designed to determine the hip mechanics by means of four standard angles. **1** *Upper left:* positioning of the patient for the AP overview of the pelvis. The knees are bent to a right angle. *Lower left:* schematic representation of the X-ray with reference points on the acetabulum and on the proximal femur, CE angle, and projected CCD angle. *Upper right:* positioning of the patient for the determination of anteversion. The hips are bent to 90° and the legs are abducted 20°. *Lower right:* representation of the X-ray with the AC angle and the projected AT angle. **2** Table for determining the real CCD and AT angles

◁ **Fig. 22.** Simultaneous shortening on left and lengthening on right. W.B., 20-year-old male. **1** Tuberculous arthritis of the hip resulted in an ankylosis in abduction and flexion with a functional shortening on the right of 4 cm (effectively 7 cm). **2** The result 2 weeks after a shortening intertrochanteric osteotomy on the left of 3 cm and insertion of the resected slice of the femur between the two fragments of the intertrochanteric osteotomy on the opposite side. The patient was treated without a spica and was able to get about with two crutches. **3** Two years later, the patient is able to walk without a cane and is symptom-free. **4, 5** Preoperative planning: full correction of the tilted pelvis could not be achieved

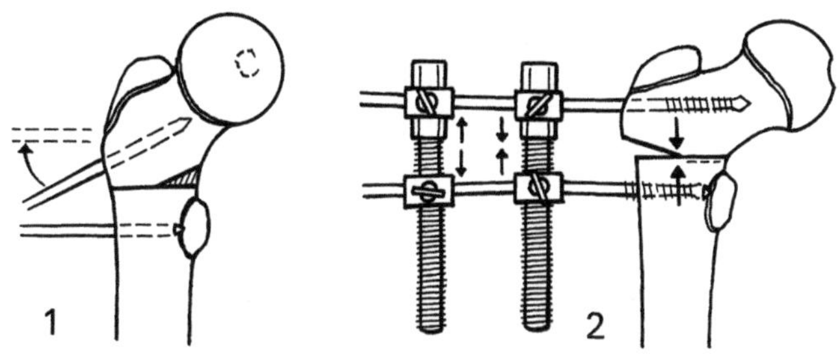

Fig. 24. Fixation of intertrochanteric osteotomy in a child of less than 4 years with external fixators. **1** Two Schanz screws are inserted, one into the neck and one into the shaft, in such a way that when they are parallel, correction of the anteversion and of the valgus will have been achieved. **2** The two clamps are fixed in a specific way. The clamp closest to the bone is under compression, i.e., it is compressing the two screws, and the outer clamp is under tension, i.e., it is pushing the screws apart. This results in interfragmental compression of the osteotomy and impaction of the fragment

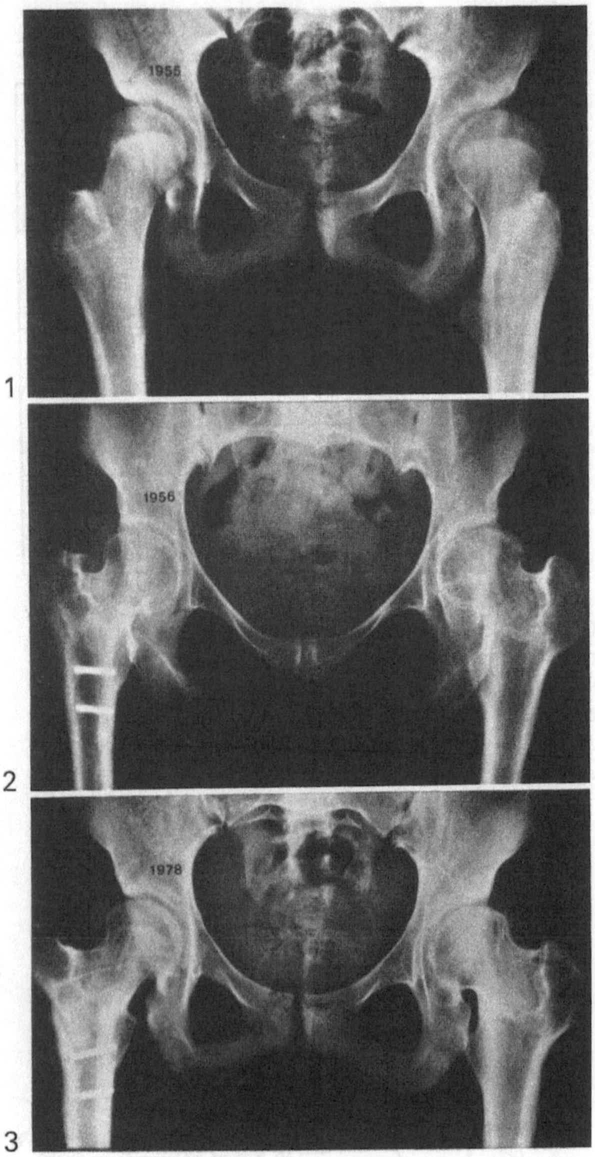

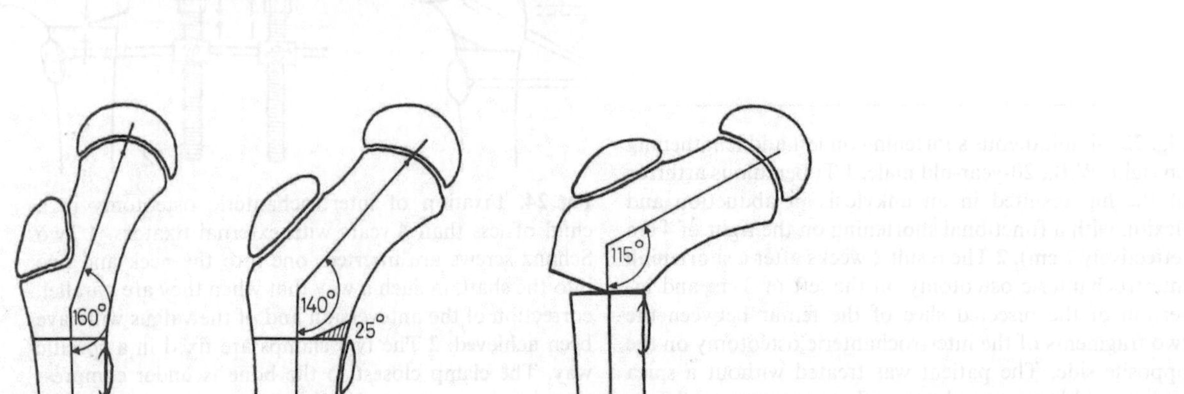

Fig. 25. Coxa valga luxans. S.M., 14-year-old girl. **1** Residual hip subluxation, more pronounced on the right than the left. CCD 145°, AT 50°, CE 0°. **2** One year after an intertrochanteric osteotomy of 25° adduction, 40° derotation, and fixation with a straight plate (which had already been removed). **3** The result after 23 years. The patient is symptom-free and has a full range of movement. Note the excellent coverage of the femoral head. CCD 120°, AT 10°, CE bilaterally 20°. **4** Preoperative drawings. **a** Preoperative contours of the AP projection. **b** Outline of the X-ray taken with the patient prone and the legs maximally abducted and internally rotated (see Fig. 2.6). The intertrochanteric line has been marked, as well as a small medial wedge. **c** Proximal fragment of **b** is joined to distal fragment of **a**

1 2 3 4

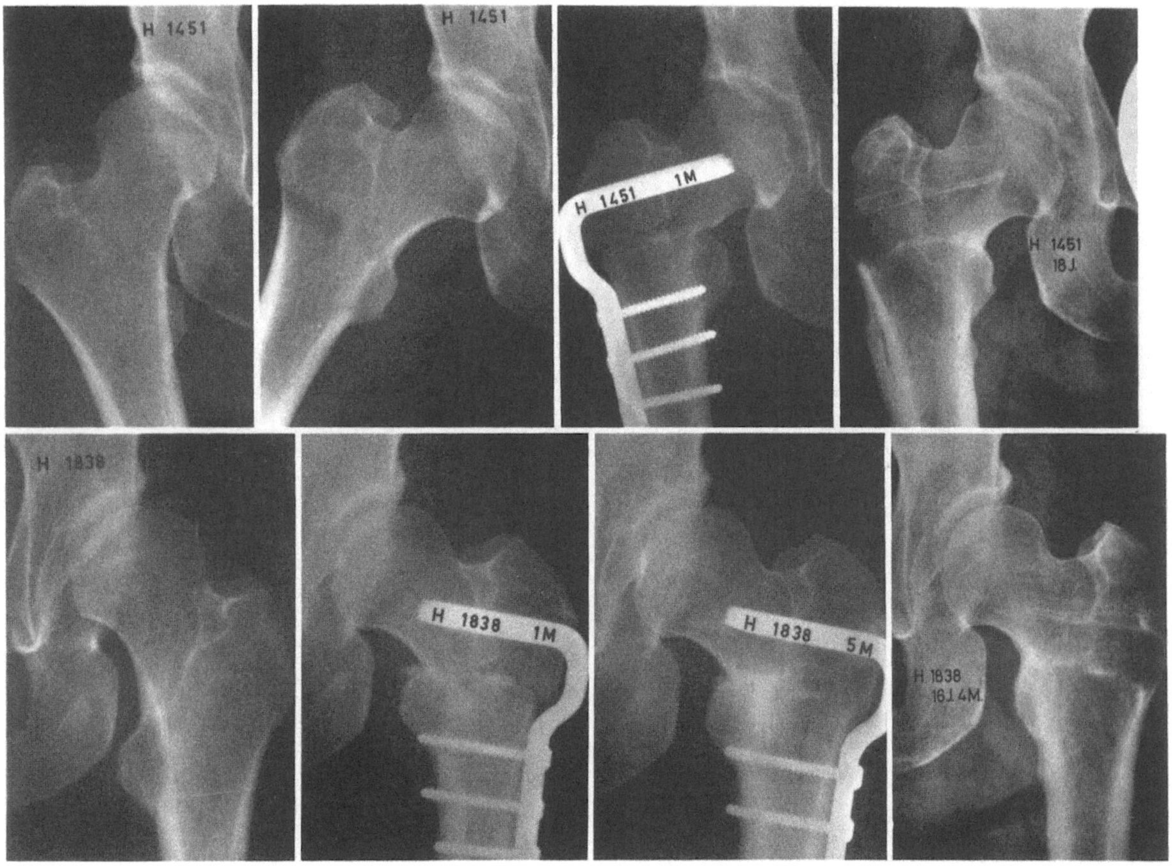

5 6 7 8

Fig. 26. Coxa valga luxans in the adult. K.H., 45-year-old woman. **1** Painful coxa valga luxans on both sides, more pronounced on the right than on the left. **2** The functional X-ray shows a better congruency and an improvement of the CE angle from 10° to 20°. **3** One month after intertrochanteric varus or adduction osteotomy of 25° with extension of 20°. **4** After 18 years, no arthritic signs, the hip is fully mobile and pain-free. **5–8** The left hip 1 and 5 months and 16 years after intertrochanteric varus osteotomy. The CE angle shows no improvement, but the patient is symptom-free

Complex Intertrochanteric Osteotomy in the Treatment of Coxa Valga Luxans. A varus osteotomy with a medial wedge results frequently in a hip which sticks out, in weakness of the abductors, in genu varum, and in shortening of 2–3 cm. If, on the other hand, rather than just resecting a medial wedge, one carries out a complex osteotomy, the hip will not stick out, the length of the femoral neck will remain the same, and the tip of the greater trochanter, because of its distal transposition, will remain a normal distance from the center of rotation of the femoral head. The same will apply to the femoral shaft axis. If prior to the osteotomy the axis of the knee joint was at right angles to the sagittal plane, it must be at right angles to the sagittal plane after the osteotomy, and the anatomical axis must be the same distance from the midsagittal plane of the body. If these points are observed, genu varum will be prevented. In order to prevent shortening greater than 8–12 mm, we do not resect a medial wedge. Instead, the neck segment removed for shortening is inserted laterally to fill the gap in the intertrochanteric area.

The preoperative planning, the final result, and the steps of the procedure are illustrated and described in Fig. 7.

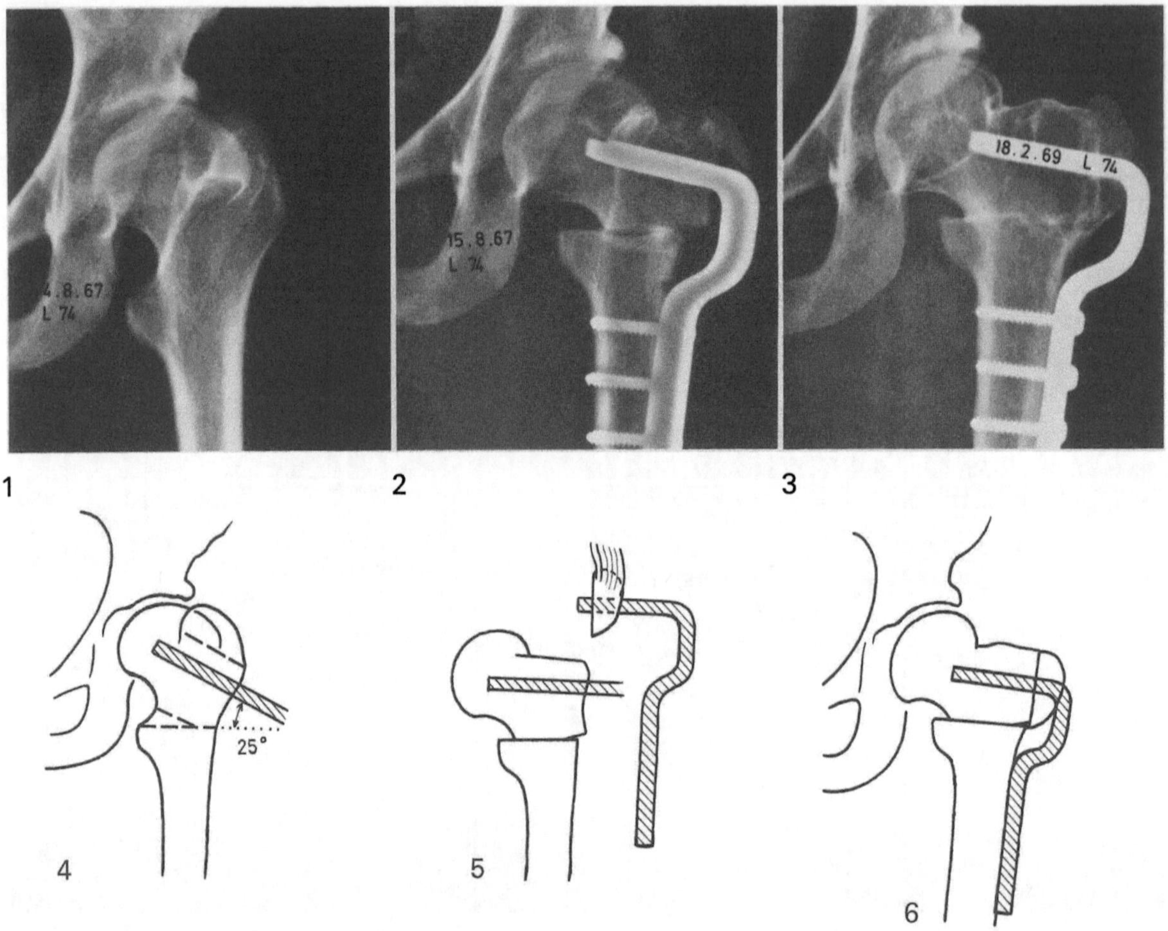

Fig. 27. Combination of intertrochanteric osteotomy with transposition of greater trochanter. F.E., 20-year-old girl. **1** Coxa valga luxans. **2** Adduction osteotomy of 25° and transposition of the greater trochanter. **3** Two years later. Note the reconstruction of normal physiological relationships. **4–6** The preoperative planning and drawing

In a complex intertrochanteric osteotomy, injury to the vessels supplying the femoral head, resulting in the dreaded complication of avascular necrosis, can come about in three ways (Fig. 8). First, if the greater trochanter is resected, the segment must not be more than 1 cm in thickness. If it is thicker, one can enter the intertrochanteric fossa and damage the retinacular vessels. Second, the vessels can also be damaged with the seating chisel if it is improperly inserted; it must be inserted as far anteriorly as possible.

Third, there is a possibility of damage if one looses control of the proximal fragment after extraction of the seating chisel. If this should occur when the blade of the osteotomy plate on which the greater trochanter has been threaded is being inserted, it may not follow the course precut with the seating chisel, but cut a new course in the bone. I have found the following tricks to be useful: The seating chisel should be knocked out 10–15 mm right after its inser-

Fig. 29. Coxa valga luxans and abduction intertrochanteric osteotomy. F.H., 27-year-old woman. **1** The 25° abduction and 15° extension osteotomy resulted in the capital drop osteophyte being brought under pressure. This was combined with an acetabular roof shelf-plasty which was too high and therefore useless. **2–4** Four months, 2 years, and 8 years respectively following the surgery. The excellent subjective and objective result can only be attributed to the intertrochanteric osteotomy ▷

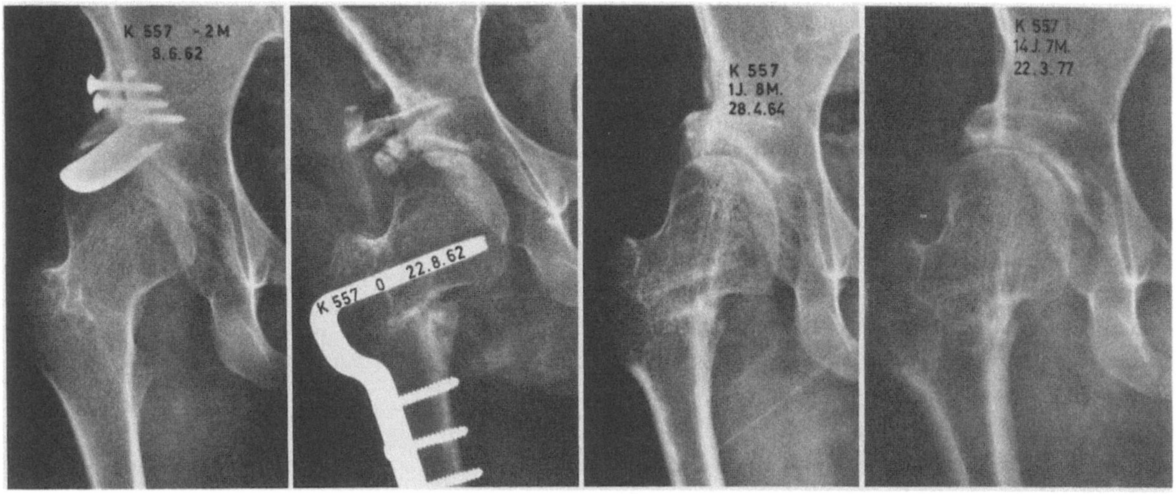

1 2 3 4

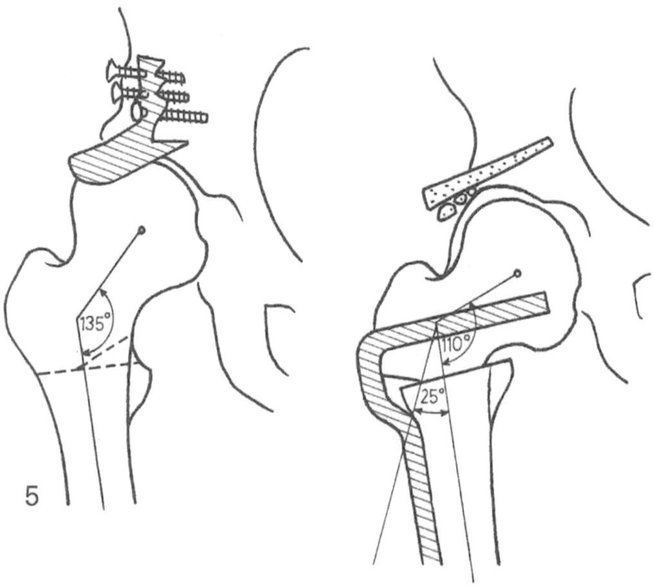

5

Fig. 28. Combination of intertrochanteric osteotomy with acetabular roof-plasty. P.M., 21-year-old woman. **1** The result of an acetabular roof-plasty buttressed with a metal plate. The patient was unable to bear weight. **2** The result 2 months after a 25° adduction and 20° derotation intertrochanteric osteotomy and a new bony shelf procedure. **3, 4** Two years and 15 years later respectively. Note the increase in the articular cartilage space. The patient is symptom-free, able to work, and has a full range of movement. **5** The preoperative drawings

---

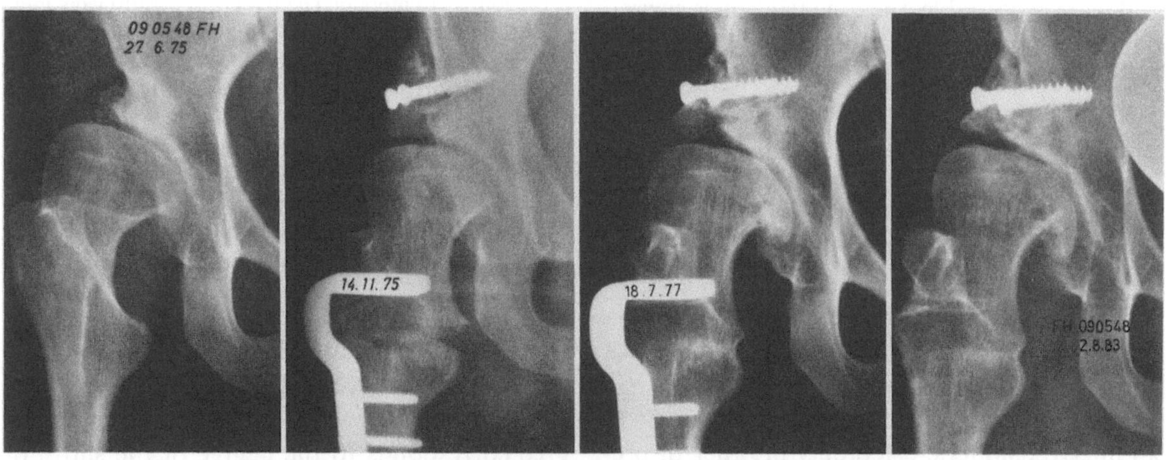

1 2 3 4

Fig. 29

tion, that is immediately prior to the execution of the intertrochanteric osteotomy. This will prevent it from becoming stuck in bone. Subsequently, the proximal fragment should be held with a bone-holding clamp from the cranial aspect to prevent any displacement.

It is extremely useful and important for the surgeon to practise the different steps of the procedure in a systematic and proper chronological order. This can be done either on cadaveric bone or on the plastic bone models which have now become available.

Complex intertrochanteric osteotomies are currently carried out by only a few surgeons. Learning their principles and the different steps necessary in their execution represents a challenge to furthering one's skills. Practise makes perfect. Once these complex osteotomies have been practised a few times on bone, their complexity vanishes; they appear to be simpler and simpler as one gains experience and skill.

Chronic Slipped Capital Epiphysis

To this very day, there are different schools of thought on how to treat a chronic epiphyseal slip. I have not deviated from the fundamental principles which I worked out some 30 years ago and published in 1957 [4]. If the slip is no greater than 25° and further growth is desirable, then the slip is stabilized with threaded Kirschner wires passed through the epiphyseal plate into the epiphysis. If closure of the epiphyseal plate is desirable, then the fixation is carried out with lag screws. If the slip is somewhere between 25° and 50°, then I feel it is best to execute a flexion intertrochanteric osteotomy combined with fixation of the epiphyseal plate. In slips of 50° or more, I prefer a resection osteotomy of the femoral neck. I fix prophylactically the opposite epiphyseal plate, even if it appears to be perfectly normal.

The degree of slip is determined from orthogonal AP and lateral X-rays of the femoral neck (Figs. 30, 31).

The epiphyseal plate must be fixed prior to an intertrochanteric osteotomy in order to prevent further slippage. The screws are passed

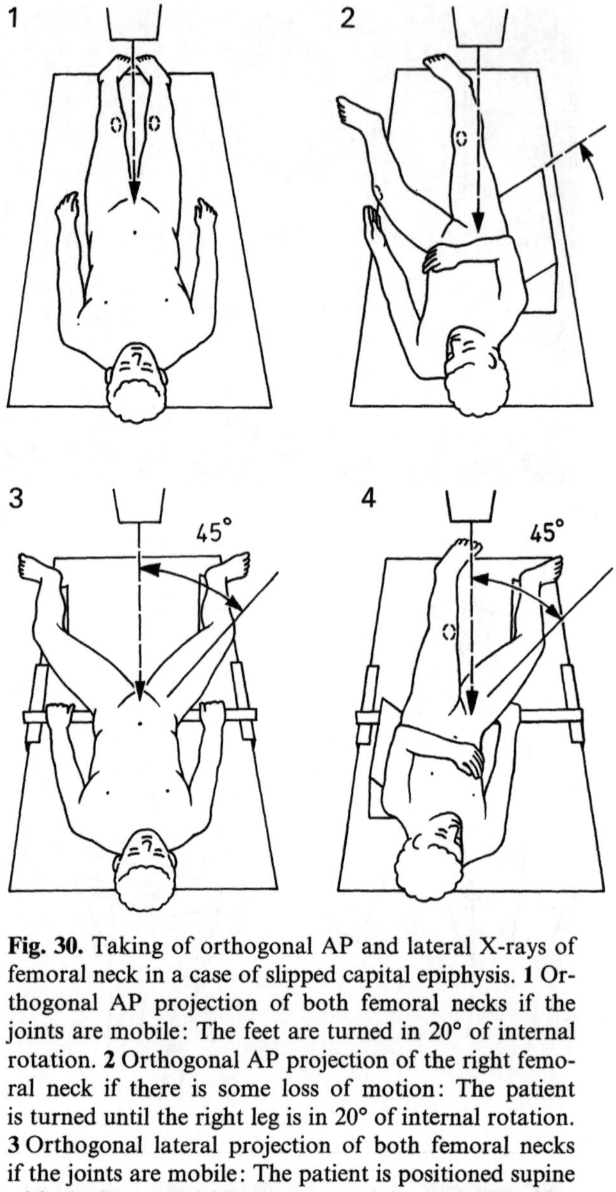

Fig. 30. Taking of orthogonal AP and lateral X-rays of femoral neck in a case of slipped capital epiphysis. **1** Orthogonal AP projection of both femoral necks if the joints are mobile: The feet are turned in 20° of internal rotation. **2** Orthogonal AP projection of the right femoral neck if there is some loss of motion: The patient is turned until the right leg is in 20° of internal rotation. **3** Orthogonal lateral projection of both femoral necks if the joints are mobile: The patient is positioned supine with the knees and hips bent to a right angle. The hips are then abducted to 45° and the legs are rested on a special support. This makes it possible to consider the real CCD angle, normally 130°–135°, in the presence of a slipped epiphysis. **4** Orthogonal lateral projection if the right joint is partially stiff: The only important change is the turned position of the body. The position of the right thigh and foot is exactly as in **3**

from front to back. Their direction is determined by the degree of slip. In the flexion osteotomy the wedge is based anteriorly and its degree corresponds to the degree of the slip. For the technique of the procedures see Figs. 32–35.

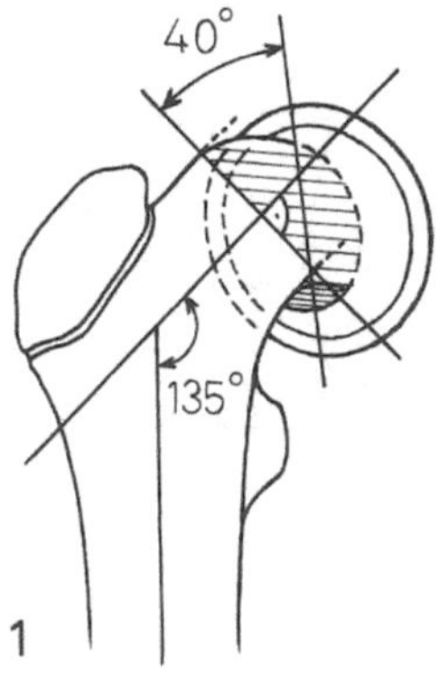

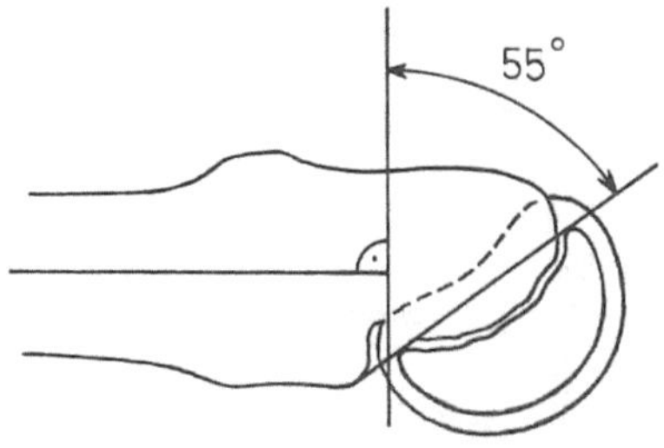

Fig. 31. Interpretation of X-rays. **1** From the AP projection: Note the extent of the callus, not only cranially but also caudally. Once this callus mass is removed, it becomes apparent that the real CCD angle is 130° or more. **2** The orthogonal lateral projection of the femoral neck allows one to measure the dorsal slip (in this instance 55°). It is measured between the perpendicular to the neck axis and a line which joins the ends of the epiphyseal plate. The real angle of the slip is 10°–15° less. It is on the basis of the real angle that one determines the correct treatment

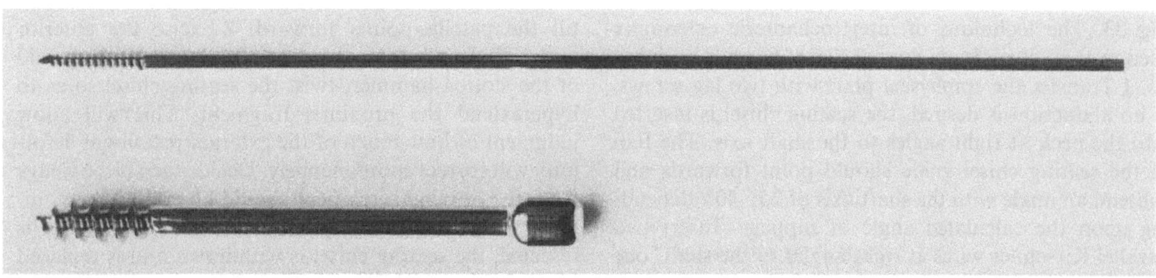

Fig. 32. Fixation devices for epiphyseal plate. **1** A 2.5-mm-thick Kirschner wire with a 16-mm threaded end. **2** A lag screw for fixation of the epiphyseal plate with a short thread and an 8-mm elongated head. The elongation makes it much easier to find the screw head if it becomes overgrown by bone

Observation. After the intertrochanteric osteotomy is made at 90° to the shaft, only half of the calculated anterior wedge should be resected from the distal fragment. When the proximal fragment is now rotated into hyperextension to an extent corresponding to the angle of correction (this is done with the help of the seating chisel and the slotted hammer), it often internally rotated. This results in the resection of the wedge more laterally. Therefore, one must check the rotational alignment before the proximal wedge is resected; since after resection of the wedge, any rotational malalignment can be corrected only through an osteotomy in the supracondylar area of the femur.

Thus, before one carries out the definitive fixation of the plate to the shaft, one must check the range of movement in all planes. An intertrochanteric osteotomy cannot give an excellent result if the slip of the capital epiphysis is more than 50°.

Subcapital Cervical Resection Osteotomy

This procedure is best carried out in combination with an extra-articular osteotomy of the greater trochanter. This has two advantages. First, once the capsule has been opened and the synovium and retinacular vessels reflected from the neck, one gains direct view of the slipped femoral head and one can easily judge the degree of slip without endangering the posterosuperior retinacular vessels. Second, it is easy

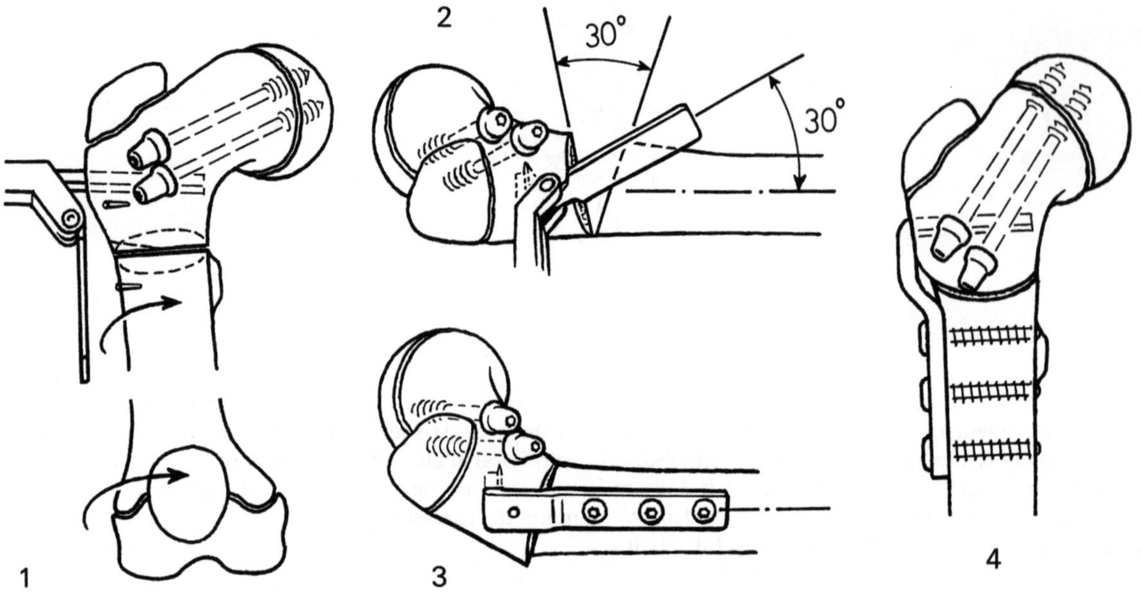

Fig. 33. The technique of intertrochanteric osteotomy used to treat chronic epiphyseal slip of a capital epiphysis. **1** Transfix the epiphyseal plate with two lag screws. If no abduction is desired, the seating chisel is inserted into the neck at right angles to the shaft axis. The flap of the seating chisel guide should point forwards and subtend an angle with the shaft axis of 25°–40°, depending upon the calculated angle of slippage. Insert two parallel Kirschner wires at right angles to the shaft, one on each side of the osteotomy, so that an exact correction of the rotational malalignment can be carried out after the intertrochanteric osteotomy at right angles to the long axis is performed. Internal rotation of the leg till the patella points forward. **2** Excise the anterior wedge first only from the distal fragment. With the aid of the slotted hammer, twist the seating chisel so as to hyperextend the proximal fragment. This will allow judgment of how much of the external rotational deformity will correct spontaneously. Decide then if the wedge from the proximal fragment should be excised more anteriorly or more laterally. Once the proximal wedge is resected, the seating chisel is withdrawn and is replaced by the plate. **3, 4** The final result as seen on AP and lateral projections. The flexion through the osteotomy results in the femoral head being relocated in the acetabulum as the leg is extended

to lateralize the greater trochanter at the end of the procedure (see Figs. 36, 38).

Particular attention must be paid to the following points: The procedure should be carried out only in the absence of any unreasonable preoperative treatment. Even in treating an acute slip, the success of the procedure is at considerable risk if one notes on the axial projection any gross change in the shape of the femoral head or a narrowing of the articular cartilage space. The epiphyseal slip occurs during the prepubertal growth spurt, and for this reason is associated with a transient coxa valga. This can always be noted on the opposite side. The coxa vara is the result of the slip, and the key to success lies in one's ability to recreate the configuration of the femoral neck prior to the slip. This is achieved through the resection of a caudal mass of callus which forms between the slipped head and the calcar. The resection of this callus is a pivotal point in the procedure and we rank it equal with the direct resection of an appropriate wedge as a prerequisite for easy and atraumatic reduction of the femoral head. It is easiest to resect this mass of callus if the hip is flexed to 60° and maximally externally rotated.

One must also resect the whole ventrocranial mass of callus. The wedge which is resected must usually have a 1.5-cm-wide base anteriorly. If the dislocation is more than 60°, one must resect an even greater wedge, so that the dorsal synovial reflection will not be placed under tension after reduction. If the slipped capital epiphysis is very loosely connected, then the whole proximal segment of the neck must be

1 2 3

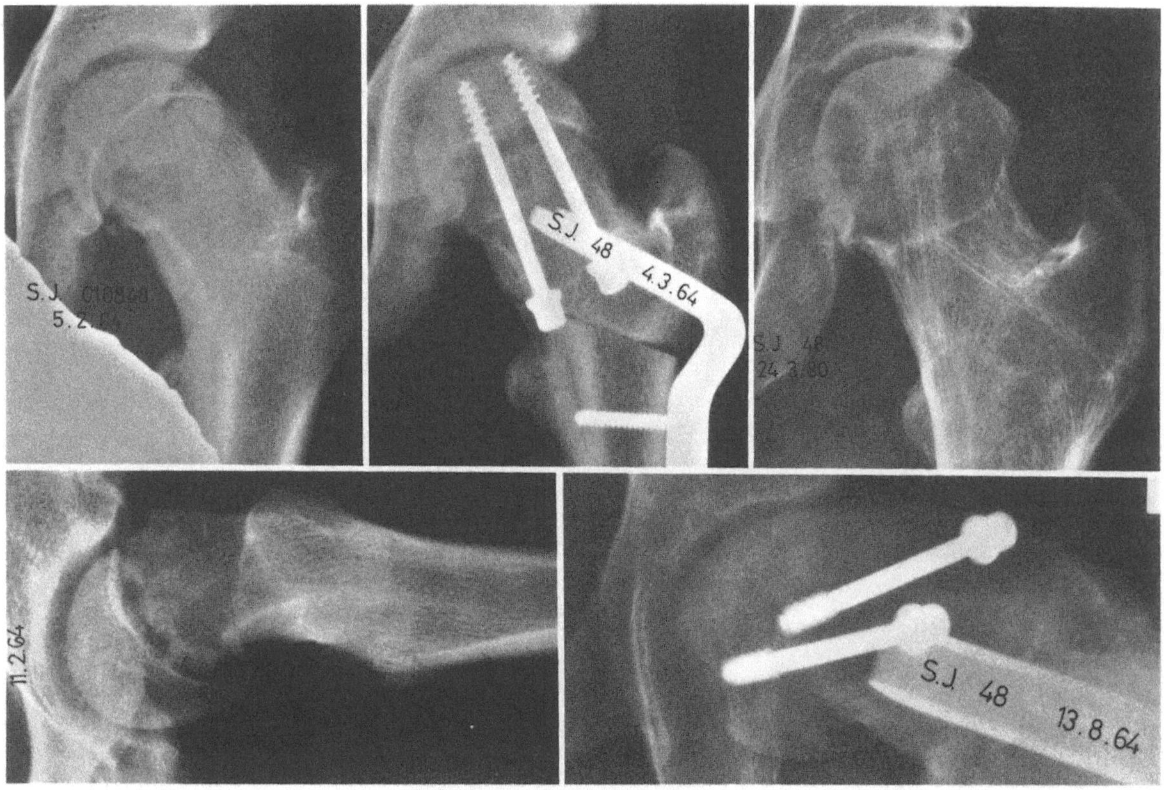

4 5

Fig. 34. Intertrochanteric osteotomy for chronic epiphyseal slip. S.J., 16-year-old male. **1, 2** Dorsal slip of 30° with a 20° external rotational deformity. No internal rotation possible. **3, 4** Six months and 9 months after a 30° flexion and 20° derotation osteotomy. Note the fixation of the epiphyseal plate with two lag screws. **5** Sixteen years after surgery. The patient is symptom-free and has full function of the hip. The slip was only partially corrected

resected up to the epiphyseal plate. Otherwise, it is sufficient simply to resect a wedge from the neck.

When the wedge is being resected, one must exercise extreme care to protect from injury the posterior synovial reflection with the retinacular vessels which supply the femoral head. We feel, therefore, that it is wisest not to resect a simple wedge, but rather a *trapezoidal segment* of bone. The posterior cortex of this trapezoidal segment is best removed piecemeal with a rongeur. This has proved to be the safest technique with the least danger to the retinacular vessels.

The lateral osteotomy line should not be made at right angles to the neck axis, but more horizontally, so that the neck osteotomy will be at right angles to the resultant after reduction (Fig. 1.1).

The reduction must be carried out under complete muscle paralysis with very gentle traction, very slowly and very carefully. Usually it is enough to apply some traction and only light pressure on the front of the neck in order to achieve proper reduction of the femoral head. Occasionally, particularly in those cases where one has resected the whole metaphysis, it is of advantage to stabilize the femoral head with the tip of a retractor while the reduction is being carried out. It is extremely important to prevent any rotational displacement between the femoral head and neck, because rotation could be most dangerous to the retinacular vessels. If the re-

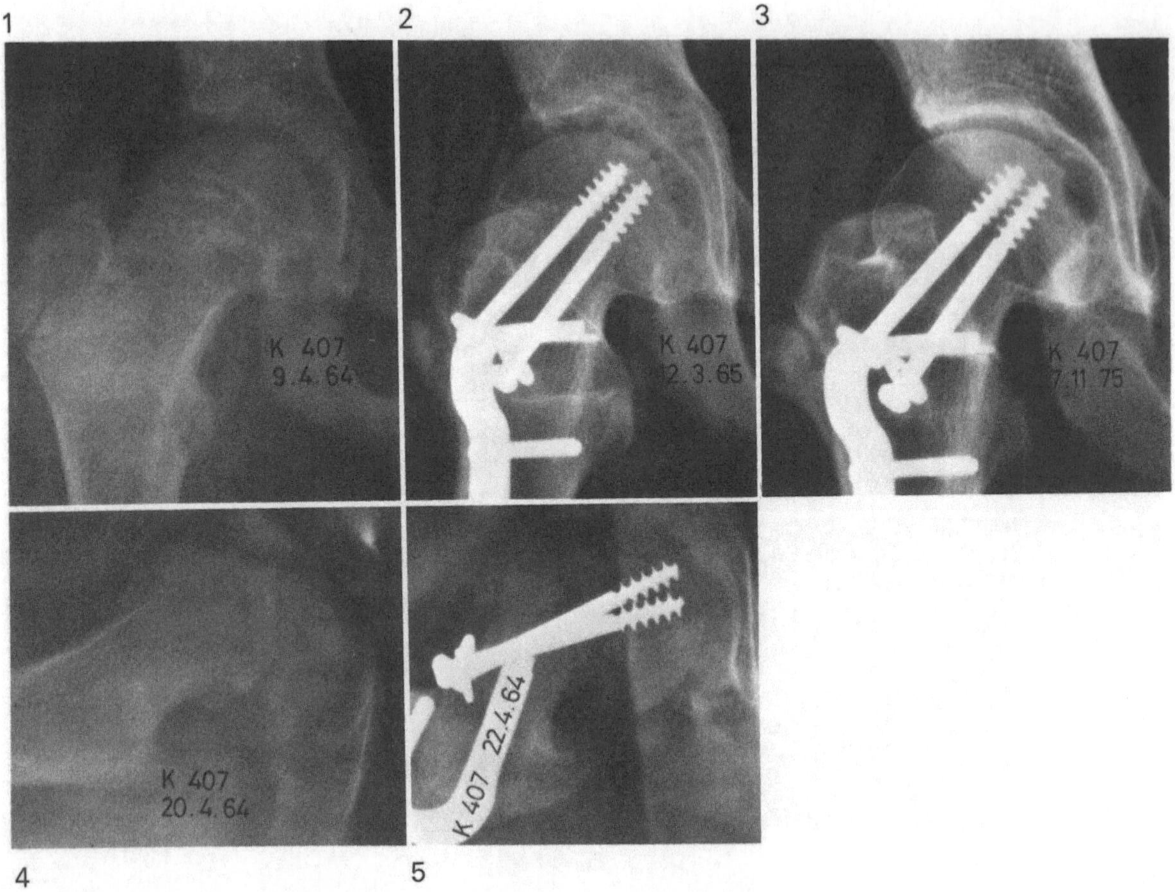

Fig. 35. Intertrochanteric osteotomy for chronic epiphyseal slip. F.H., 12-year-old male. **1, 2** Prior to surgery, slip of 40°. **3, 4** Postoperative X-rays after intertrochanteric osteotomy of 30° flexion, 20° internal rotation, and 10° abduction. **5** Eleven years after the flexion intertrochanteric osteotomy. The patient is symptom-free but has lost internal rotation

duction has been properly executed, there will be at least an 8–10 mm projection of the femoral head ventrally and laterally beyond the neck. Before the definitive fixation is achieved with lag screws, one must check the reduction with an axial X-ray of the femoral head. The fixation must be secure. If lag screws are used, their threads must be entirely within the capital epiphysis. The screws should be inserted parallel to one another in order to exert compression on the osteotomy.

Technical Steps of the Procedure. The patient is positioned supine. A lateral approach is used. The incision is 15 cm long and runs distally from the tip of the greater trochanter. The fascia lata is opened in line with the skin. The hip joint is approached between the tensor fascia lata and the anterior border of gluteus medius. A periosteal elevator is placed between the gluteal musculature and the capsule of the joint and the greater trochanter is osteotomized extra-articularly with an oscillating saw. In this way one gains a wide exposure of the joint capsule, which is now opened anteriorly all the way to the limbus. This exposes the anterior acetabular edge and the inferior aspect of the femoral neck. With the hip in 60° of flexion, and maximal external rotation, and abduction, one proceeds to the resection of the caudal mass of callus between the calcar and the slipped capital epiphysis. This is accomplished with an osteotome and rongeurs.

The ventral trapezoidal segment of bone is resected with the hip in maximal abduction and external rotation. The first step is a transverse

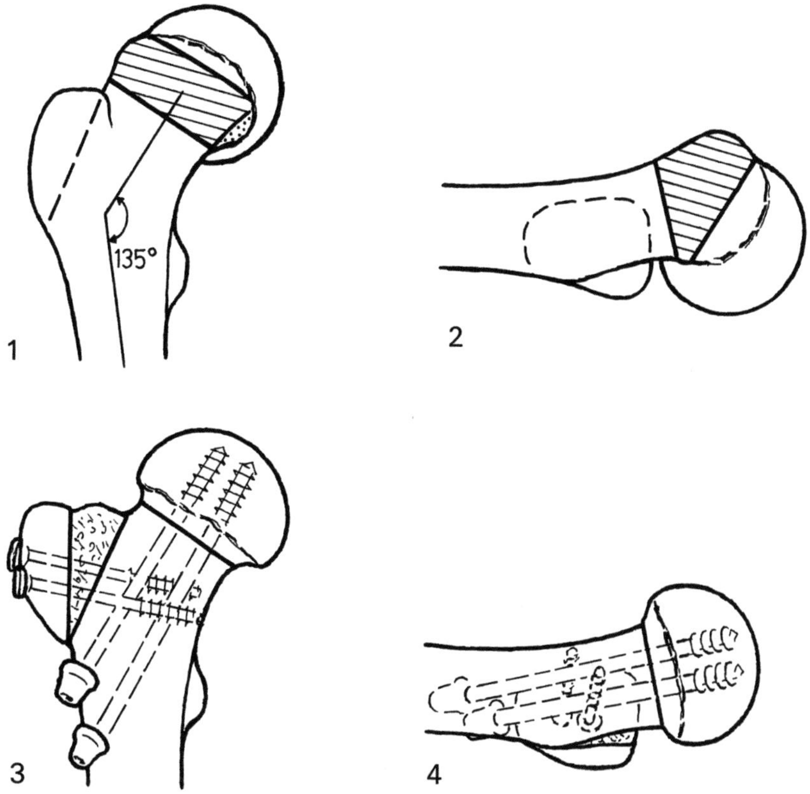

Fig. 36. Principles of cervical osteotomy. First osteotomize the greater trochanter extra-articularly, remove the caudal mass of callus (*a*) in flexion of the hip, and osteotomize three-quarters of the neck somewhat more horizontally than the right angle to the true neck axis. **2** Resect a trapezoidal wedge from the ventral mass of callus. Both osteotomy surfaces must be even. Particular care must be taken not to damage the dorsal blood vessels. Before the trapezoidal wedge is completely resected with a rongeur, three threaded Kirschner wires are inserted up the neck until their tips poke through the lateral osteotomy surface. The reduction is then accomplished by traction, internal rotation, abduction, and light pressure on the anterior aspect of the femoral neck. **3, 4** Note on the AP and lateral projection that the epiphysis projects 1 cm beyond the neck. After the check X-ray, if everything is alright the osteotomy is fixed with three lag screws

lateral osteotomy, made with the oscillating saw. Great care must be taken not to cut all the way through the neck. With a curved osteotome, beginning medially and working towards the osteotomy line, about two-thirds of the planned trapezoidal wedge of bone are resected. Three 2.5-mm-thick Kirschner wires with a short threaded end are inserted through the lateral cortex of the femur and pushed in until they appear at the osteotomy line. The excision of the trapezoidal segment is then completed piecemeal with a small rongeur. Extreme care must be taken to protect the dorsal periosteum, the synovial reflection, and in particular the retinacular vessels.

Once the neck is transected and the segment of bone removed, reduction of the capital epiphysis must follow easily with slight traction and abduction and internal rotation. At times, it is necessary to smooth out the osteotomy surfaces so that they come together. If the reduction cannot be performed with great ease, then something is blocking it. Usually the problem is either a small spicule of bone or the fact that the tip of the trapezoidal segment of bone was not sufficiently wide at the back of the femoral neck. If the reduction is correct, then the femoral head protrudes about 1 cm in front and at the back beyond the neck.

The reduction is maintained by maximal internal rotation of the leg. The Kirschner wires are then inserted a further 2 cm. The reduction and the position of the Kirschner wires is then checked on orthogonal X-rays, taking both AP

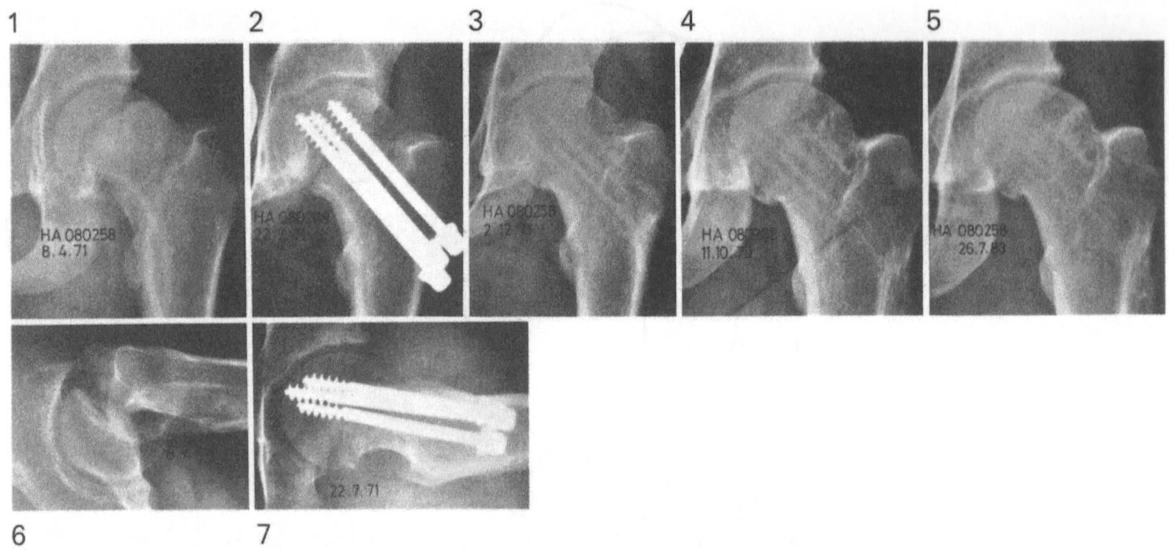

Fig. 37. Cervical osteotomy for chronic epiphyseal slip. H.A., 13-year-old girl. **1, 2** Dorsal slip of a capital epiphysis of 65°. **3, 4** Two months after a trapezoidal resection osteotomy of the neck. The neck is somewhat shortened, but otherwise all relationships are physiological. **5** After 8 months the screws were removed. **6, 7** The result 8 and 12 years later: femoral neck shorter but otherwise radiologically and clinically physiological conditions

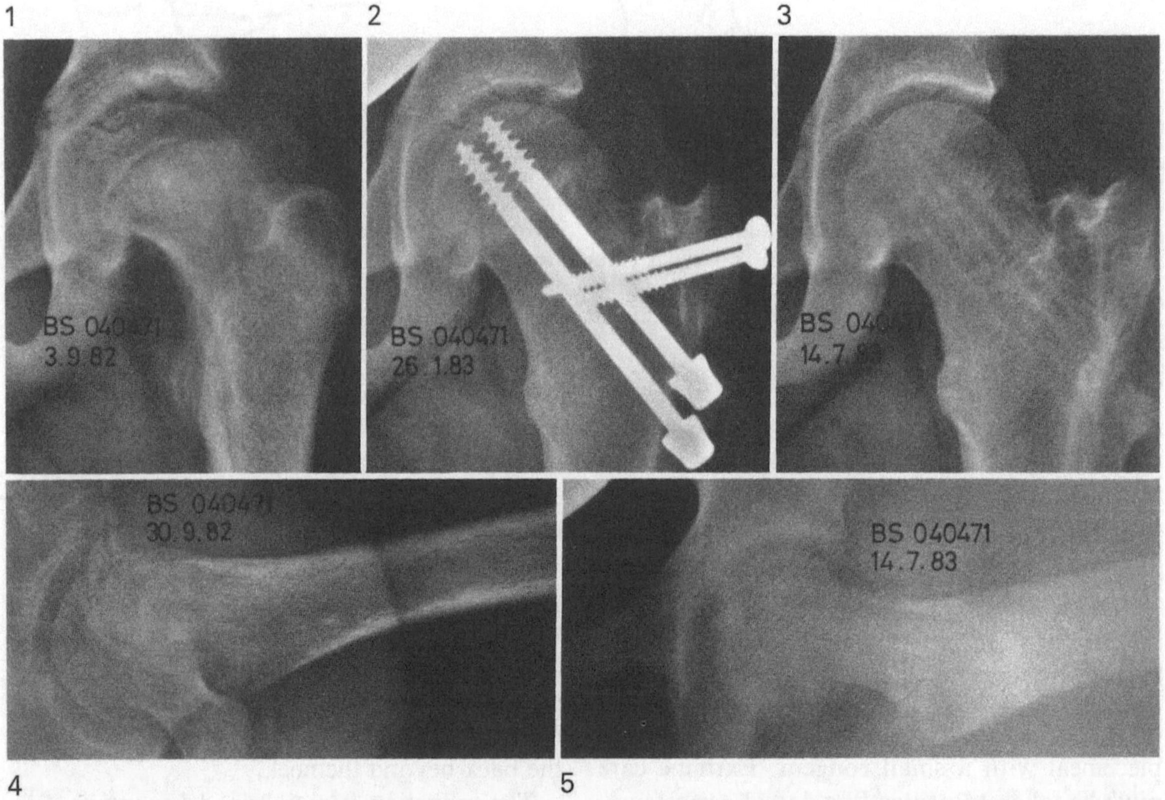

Fig. 38. Subcapital osteotomy with lateral transposition of greater trochanter. B.S., 12-year-old girl. **1, 2** Slip of 60°. **3** Three months after a resection osteotomy of the neck with lateralization of the greater trochanter, accomplished by inserting the resected callus as a graft into the osteotomy of the trochanter. **4, 5** Ten months after removal of the implant. The reduction is perfect and the head is viable. Note that both clinically and subjectively, the patient has right/left symmetry. The patient has returned to full participation in athletics

and axial projections of the femoral neck. The length of the screws is then determined. The Kirschner wires are replaced by special cancellous screws with extra-long heads. At the end of the procedure, the osteotomy should be barely discernible and one should be able to put the hip through a full range of passive motion.

At the end of the procedure, the extremity is maintained in abduction and internal rotation with the aid of boots and bars. Mobilization is begun 6 or 7 days after surgery. On the 10th postoperative day the patient is allowed up, but is permitted only minimal weight-bearing. Full weight-bearing is allowed usually only after 6 months. The screws are removed at 8–12 months.

The example of cervical osteotomy without transposition of the greater trochanter (Fig. 37) shows a much shorter neck than that with lateralization of the trochanter (Fig. 38).

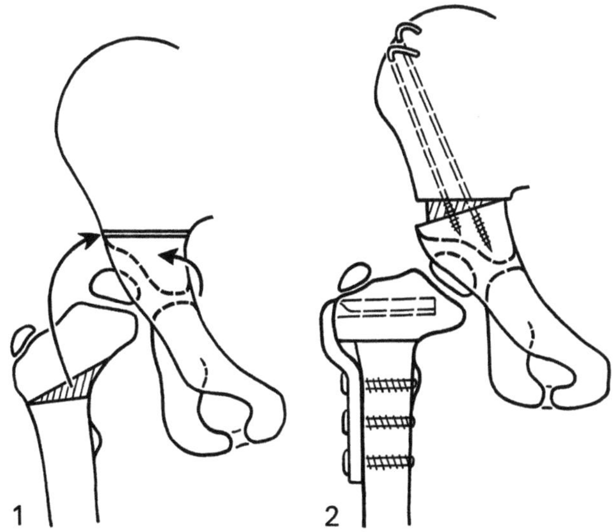

Fig. 39. Combination of pelvic osteotomy as described by Salter with intertrochanteric osteotomy. Two ventrolateral incisions are made approximately 8 cm in length. One begins at the anterior superior spine and extends ventrodistally, the other begins at the tip of the greater trochanter and extends distally in line with the femoral shaft. The approach to the pelvis is between tensor fascia lata and sartorius. The abductors, such as the gluteus minimus, are reflected together with the tensor fascia lata. Retractors with broad tips are inserted into the greater sciatic notch, one medially and one laterally, to protect the soft tissues. **1** The pelvic osteotomy is carried out between the anterior superior and anterior inferior spine and should be at right angles to the body axis. It is carried out with an oscillating saw. The intertrochanteric osteotomy is then completed and the wedge with the base medially is resected. **2** The wedge is used as a graft which is inserted into the pelvic osteotomy once the distal fragment is displaced forwards, downwards and laterally. The pelvic osteotomy is fixed with two to three threaded Kirschner wires and the intertrochanteric osteotomy with the special hip plate for children. Note that the anteversion has been also corrected

Combination of Intertrochanteric Osteotomy with Pelvic Osteotomy

Frequently, some years after a Salter pelvic osteotomy, persistent anteversion has to be corrected by means of a derotation osteotomy. Therefore, if we find an excessive degree of anteversion at the time of an open reduction, we combine the Salter osteotomy with a derotation varus intertrochanteric osteotomy. The resected femoral wedge is then used to graft the opening wedge in the pelvis. This prevents any damage to the pelvic apophysis (Fig. 39, 40).

If after an innominate osteotomy the head is still subluxed the reason often lies in an intraarticular incongruency, the head being too large for the narrow acetabulum. A correction of the anteversion will then not lead to a correction of the deformity (Fig. 41).

Legg-Calvé-Perthes Disease

Legg-Calvé-Perthes disease is caused by an avascular necrosis of the femoral head. In its treatment, we are concerned more with the prevention of premature secondary osteoarthritis of the hip than with the question of revascularization. Thus, we must concentrate our efforts on the prevention of deformity of the diseased femoral head and on the maintenance of congruency of the joint.

In earlier years, a simple intertrochanteric osteotomy was proposed as the solution. It was felt that the reactive hyperemia would accelerate the revascularization of the head. An analysis of patients so treated did not demonstrate any

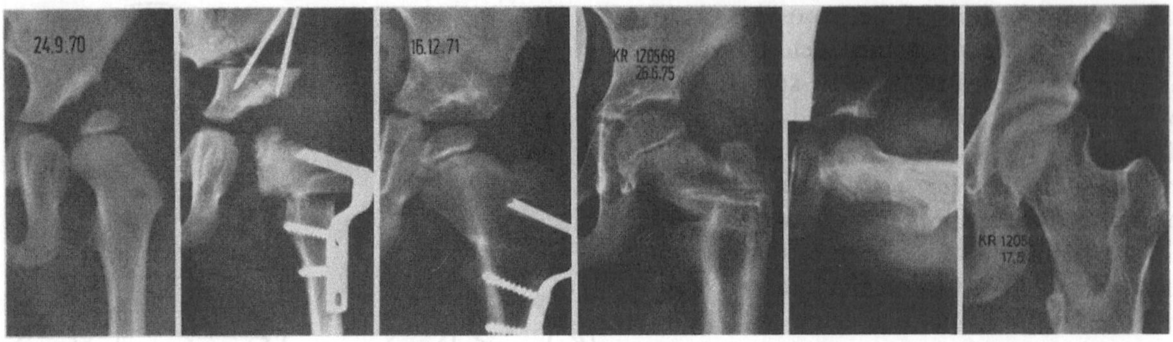

Fig. 40. Combination of intertrochanteric osteotomy with Salter pelvic osteotomy. K.R., $2^1/_3$-year-old girl. **1** The X-ray is similar to that of the patient in Fig. 41. An open reduction was carried out after pelvic osteotomy and intertrochanteric osteotomy. **2** Note the good reduction at 1 month. **3** Note the excellent coverage of the femoral head after $1^1/_4$ years. **4, 5** After 5 years, the clinical and radiological result is excellent. The anteversion has been reduced to 10°. **6** Result still excellent after 13 years

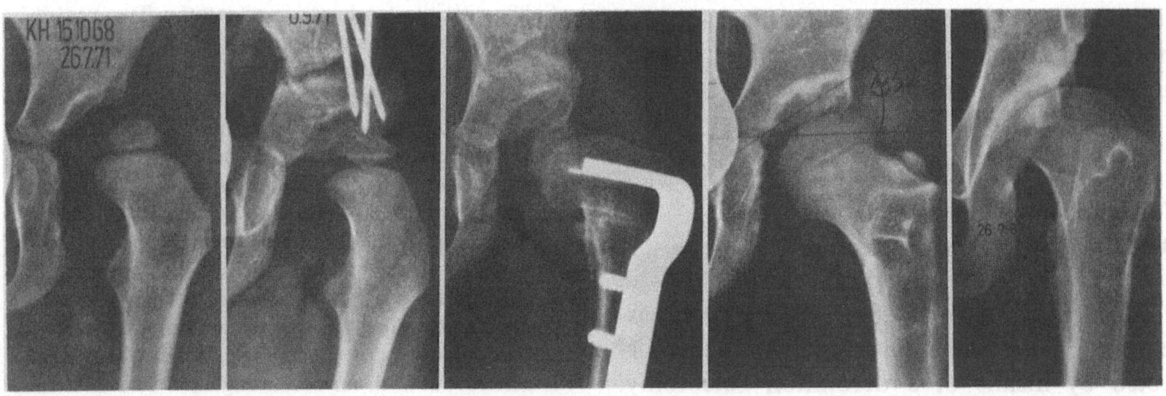

Fig. 41. Intertrochanteric osteotomy after unsuccessful pelvic osteotomy. K.H., $2^3/_4$-year-old girl. **1** Dislocated hip with a steep acetabular roof. **2** After Salter pelvic osteotomy and an incomplete open reduction. **3, 4** After an intertrochanteric osteotomy of 20° of adduction and 50° of derotation the residual subluxation was only partially corrected. The prognosis was uncertain. **5** Twelve years later the hip is still subluxated and a Chiari type pelvic osteotomy has been recommended

improvement in the natural history of the disease. Today, we carry out an extreme varus of 30°, which brings the lateral portion of the enlarged epiphysis under pressure (Fig. 42). The patients can begin ambulation with two crutches 6 weeks after surgery, and at 3 months can begin walking unaided. If this excessive varus intertrochanteric osteotomy is carried out early in the course of the disease, it appears to result in spherical and congruous femoral heads (Figs. 43, 44). A valgus osteotomy is sometimes necessary 4–5 years after surgery to correct the excessive varus.

Pelvic and Acetabular Fractures

Central fracture dislocations of the acetabulum which are allowed to heal without reduction frequently result in painful abduction and flexion contractures and in an unsightly gait disturbance. These patients can usually be helped a great deal by a simple varus extension osteotomy (Fig. 45). If the joint space is irregular but still visible and the hip adducted years after a posttraumatic avascular necrosis, I always advocate an intertrochanteric abduction osteotomy (Fig. 46).

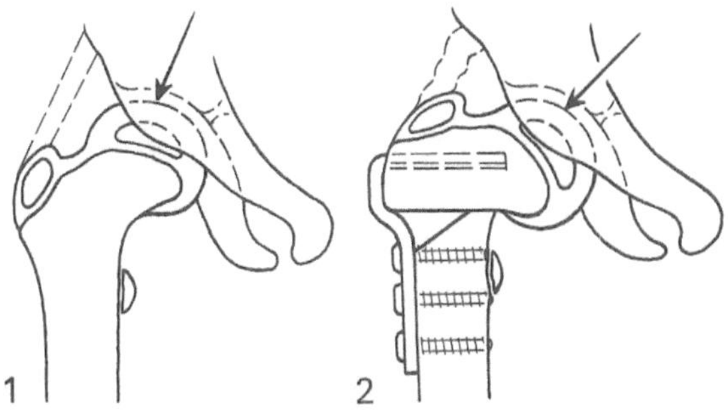

Fig. 42. Technique of intertrochanteric osteotomy and its mode of action in treatment of Legg-Perthes. **1** The femoral head is both wider and flatter. **2** The broad, lateral portion of the femoral head is brought under the weight-bearing portion of the roof by carrying out a simple adduction opening wedge osteotomy. The CCD angle is usually reduced to 95°–100°

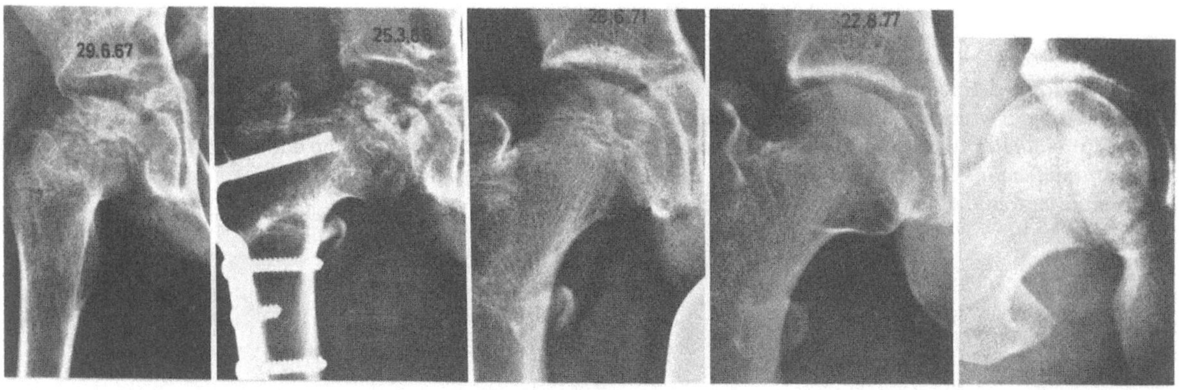

1 2 3 4 5

Fig. 43. Intertrochanteric osteotomy for Legg-Perthes disease. C.P., 6-year-old boy. **1** Legg-Perthes disease with slight subluxation. **2** The result after a 25° adduction osteotomy. Note that the lateral portion of the femoral head has been brought under the acetabular roof. **3, 4** The results at 4 and 10 years after the intertrochanteric osteotomy. Note that the cartilage space has slightly narrowed. **5** The orthogonal lateral projection demonstrates excellent concentricity of the head. The patient is subjectively and clinically symptom-free

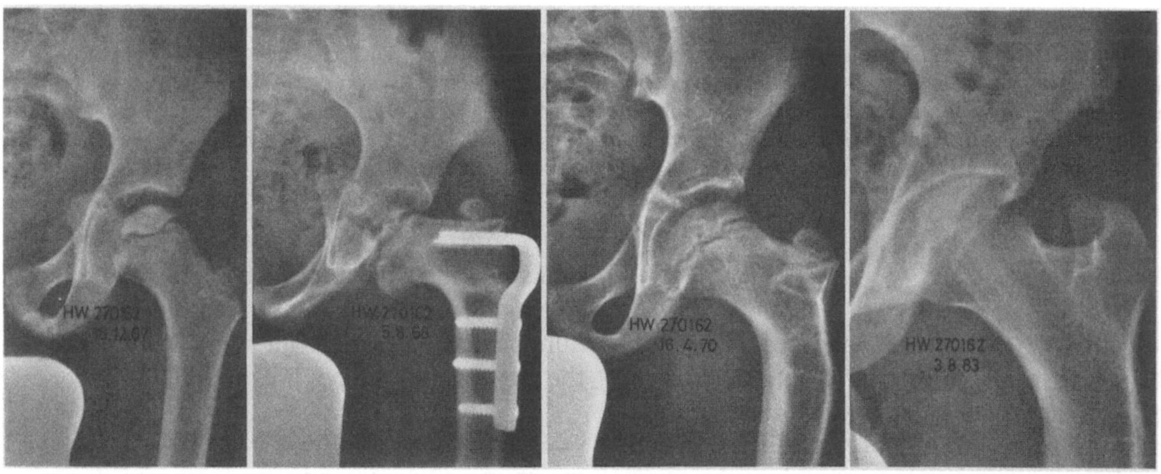

1 2 3 4

Fig. 44. Intertrochanteric osteotomy for Legg-Perthes and subluxation. H.W., 5-year-old boy. **1** Unilateral Perthes disease. The epiphysis of the femoral head is totally involved in the necrotic process and the epiphyseal plate shows some irregularities. **2** Eight months after adduction osteotomy of 40° degrees. **3, 4** $2^1/_2$ and 16 years after intertrochanteric osteotomy. Clinically and radiologically, conditions almost identical to those on the normal right side. Only the joint space appears slightly narrower on the operated side

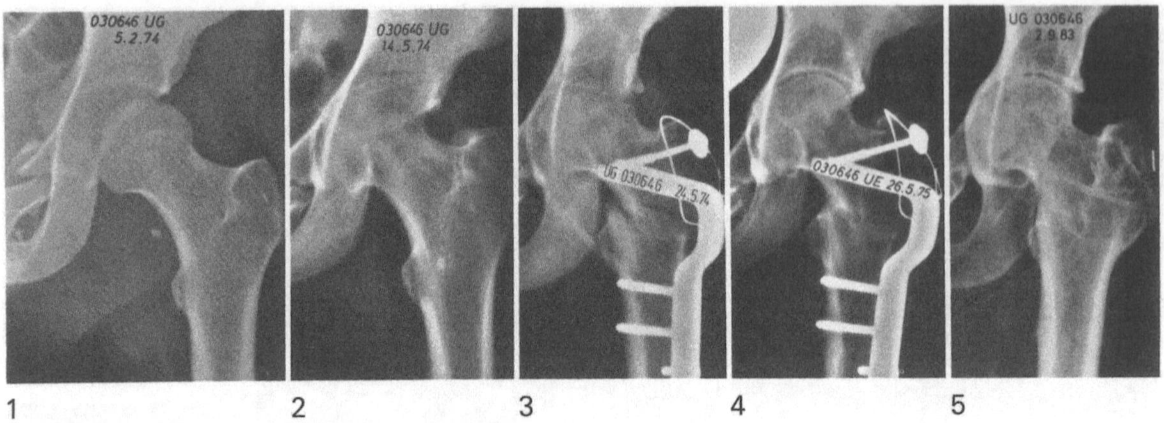

Fig. 45. Malunited fracture dislocation of acetabulum. U.G., 28-year-old woman. **1** Central fracture dislocation of the hip treated in traction. **2** The hip stiffened in abduction and flexion. **3** After a 20° adduction and 20° extension osteotomy. **4** The result after 1 year. **5** The result after 6 years. The patient is almost pain-free despite signs of early osteoarthritis and reduced mobility (flexion only 75°, abduction and adduction 5° and 10° respectively, no rotation)

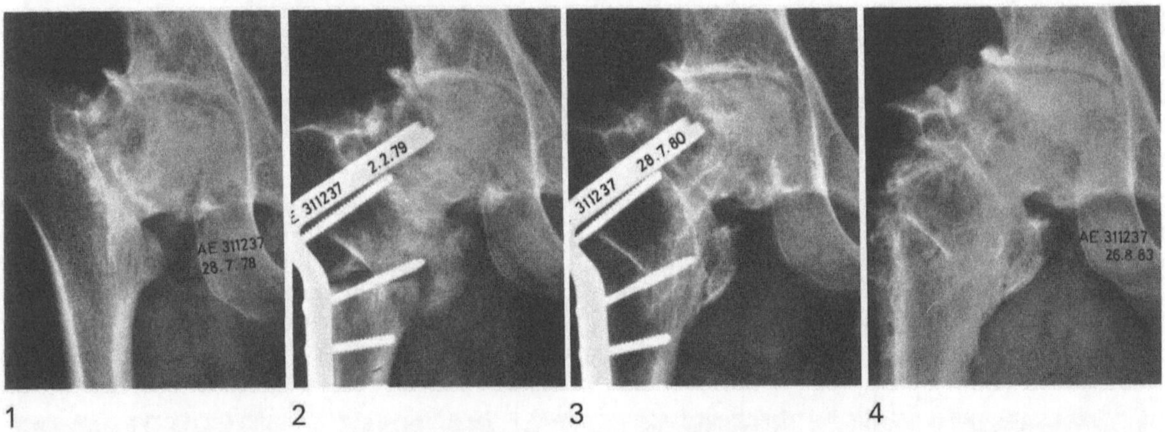

Fig. 46. Intertrochanteric osteotomy in malunion and avascular necrosis of femoral head. A.E., 41-year-old man. **1** We see what appears to be hopeless destruction of the joint 3 years after nailing of a subcapital fracture. The patient had an abduction contracture and was able to get about only with crutches. **2** Two years after an adduction and extension osteotomy. **3, 4** The result $1^1/_2$ years and 5 years after the intertrochanteric osteotomy. The patient is able to walk for 8 h without crutches and is completely free of pain

Cerebral Palsy

Twenty-five years ago, I published extensively [4] on the influence of intertrochanteric osteotomy on the spastic gait of patients with cerebral palsy. An overcorrection of the anteversion with simultaneous varus gives a surprising improvement of their gait. The varus results in shortening of the femur, which leads to relaxation or effective lengthening of the muscles in the region of the hip and considerable lessening of the knee flexion contractures. The equinus frequently diminishes, and sometimes we see a plantigrade gait right from the start. We feel that this procedure should be carried out somewhere between the 4th and 8th years of life, but only in children

Fig. 47. Cerebral palsy. B.V., 4-year-old girl. **1, 2** The child was able to walk only if held by the hand. She walked with severe equinus. Her CE angle on both sides was 5°. Anteversion was bilaterally 70°. **3, 4** One year after intertrochanteric osteotomy and derotation of 60°. **5, 6** At 5 years from surgery the child is able to walk well independently ▷

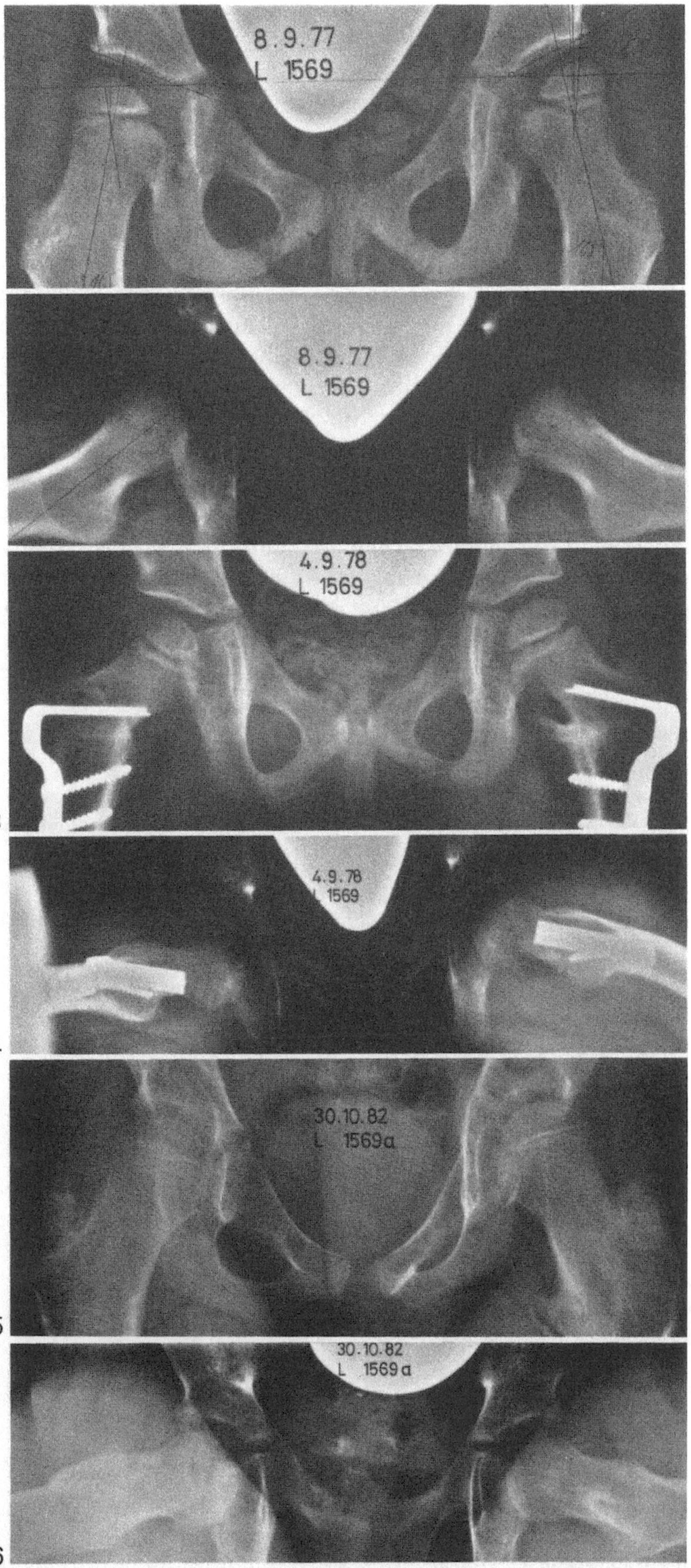
8.9.77
L 1569
1
8.9.77
L 1569
2
4.9.78
L 1569
3
4.9.78
L 1569
4
30.10.82
L 1569a
5
30.10.82
L 1569a
6

Fig. 47

who are able to walk if held by the hand. We have found that the results are best if no previous tendon or nerve procedures have been carried out.

As long as the child is continent of urine, we have found that a fixation of the intertrochanteric osteotomy by means of the external fixators (Fig. 25) combined with a spica has given very good results, and we use this method up to the 4th year of life. In older children, we employ the 90° blade plate. In contrast to the usual derotation intertrochanteric osteotomies in children, where we do not remove any wedges, in the treatment of spastics we aim at resection of wide wedges to achieve muscle decompression and attempt to lateralize the femoral shaft in order to overcome the genu valgum. The CCD angle is reduced to less than 100°.

The case which we have illustrated in Fig. 47 is that of a 4-year-old child with severe spasticity and equinus who could walk only with great difficulty when supported by one hand. The anteversion was completely corrected. The right-angle plate was used for fixation and a hip spica was used for $1^1/_2$ months. Rehabilitation was then begun, and for 6 weeks the child used parallel bars and a walker. At the end of 6 months the child was able to walk unaided. Two years later the child could run, jump, and walk for hours with a plantigrade gait. A pes planus developed on one side and was treated by a tibialis anterior transfer to support the navicular.

Fresh Fractures in the Proximal Femur

If the decision is made to perform internal fixation of a subcapital fracture in a patient with severe osteoporosis, we feel that the procedure should be combined with a repositioning osteotomy in order to convert all shearing forces into compressive forces and thus minimize the forces of displacement. Impaction of the fragments is not necessary, and the open reduction combined with intertrochanteric osteotomy becomes quite simple.

Intertrochanteric osteotomy can also be used in the treatment of comminuted intertrochanteric fractures. It can result in a good medial buttress and thus stability [9]. The marked valgus of the proximal fragment results in medialization of the femoral shaft which makes the proximal femur look very similar to the humerus (Figs. 48, 49). It is extremely difficult in these resection osteotomies to achieve correct rotational alignment.

Idiopathic Osteoarthritis of the Hip

The use of intertrochanteric osteotomy in this context is discussed in this volume at great length by Schneider. I have found that the adduction or varus osteotomy is indicated only in those patients in whom the X-rays of the hip taken in abduction show an improved con-

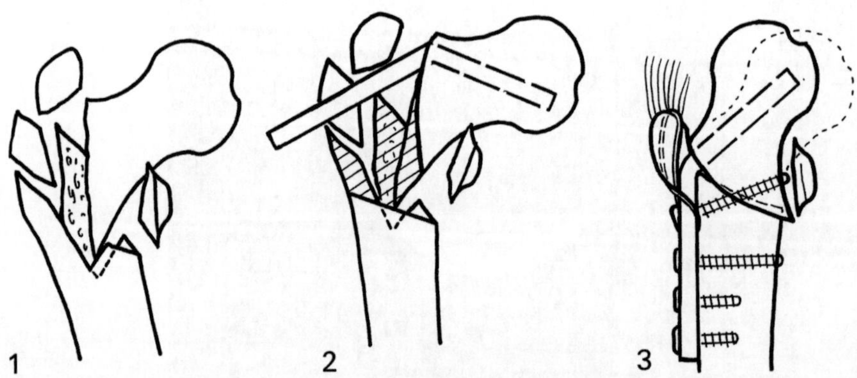

Fig. 48. Valgus osteotomy in a fresh fracture. **1** A comminuted intertrochanteric fracture. **2, 3** Repositioning of the fragments and fixation with a 130° plate. Note that the most proximal screw inserted through the plate, acts as a lag screw between the head and shaft fragments, and imparts great rotational stability to the fixation. The greater trochanter was fixed by means of a tension-band wire

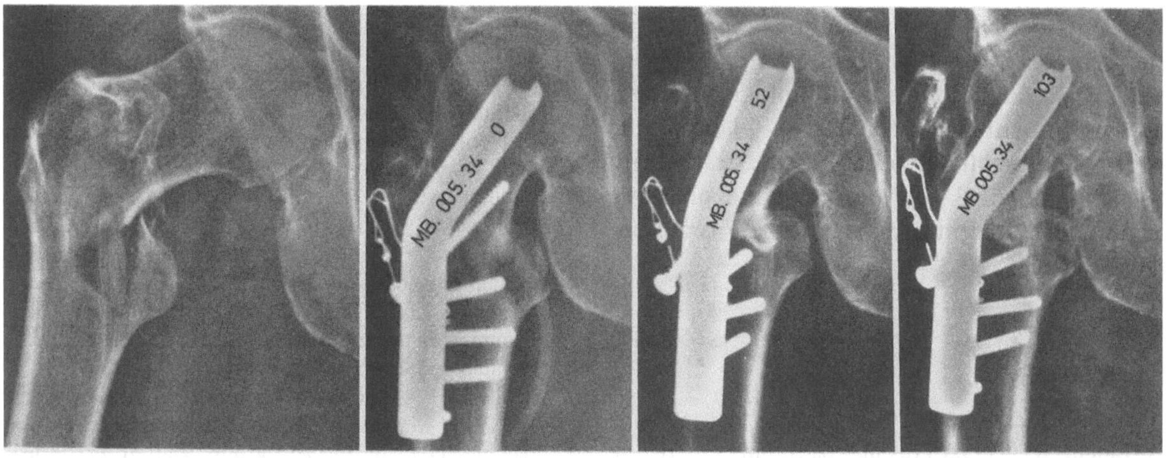

1 2 3 4

Fig. 49. Unstable intertrochanteric fracture. T.C., 82-year-old woman. **1** At the time of the accident. **2** The X-ray picture after valgus osteotomy. **3, 4** Respectively 1 and 2 years after the intertrochanteric osteotomy. Note that the greater trochanteric fragment has redisplaced

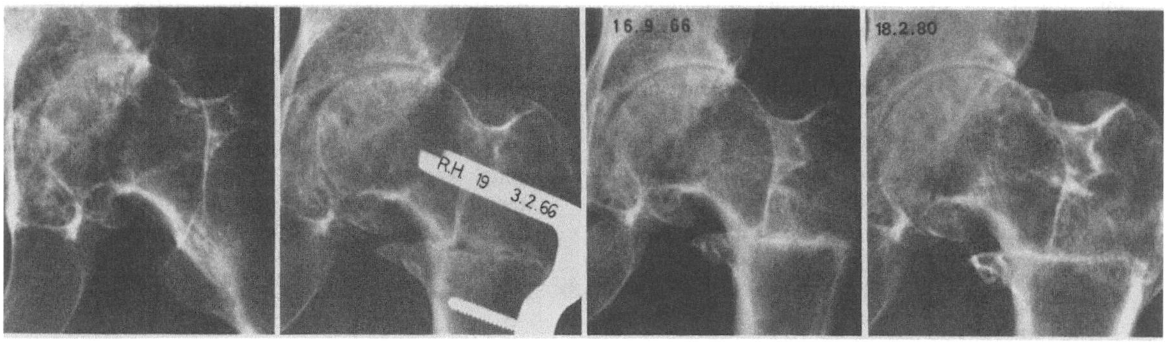

1 2 3 4

Fig. 50. Intertrochanteric osteotomy in idiopathic osteoarthritis of the hip. R.H., 47-year-old man. **1** Abduction contracture. Note that the cartilage space has vanished. **2, 3** Note the slow recovery of the cartilage space over 14 years. **4** Slight recurrence of symptoms at 16 years following the osteotomy. Once the symptoms reach the point of complete disability, a total replacement arthroplasty will be necessary

gruence and no narrowing of the articular cartilage space laterally. Spherical heads lend themselves much more to this osteotomy than deformed heads, and the results are better in those with some abduction contracture (Fig. 50). On the other hand, an abduction intertrochanteric osteotomy is usually indicated in elliptic heads and in deformed heads with some adduction contracture. These intertrochanteric varus and valgus osteotomies have to be combined with an extension osteotomy.

Conclusions and Summary

Intertrochanteric osteotomy is a rational surgical procedure for most structural disorders of the hip. Even in early arthrosis, a reversal of the disease process may be brought about by proper application of the principles of this operation. Intertrochanteric osteotomy is also of value in a few carefully selected patients with advanced degenerative joint disease.

In this chapter the indications of intertrochanteric osteotomy for 25 different conditions are discussed and long-term radiological follow-up is presented. Preoperative planning is stressed as essential in obtaining the desired end result. A detailed description of the planning technique is presented by means of 17 representative cases.

References

1. Blount WP (1952) Proximal osteotomies of the femur. American Academy of Orthopedic Surgeons Instruction Course Lectures, vol. IX
2. Ganz R, Jakob RP (1980) Segmental vascular necrosis of the femoral head: flexion osteotomy combined with cancellous bone grafting of the lesion. Orthopade 9:265
3. v Lanz T, Wachsmuth W (1938) Praktische Anatomie. Ein Lehr- und Hilfsbuch der anatomischen Grundlagen ärztlichen Handelns. 1. Bd, 4. Teil: Bein und Statik. Springer, Berlin
4. Müller ME (1971) Die hüftnahen Femurosteotomien. 2. Aufl mit Anhang: 12 Hüfteingriffe. Thieme, Stuttgart
5. Müller ME (1975) Intertrochanteric osteotomies in adults: planning and operating technique. In: Cruess RL, Mitchell NS Surgical management of degenerative arthritis of the lower limb. Lea & Febiger, Philadelphia
6. Müller ME (1979) Planung einer komplexen intertrochanteren Osteotomie. Z Orthop 117:145–150
7. Müller ME (1983) Intertrochanteric osteotomies. In: McCollister Evarts C (ed) Surgery of the musculoskeletal system. Churchill Livingstone, New York
8. Müller ME (1984) Indikation, Lokalisation und zeichnerische Planung hüftgelenknaher Femurosteotomien bei posttraumatischen Zuständen. In: Hierholzer G, Müller KH: Korrekturosteotomien nach Traumen an der unteren Extremität. Springer, Berlin Heidelberg New York Tokyo
9. Müller ME, Allgöwer M, Schneider R, Willenegger H (1979) Manual of internal fixation. Techniques recommended by the AO group. 2nd ed, expanded and revised. Springer, Berlin Heidelberg New York
10. Pauwels F (1973) Atlas zur Biomechanik der gesunden und kranken Hüfte. Prinzipien, Technik und Resultate einer kausalen Therapie. Springer, Berlin Heidelberg New York
11. Schenk RK, Müller J, Willenegger H (1968) Experimentell-histologischer Beitrag zur Entstehung und Behandlung von Pseudarthrosen. Hefte Unfallheilkd 94:15–24
12. Schneider R (1979) Die intertrochantere Osteotomie bei Coxarthrose. Springer, Berlin Heidelberg New York
13. Sugioka Y (1978) Transtrochanteric anterior rotational osteotomy of the femoral head in the treatment of osteonecrosis affecting the hip: a new osteotomy operation. Clin Orthop 130

Biomechanical Classification of Osteoarthritis of the Hip with Special Reference to Treatment Techniques and Results

R. BOMBELLI and J. ARONSON

Biomechanical Analysis of Normal and Abnormal Hip Geometry

From our experience, a hip is geometrically *normal*, and therefore able to withstand the stress acting in it without damage, only when all the following prerequisites are observed:

1. The acetabular weight-bearing surface (WBS) horizontal in the coronal plane
2. The shape of the femoral head is spherical within limits (the vertical diameter a few millimeters less than the horizontal diameter), in order to achieve dynamic congruence with the acetabulum (congruent incongruity)
3. The femoral neck-shaft angle is about 130° and anteversion about 12°

If one or more of these conditions are not fulfilled, the hip is *abnormal*.

Before we can consider each prerequisite separately, we must discuss the normal biomechanics of the hip. In order to plan effective treatment, one must understand the consequences of abnormal geometry.

Pauwels [23], describing the forces acting about the hip in monopodal stance, defined K as the weight of the body less the weight of the limb in stance. Force K, acting with a lever arm b on the center of rotation (CR) of the femoral head, would rotate the pelvis medially and downward, were it not counteracted by an equal and opposite force, the abductors (M) acting on CR with a lever arm a, which rotate the pelvis laterally and downward. From this basic principle, two component forces of the abductors may be derived, i.e., the vertical (downward directed) force P_M and the horizontal (laterally directed) force Q_M (Fig. 1) [6].

In the hip joint, during monopodal stance forces K and P_M are directed vertically downward and combine with the horizontal force Q_M acting laterally to form resultant force R. This resultant force is identical to the R that Pauwels calculated in a different way [23]. The sum of K and P_M may be considered as P_R (the vertical component of R) and force Q_M as Q_R (horizontal component of R) (Fig. 2) [6].

Force R, the "acting" force, is resisted by the counterthrust from the ground, which we designate R_1 (reacting force), equal in magnitude but opposite in direction to force R. In the coronal plane, force R_1 pushes the femoral head obliquely against the WBS of the acetabulum, which lies normally in a horizontal direction. The direction of the WBS is determined by a line joining the lateral and the medial edges of the sourcil or by a line traced perpendicularly to the line bisecting the Gothic arch. In a normal hip joint these two lines are horizontal (Fig. 3). A proof that the hip forces require only a horizontal WBS is illustrated in Fig. 4.

We can therefore imagine a shearing component of R_1 parallel to the direction of the WBS, force Q, and a compressive component of R_1 perpendicular to the direction of the WBS, force P (Fig. 5). A composite diagram of the forces is shown in Fig. 6.

Three fundamental points in the hip are CR, T, and H (Fig. 7). Point T corresponds to an ideal point where force P passes through the acetabulum, point H is the ideal point where the counterresultant force R_1 passes through the acetabulum, and CR is the center of rotation of the femoral head. Force R_1 is directed from CR to H, force P from CR to T, and force Q from T to H.

Only when the acetabular WBS is horizontal do the vertical forces $P_R(P_M+K)$ and P have the same magnitude and opposite directions.

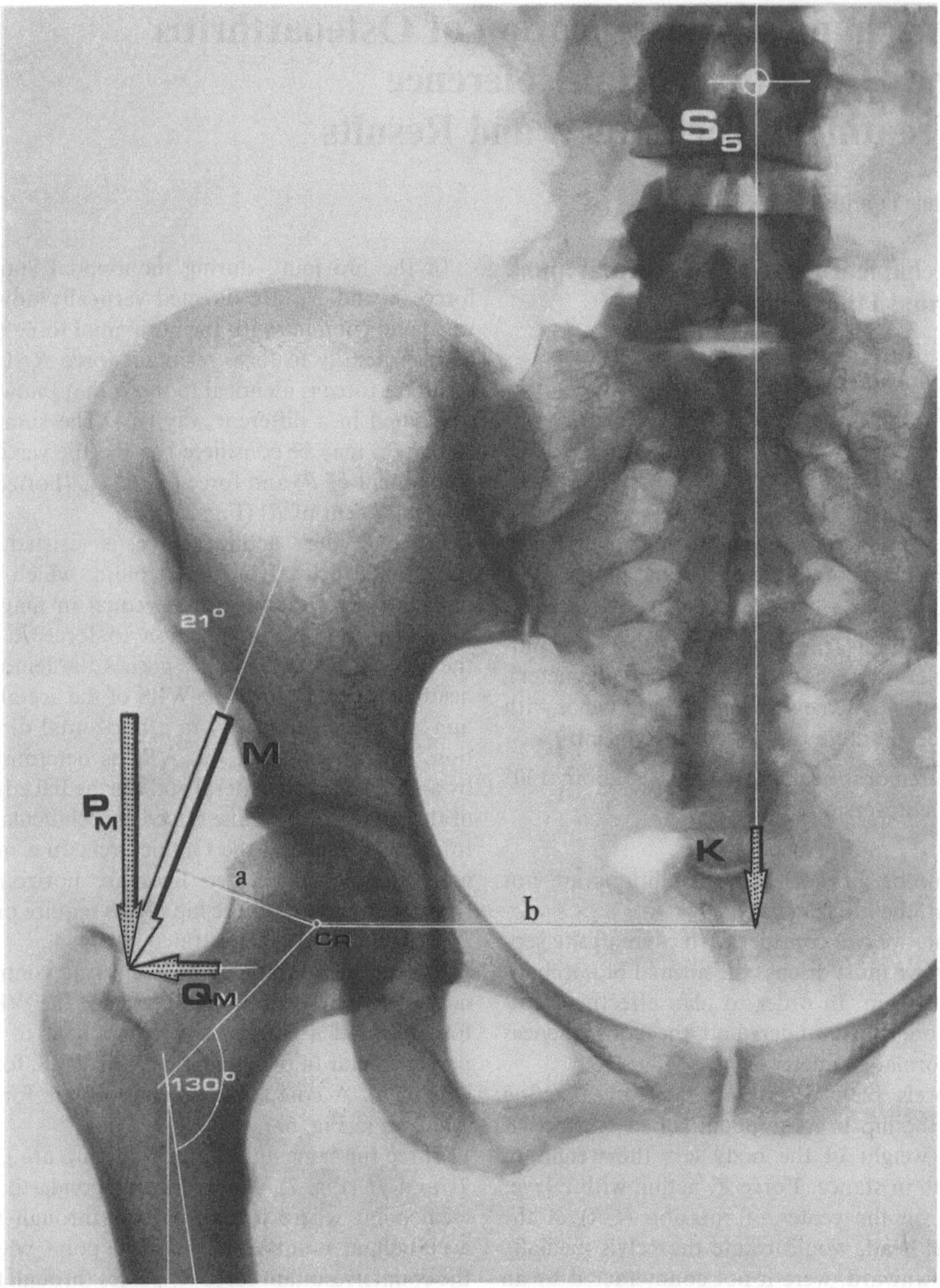

Fig. 1. Forces acting in the normal hip in right monopodal stance. The weight of the body S_5 acts by force K (gravity) on lever arm b. The pelvis is kept level by the action of the abductors working through lever arm a. Force M is resolved into vertical component P_M and horizontal component Q_M

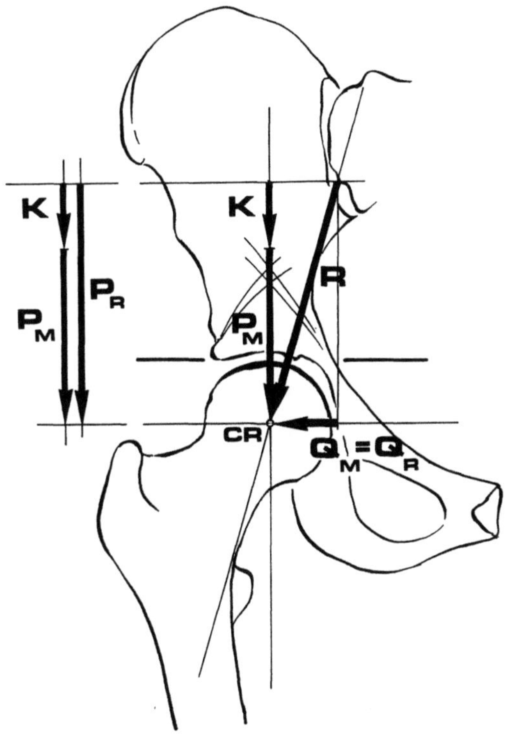

Fig. 2. Derivation of force R from the forces acting in the normal hip in monopodal stance. To simplify, the vertical forces K and P_M are combined as P_R and the horizontal component of M, Q_M, is renamed Q_R

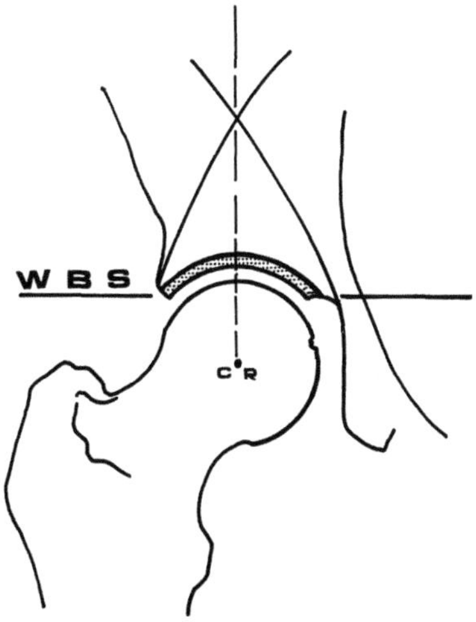

Fig. 3. Determination of direction of the acetabular WBS. If a line cannot be drawn across the medial and lateral margins of the sourcil, a perpendicular from the line bisecting the Gothic arch provides the inclination of the WBS from the horizontal

The horizontal forces $Q_R(Q_M)$ and Q are also equal in magnitude and opposite in direction. We have previously discussed the effect of these forces on the trabecular structure of the pelvis and on the upper part of the femur (Fig. 8) [4].

Force P_R, a gravity force, is always directed downward and force Q_R, perpendicular to P_R, is always horizontal. Their directions do not change during gait and are not affected by different inclination of the WBS. Conversely, forces P and Q are derived from the impact of force R_1 on the acetabular WBS and must modify their magnitude and direction according to the direction of the WBS (Fig. 9) [2].

WBS of Acetabulum

The direction of the WBS plays a paramount role in determining the direction and the magnitude of the component forces P and Q of the counterresultant force R_1. Let us consider what happens to forces P_R and P and to forces Q_R and Q when the WBS inclines craniolaterally or craniomedially[1].

Craniolateral Inclination of WBS

Forces P_R *and* P. The more the WBS inclines craniolaterally, the greater the magnitude of force P becomes (Fig. 10a), until a magnitude equal to that of force R_1 is achieved when the WBS reaches an inclination perpendicular to R_1 (Fig. 10b). We call this the *point of reversal.* The clinical correlate is a progressive increase in joint pain.

Flattening of the entire WBS of the femoral head and of the lateral part of the acetabulum due to the increasing force P is responsible for a further inclination of the WBS. When the point of reversal is surpassed, the magnitude of force P diminishes proportionately, and clinically the patient experiences a regression in pain (Fig. 10c).

Forces Q_M *and* Q. Increasing craniolateral inclination of the WBS produces a reduction in the

1 Here we have used "cranio" rather than "supero" for anatomical clarity. The meaning is identical in every case to "supero" as used previously [2–5, 7].

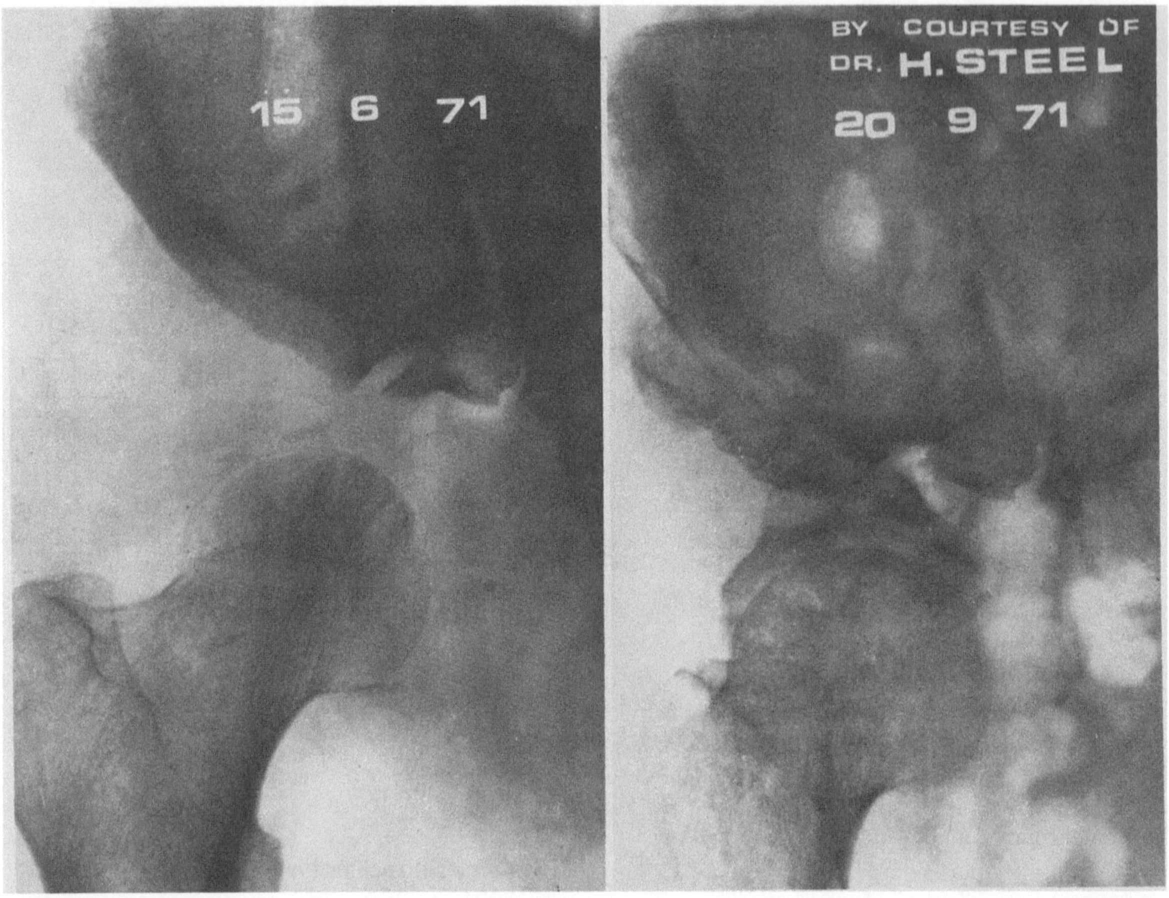

Fig. 4. This patient underwent complete resection of the acetabulum for tumor. The radiographic follow-up demonstrates remarkable regeneration of a new WBS extending from the ilium, stimulated by partial weight-bearing gait with crutches for 3 months. Note that this new WBS is horizontal and bears significant similarity to the sourcil. Trabeculae resembling the Gothic arch are present. (Courtesy of Dr. H. Steel)

magnitude of force Q (Fig. 10a), which completely disappears at the point of reversal (Fig. 10b). Therefore, when the WBS presents a craniolateral inclination, force Q can never counteract force Q_M, either in magnitude or in direction. The femoral head is compelled to move progressively out of the acetabulum in an anterocraniolateral direction, producing incongruency between the femoral head and the acetabulum. As the surface of the acetabulum–femoral head contact area decreases, the stress both in the femoral head and in the acetabulum increases. Under this heightened stress the bone reaction (cysts and eburnation) produces flattening of the head and further inclines the craniolateral part of the acetabulum (Fig. 12).

When the point of reversal is surpassed by progressive inclination of the WBS, the magnitude of force P decreases but a new force appears, opposite to the original force Q. We call it force S (shearing, *Schub, spinta*). Force S augments force Q_M to accelerate the subluxation of the femoral head (Figs. 10c, d, 11). Progression of this anterocraniolateral subluxation is limited by the tension in the craniolateral fibers of the capsule and ligaments. Early on, in the young patient, the elasticity in the soft tissues can resist the abnormal stress, but with continuous and increasing stretching they eventually give way. Later on the capsule becomes sclerotic and transmits stress to its bony origin, thus creating traction osteophytes (Fig. 13).

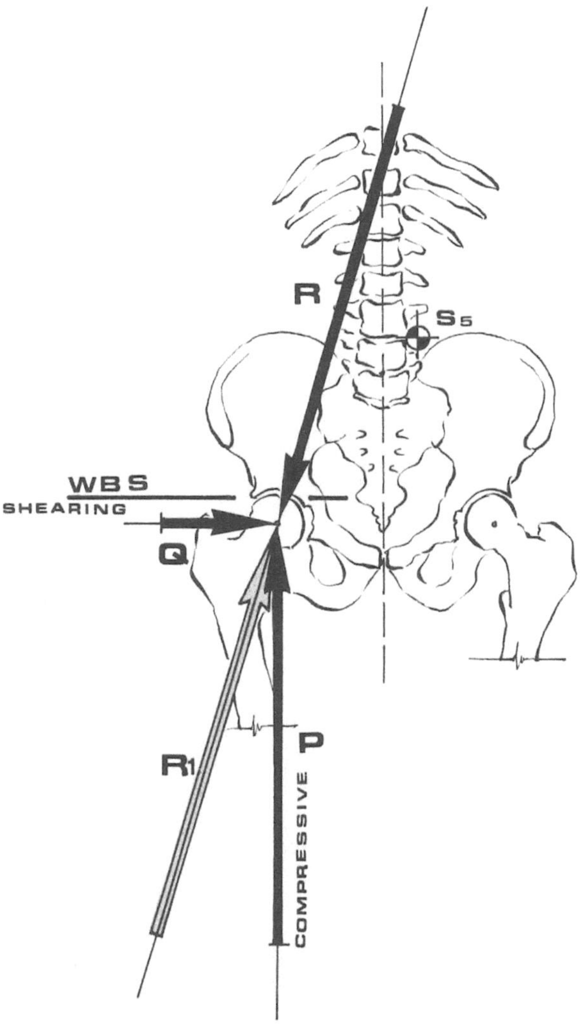

Fig. 5. The shearing and compressive components of the reacting force R_1. The compressive component P is always defined as perpendicular to the WBS. Force Q is always parallel to the WBS. Together, P and Q must result in R_1, equal and opposite to R

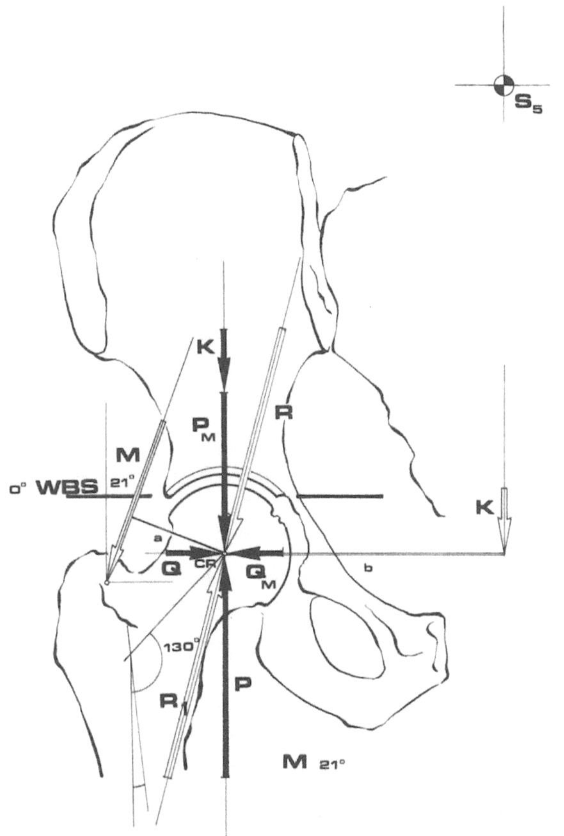

Fig. 6. The balanced forces acting in the normal hip joint (neck-shaft angle of 130° and WBS of 0°) during monopodal stance

When the WBS slants craniolaterally, point T moves toward point H; when the distance between T and H is reduced, the magnitude of Q decreases. When the WBS is perpendicular to R_1, points T and H coincide, i.e., there is no distance between T and H (Fig. 14). Force Q disappears, and force P, being equal to force R_1, is at its maximum and pain reaches its peak. With further inclination of the WBS, point T moves medially and posteriorly to point H, and force S, directed from T to H, appears (Fig. 15).

Effect of Antalgic Gait. As soon as the patient experiences pain, he limps, because of an antalgic reflex. The antalgic gait reflex means trunk shift without pelvic tilt. In monopodal stance the patient shifts the center of gravity of the body (S_5) laterally toward the painful hip, and by doing so shortens the lever arm b of the weight K. Since the force of abductors (M) varies in direct proportion to b, as b is decreased M is also decreased, according to the equation $M=\frac{Kb}{a}$. The two components of M, P_M and Q_M, are both reduced, thereby reducing the magnitude of R and R_1, which assume a more vertical direction. The overall force on the hip is reduced and pain is relieved. When S_5 is shifted above CR, theoretically the abductors M no longer need to exert a force, therefore P_M no longer exists, and pain is maximally re-

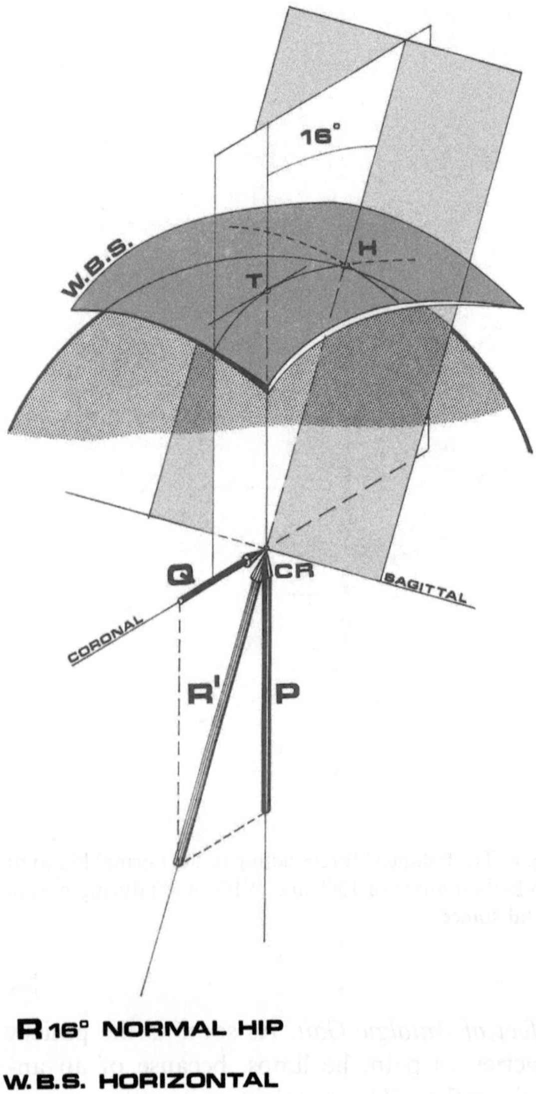

Fig. 7. Three-dimensional diagram of the right hip joint during monopodal stance. The WBS (*dark gray*) is horizontal. Reacting force R_1 is inclined 16° in the coronal plane (*white*). Compressive force P passing through CR ends at point T perpendicular to the WBS. H is the contact point as force R_1 extends from CR to the joint surface. Shearing force Q parallel to the WBS is also parallel to a line from point T to point H. The sagittal plane is shown in *light gray* and the femoral head is dotted

lieved because the only compressive forces are K and K ($K_1 = R_1$) (Fig. 16).

When the WBS is horizontal, the antalgic gait moves point H toward T, thereby reducing the magnitude of Q (Fig. 17). When the WBS is craniolaterally inclined, the antalgic gait moves point H more laterally to and then beyond point T (Fig. 18). The progressive craniolateral inclination of the WBS combines with the antalgic gait (Fig. 19) to cause the swift disappearance of force Q and the precocious appearance of force S, whose presence reduces the magnitude of the painful compressive force P. In other words, pain is reduced by the overall reduction of forces R and R_1 and the early appearance of force S.

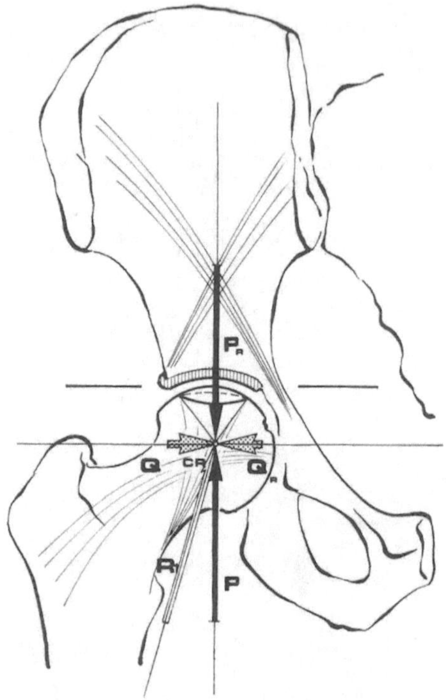

Fig. 8. *Trabecular response to stress.* The sourcil, Gothic arch, and hourglass are a response to force P. Compressive trabeculae in the femoral neck support the spherical sector in response to force P_R. Tensile trabeculae in the femoral head reflect the Q forces

When the WBS is already inclined beyond the point of reversal, the antalgic gait reduces all forces acting in the joint, but increases the proportional magnitude of force S. Consider the magnitude of force R_1 before the antalgic gait in a hip with craniolateral inclination of the WBS of 32°. Force R_1 ist 113.96 kg, force S ist 30.37 kg, and force P is 109.84 kg (Fig. 11). The magnitude of force S corresponds to 26% of force R_1, that of force P to 96 of force R_1.

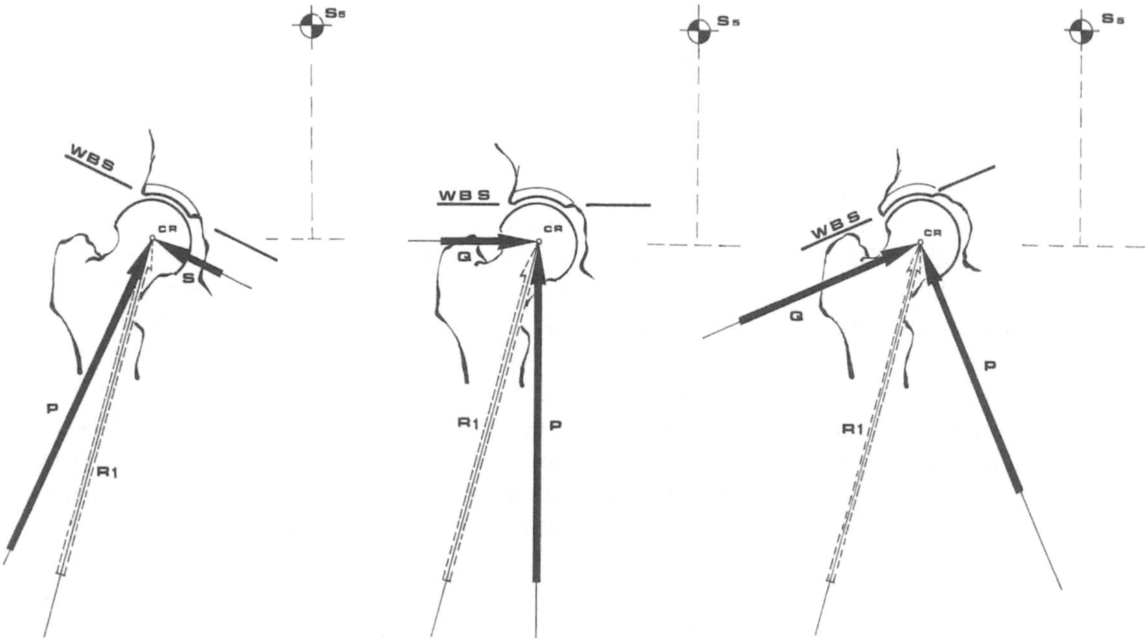

Fig. 9. Impact of the inclination of the WBS on the components of force R_1. Only when the WBS is horizontal is P vertical and Q horizontal (*center*). When the WBS is craniolaterally inclined more than 16°, the shearing force Q changes direction to force S, creating craniolateral subluxation in the coronal plane (*left*). When the WBS is craniomedially inclined, the magnitude of force Q increases, tending to push the head deep into the fundus acetabuli (*right*)

In the same hip, after appearance of antalgic gait, the magnitude of force R_1 is reduced to 47.76 kg, that of force S to 19.42 kg, and that of force P to 43.63 kg (Fig. 19). The magnitude of force S now corresponds to 44% of force R_1 and that of force P to 91% of force R_1. It seems that nature exploits the antalgic gait, not only reducing the magnitude of the painful force P from 109.84 kg to 43.63 kg, but also transferring a portion of it to nonpainful tissues (capsule and ligaments) through the proportional increase in force S. Force S plays an important role in osteophyte formation (Fig. 20a). Now let us analyze what happens when R shifts to 0° and the WBS is 45°. Force S has achieved equality with force P, yet it has increased from 48% of R before the antalgic gait, when R is at 16°, to 71% of R at 0°, while force P has decrease from 85% (R 16°) to 71% (R 0°). When the WBS inclines 53° and R is 0° (maximal trunk shift) force S is greater than P, having increased to 80% of R when R is at 0° from 60% when is at R 16°. Force P has decreased to 60% when R is at 0° from 80% when is at R 16°.

Static anatomical inclination of the WBS when combined with the antalgic gait, lessens the proportional magnitude of force P and increases that of force S. When the pelvis tilts downward toward the swing limb, as described by Trendelenburg, a dynamic craniolateral inclination of the WBS on the stance side combines with the trunk shift of antalgic gait (Fig. 20b, c). During Trendelenburg gait both trunk shift and craniolateral pelvic tilt are present in the support hip. The patient who shifts his trunk directly over the abnormal hip and drops the pelvis away appears to waddle, and may complain of lumbar pain and buttock stretch but not hip pain. The tremendous reduction of force P and the introduction of force S together unload the painful area of femoroacetabular contact.

Craniomedial Inclination of WBS

As already stated, the magnitude and direction of forces P_R and Q_R do not depend on the direction of the WBS. On the contrary, the magnitude and direction of forces P and Q depend on it.

Force P. The magnitude of force P, perpendicular to the direction of the WBS, decreases as the craniomedial inclination increases, reducing therefore the compression of the femoral head against the acetabular WBS (Fig. 9). This may explain why both the joint cartilage of the WBS of the femoral head and the corresponding cartilage of the acetabulum are preserved (Fig. 21 a). On an X-ray AP view, the weight-bearing portion of the joint space is clearly visible; on an axial view the joint space disappears posteromedially and the femoral head points posteriorly (Fig. 21 b).

Force Q. At the same time, the magnitude of force Q, parallel to the acetabular WBS, increases. In gait, force Q normally reaches its peak at the heel-strike phase, when it is posteromedially directed [6]. With craniomedial inclination of the WBS, force Q is always dominant to force Q_M and at heel strike pushes the femoral head posteromedially into the acetabulum with maximum intensity. This may explain why the cartilage covering the posteromedial aspect of the femoral head is worn out and why in the long run the head, compressing the fundus acetabuli, migrates into the pelvis. In this situation, the increased magnitude of force Q contributes to coxa equatorialis, coxa profunda, or protrusio acetabuli (Fig. 22).

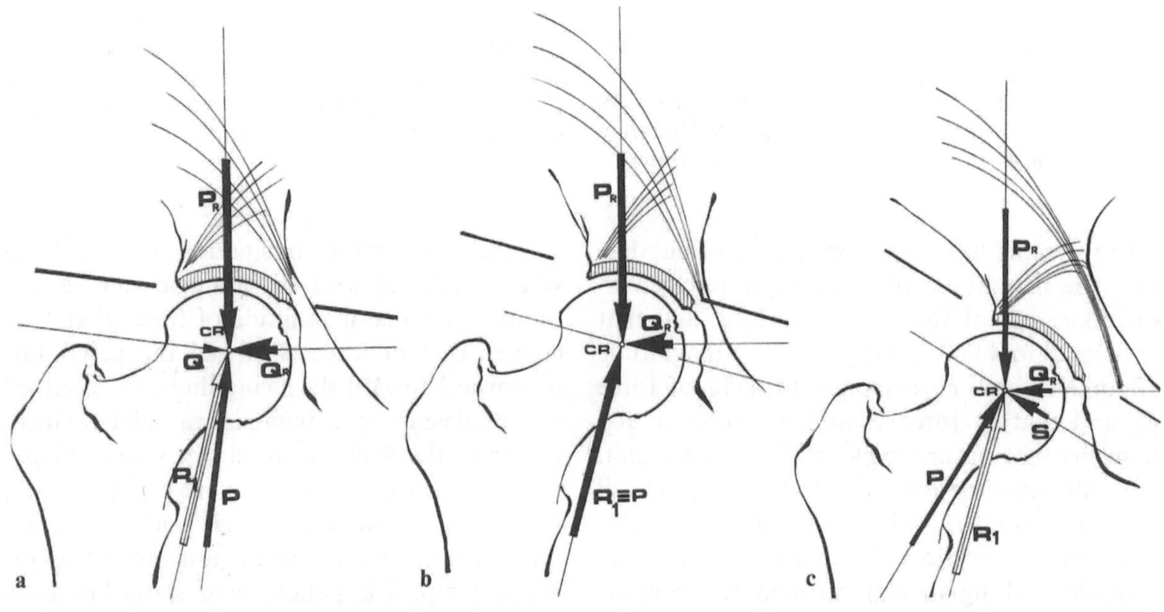

Fig. 10 a–d. Effect of increasing craniolateral inclination. **a** When the inclination is less than 16°, force Q diminishes and cannot completely counteract force Q_R, which is transmitted to the lateral capsule. Force P increases in magnitude, overcoming force P_R and adding extra stress to the acetabulum. **b** When the inclination is 16°, force Q disappears completely and force P reaches its maximum, equaling force R_1. **c** When the inclination is more than 16°, force Q reverses, transforming to force S, which, when added to force Q_R, accelerates the subluxation of the head against the lateral capsule. The magnitude of force P decreases in proportion to further inclination. **d** The comparable forces of the right hip in monopodal stance (phase 16) from a posterior view. As the WBS inclines anterolaterally, forces K, P_M, and Q_M do not change, as R remains stable at 16° (dependent on S_5 and lever arm b). However, forces P and Q change both magnitude and direction as the WBS inclines. Forces $P_{0°}$ and $Q_{0°}$ (*white*) correspond to the normal horizontal $WBS_{0°}$. Force $P_{8°}$ increases in magnitude and force $Q_{8°}$ decreases in magnitude when WBS inclines to 8°; the direction of $P_{8°}$ and $Q_{8°}$ change as illustrated. When the WBS is 16° the point of reversal is reached; $P_{16°}$ (*black*) equals R_1 in magnitude and direction, while $Q_{16°}$ is nonexistent. When the WBS inclines beyond the point of reversal to 20°, $P_{20°}$ (*dark gray*) decreases again in magnitude as a new force $S_{20°}$ (*dark gray*) appears with a direction opposite to that of the original force Q, thus augmenting the shearing effect of force Q_M

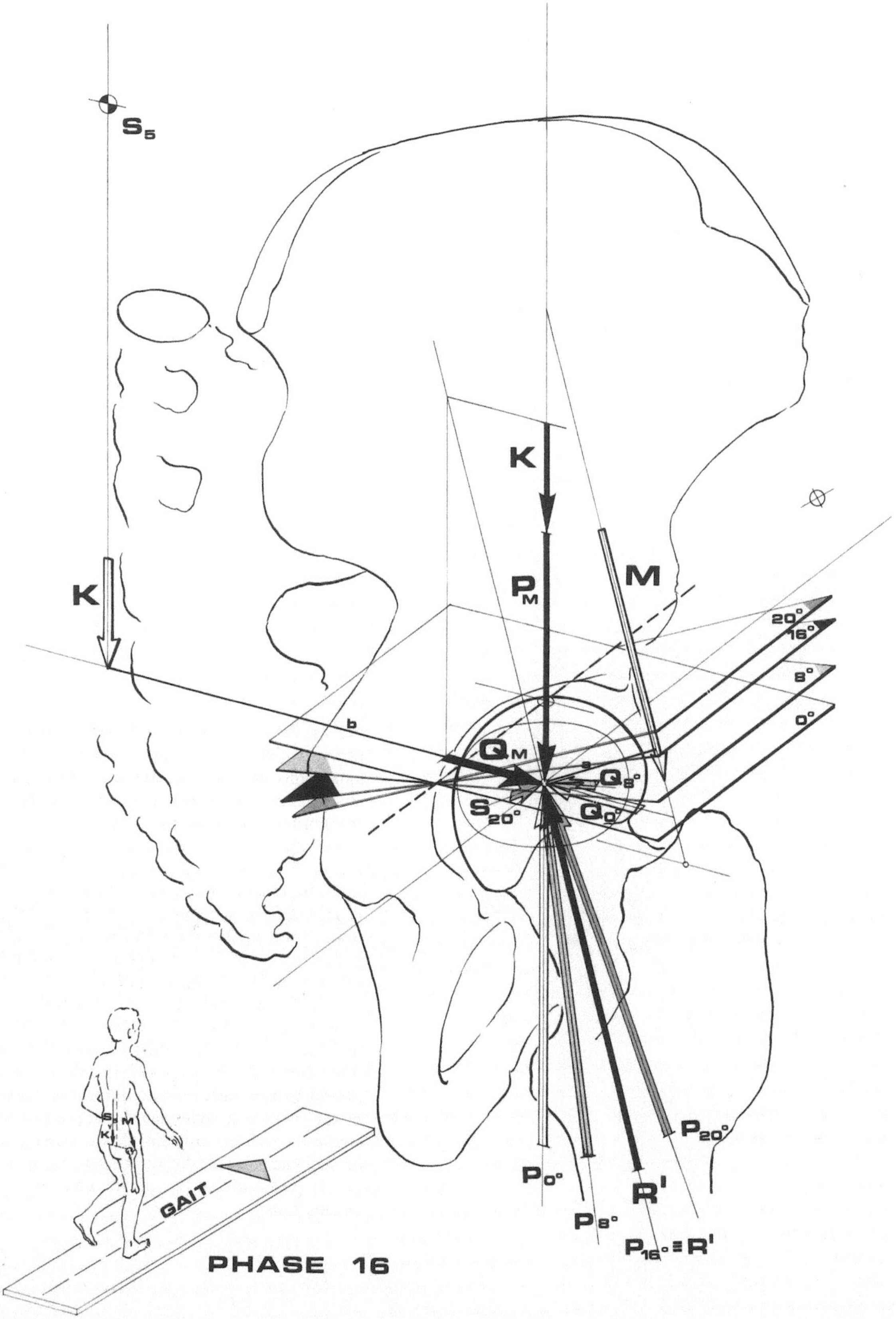

Fig. 10d

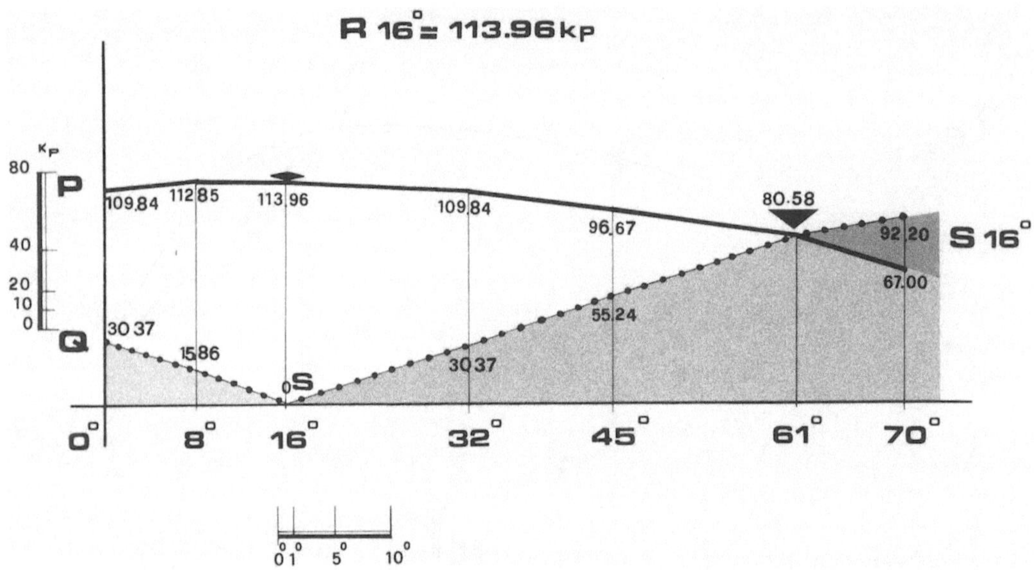

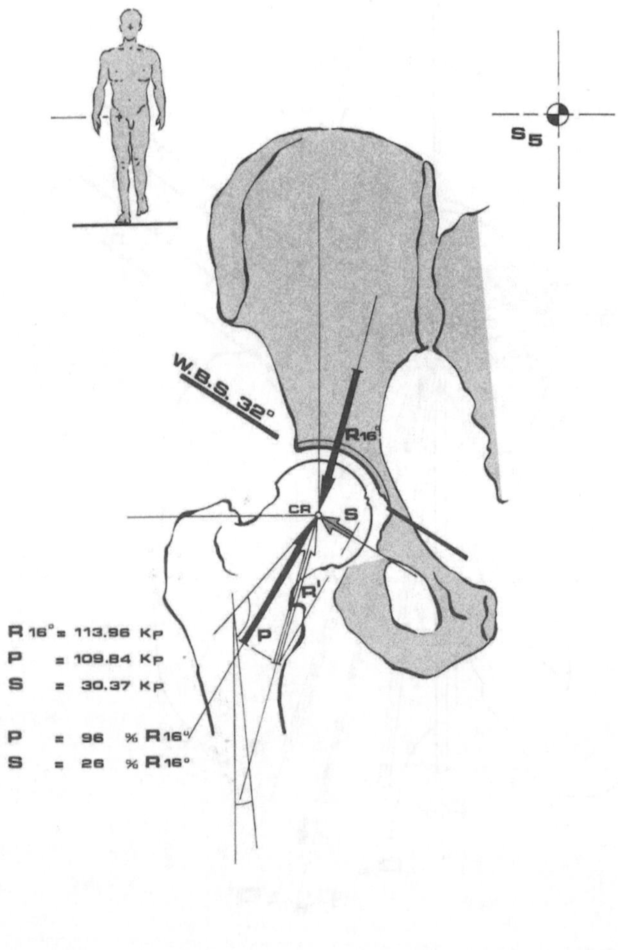

Fig. 11. Effect of WBS inclination on reaction forces P and Q (in a dysplastic hip before the appearance of pain). In dynamic phase 16, K is 30.71 kp and M, which maintains the pelvis in equilibrium, is 84.76 kp. Resultant force R is 113.96 kp, R_1 is 113.96 kp, and of its component forces, P is 109.84 kp and Q is 30.37 kp. When the WBS inclines, the magnitudes of forces P and Q are modified according to the degree of inclination. When inclination is 16°, force Q disappears and the value of force P corresponds to the value of force R: 113.96 kp (point of reversal). More accentuated inclination makes force S appear and progressively reduces the value of P. When the inclination is 61°, the values of force P and force S are equal (80.58 kp). From this degree of inclination onward, force S is dominant and the inferior cervical osteophyte may develop and take the shape of an elephant's trunk. In reality, R has an inclination of 15.43° to the vertical in the dynamic phase but is put at 16° here to simplify calculations

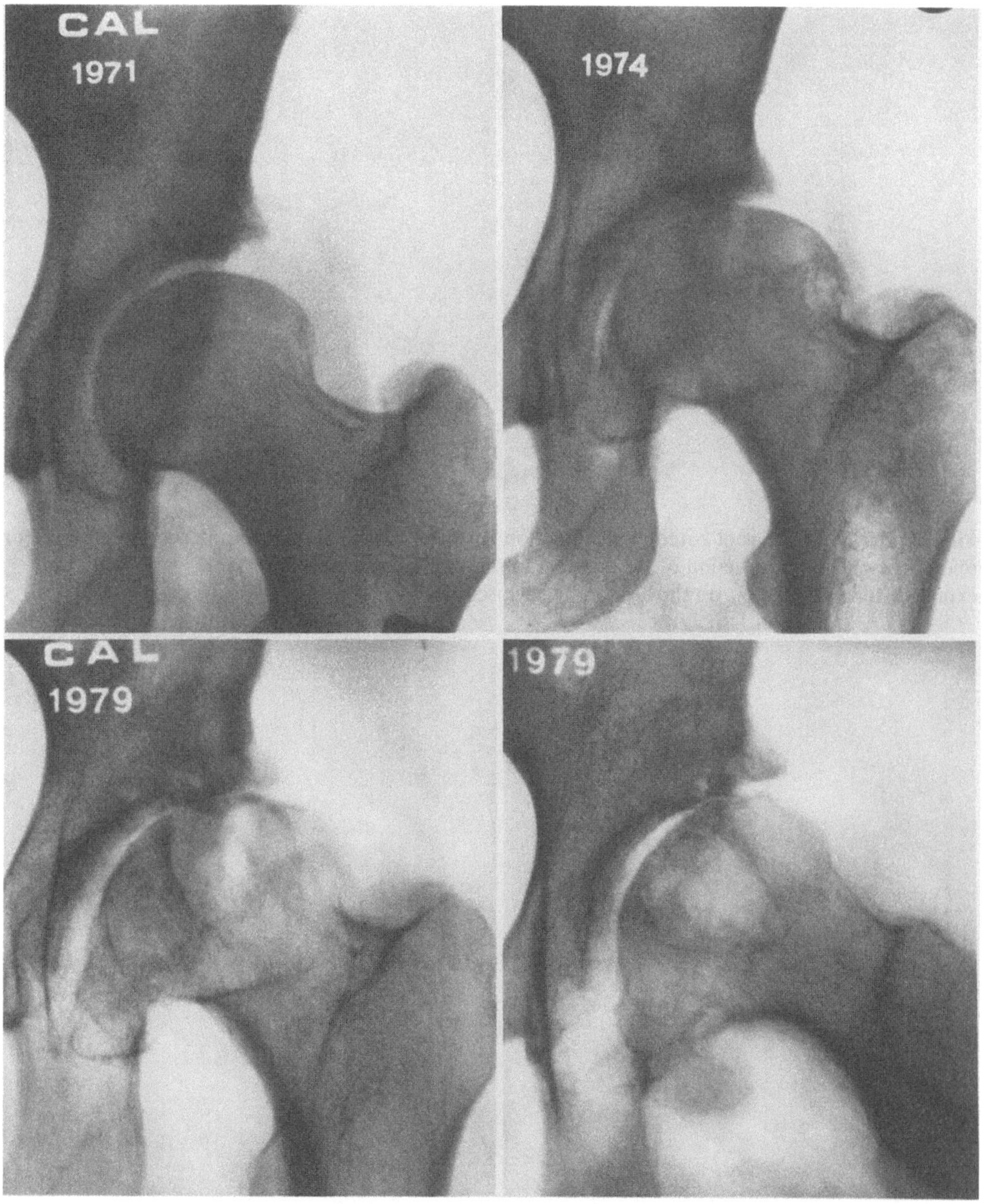

Fig. 12. Natural history of the progressive craniolateral inclination over 7 years. In 1974 eburnation of head and acetabulum reflect imbalance of the *P* forces (extra stress). Craniolateral subluxation of the head reflects the reduction of force *Q*. Five years later (1979), the combination of force *S* and force Q_R increases the subluxation. Medial osteophytes have appeared in the medial joint space. In spite of reduction in force *P*, the subluxation has markedly decreased the WBS, to the point that the unit load has increased, provoking cysts in the head

In a hip with the WBS inclined craniomedially, point *T* is located more laterally than in a normal hip. The distance from point *T* to point *H* is increased, as is the magnitude of force *Q* (Fig. 23).

Effect of Antalgic Gait. When antalgic gait appears, the magnitude of the overall forces in action are diminished, but that of the damaging force *Q* is particularly reduced. For example with force *R* at 16°, force *Q* corresponds to 80%

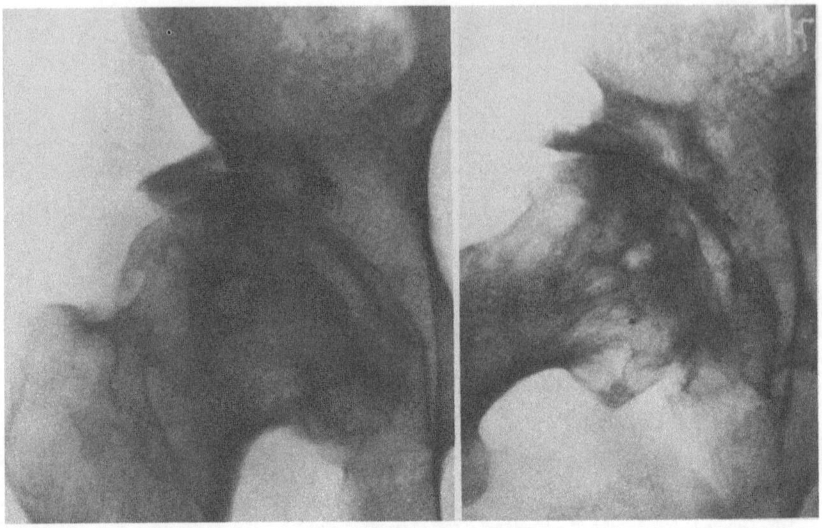

Fig. 13. Origin of the roof osteophyte. Traction on the sclerotic capsule by the action of the anterocraniolateral expulsive forces S and Q_R on the head induce neo-ossification along the anterocraniolateral border of the acetabulum

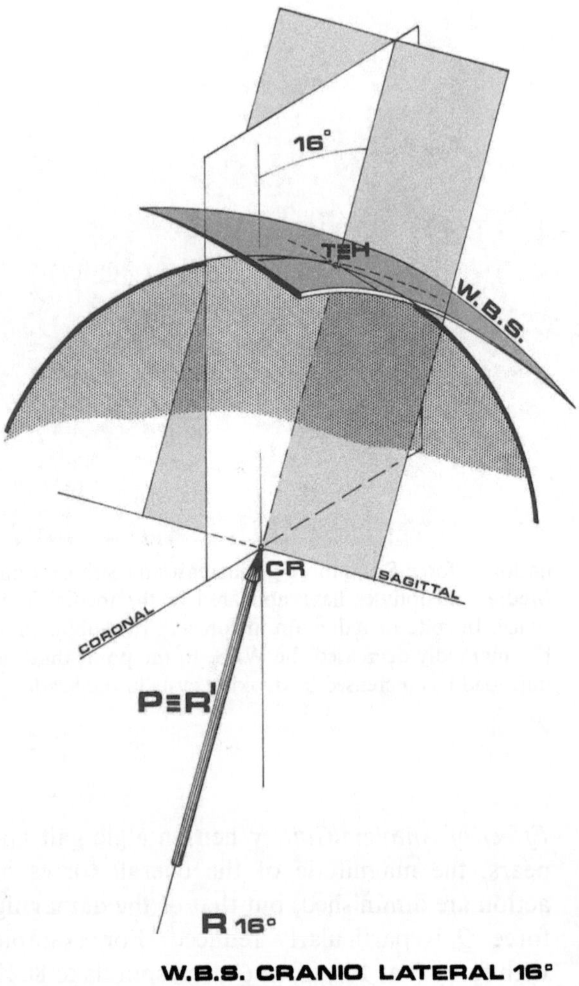

Fig. 14. Three-dimensional diagram of the point of reversal. A craniolateral shift in the WBS diminishes force Q as point T translates toward point H until they coincide at 16°, the point of reversal. Force Q has disappeared and force P is equal to R_1. Note that R of 16° indicates absence of antalgic gait

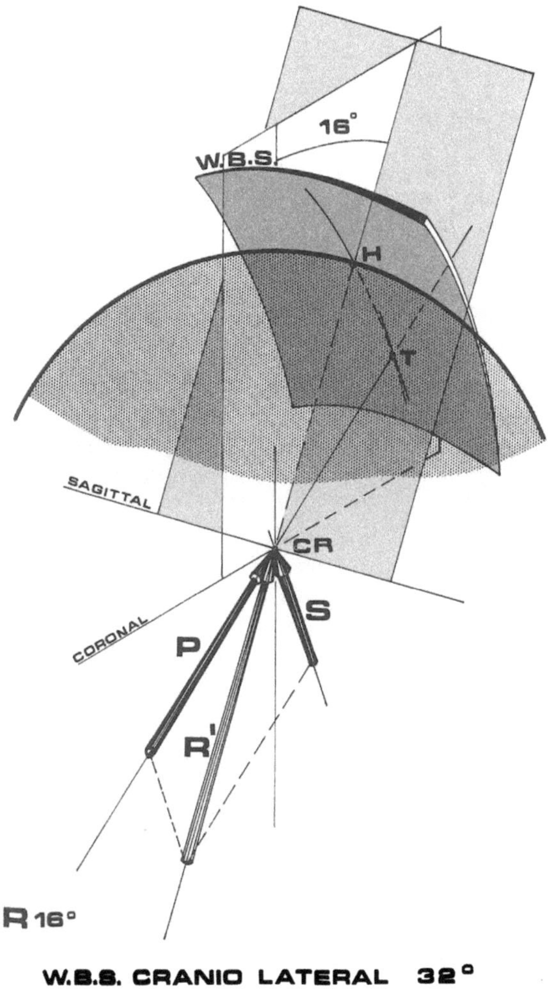

Fig. 15. Three-dimensional diagram of WBS inclined to 32°. When the point of reversal is surpassed, point T moves medially to point H. The direction of line $\overline{TH}$ corresponds to the direction of the new force S. Note that R is at 16°

of R (91.2 kg). In antalgic gait, force Q corresponds to 61% with R at 8° (29.1 kg) (Fig. 24).

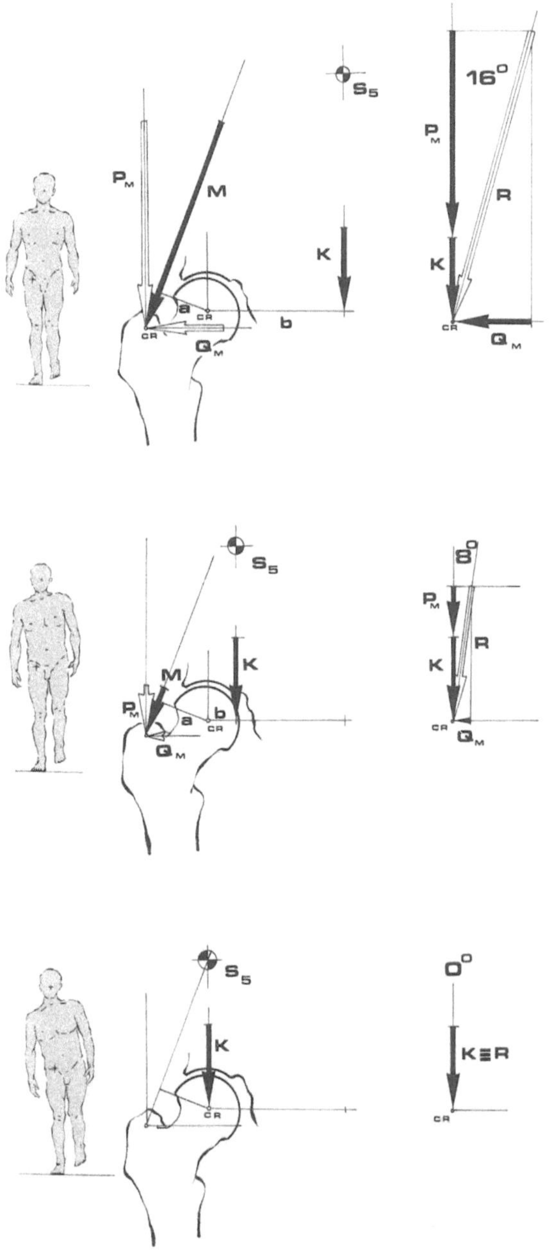

Fig. 16. Effect of antalgic gait. The trunk shift of antalgic gait directly reduces the normal inclination of R at 16°, as the center of gravity S_5 moves toward the painful hip. When S_5 is directly over CR, the magnitude of force R equals force K (R 0° to vertical). As S_5 translates horizontally toward CR, lever arm b decreases, thus reducing force M, which is necessary to balance the pelvis. Force P_M decreases accordingly. In other words, trunk shift means reduction in the magnitude of total force R (pain relief) and its verticalization

Shape of Femoral Head

The femoral head can be spherical or elliptical. When it is spherical, both the neck-shaft angle and the inclination of the WBS are critical in planning effective treatment. When the head is elliptically deformed, it always articulates with an acetabulum whose WBS is craniolaterally inclined. The elliptical head actually glides anterocraniolaterally out of the acetabulum. Choice

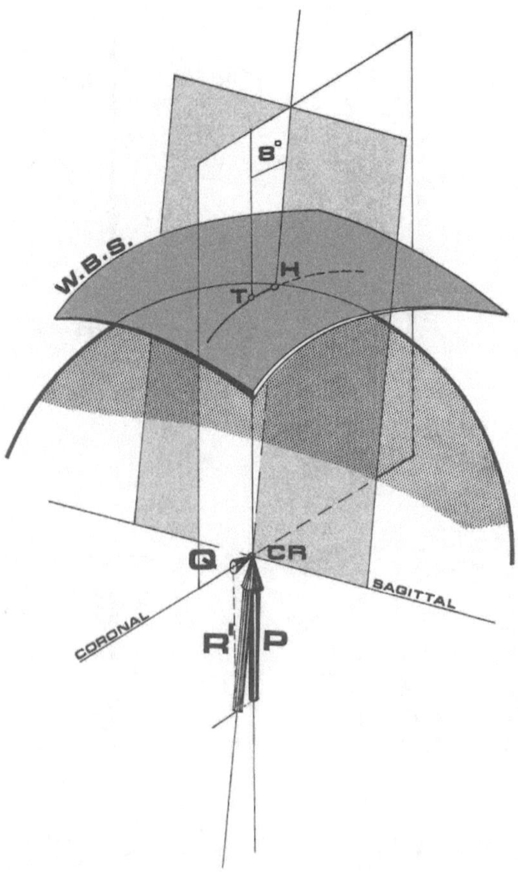

R8° ANTALGIC GAIT

W.B.S. HORIZONTAL

Fig. 17. Three-dimensional diagram of effect of antalgic gait on force Q. With a normal WBS of 0°, a trunk shift to R 8° means a displacement of H towards T that corresponds to a reduction of force Q. Force P is reduced proportional to the reduction in R_1

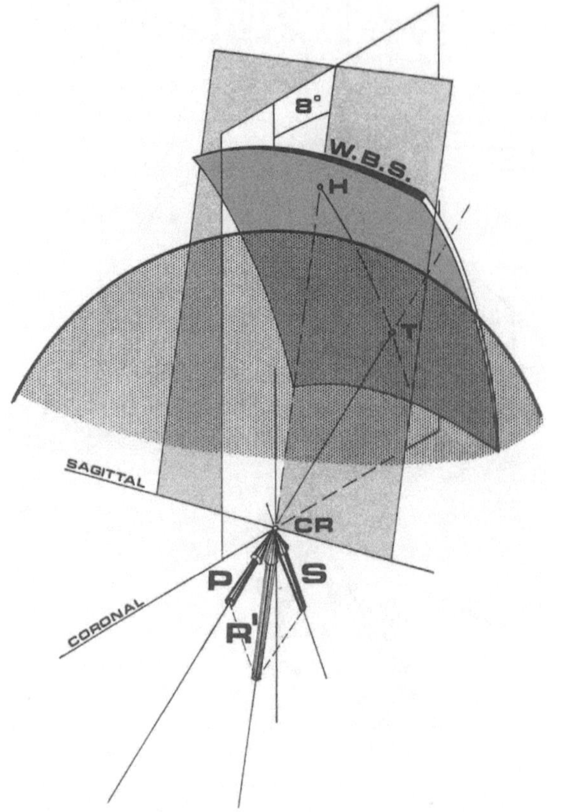

R8° ANTALGIC GAIT

W.B.S. CRANIO-LATERAL 32°

Fig. 18. Three-dimensional diagram of combined craniolateral inclination of the WBS (32°) and trunk shift (R 8°). The inclination of the WBS has moved T medially to H and trunk shift has further lateralized H. The new force S is parallel to line $\overrightarrow{TH}$. Note that the overall force magnitude is reduced, but the percentage of force S has increased when antalgic gait combines with craniolateral inclination. (See Fig. 14)

of treatment in this condition is not affected by the value of the neck-shaft angle.

Femoral Neck-Shaft Angle

Because the value of the vertical downward compressive force P_R $(K+P_M)$ depends not only on the weight of the patient (K) but also on the force P_M derived from the magnitude and direction of the abductor muscles (M), any modification in the position of the greater trochanter has a direct effect on P_R. In coxa vara the cranial position of the greater trochanter makes the abductor lever arm a longer and the direction of the abductors (M) more horizontal. The values of P_M and therefore of P_R are thus lower than in the normal hip (Fig. 25). In coxa valga, on the contrary, the caudal position of the greater trochanter shortens the lever arm a of the abductors (M) and makes their direction more vertical. As a consequence, forces P_M

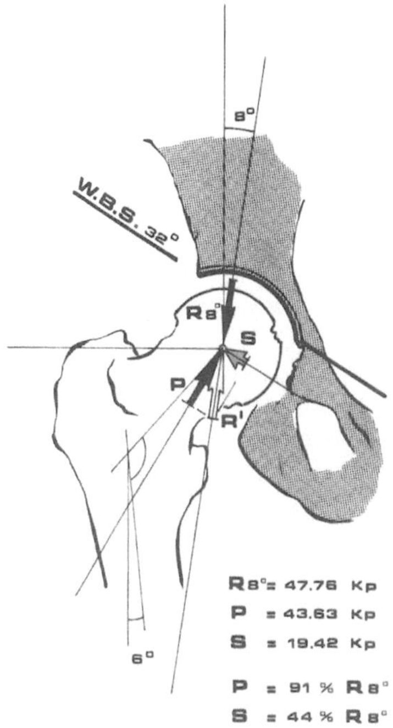

Fig. 19. Effect of combined craniolateral inclination of the WBS and trunk shift on forces *P*, *Q* and *S*. Forces *P*, *Q* and *S* are illustrated when the acetabular surface slants and the load on the hip provokes pain. In the case of a painful hip the patient is compelled by the pain reflex to shift the center of gravity of his body toward that side, and therefore the inclination of resultant force *R* in the frontal plane is reduced (e.g. 8°). By this simple reflex, the value of force *R* is reduced to 47.76 kp. The muscular force of abductors (*M*) is 17.81 kp, counter-resultant force R_1 is 47.76 kp. When the WBS is horizontal, its component forces are *P* (47.33 kp) and *Q* (6.38 kp). When inclination of the WBS increases to 8°, force *Q* disappears and the value of force *P* corresponds to the value of force R_1: 47.76 kp (point of reversal). More accentuated inclination makes force *S* appear and progressively reduces the value of force *P*. The values of force *P* and force *S* are equal (33.77 kp) when the WBS has an inclination of 53°. From this point on, force *S* is dominant and an inferior cervical osteophyte may develop in the shape of an elephant's trunk

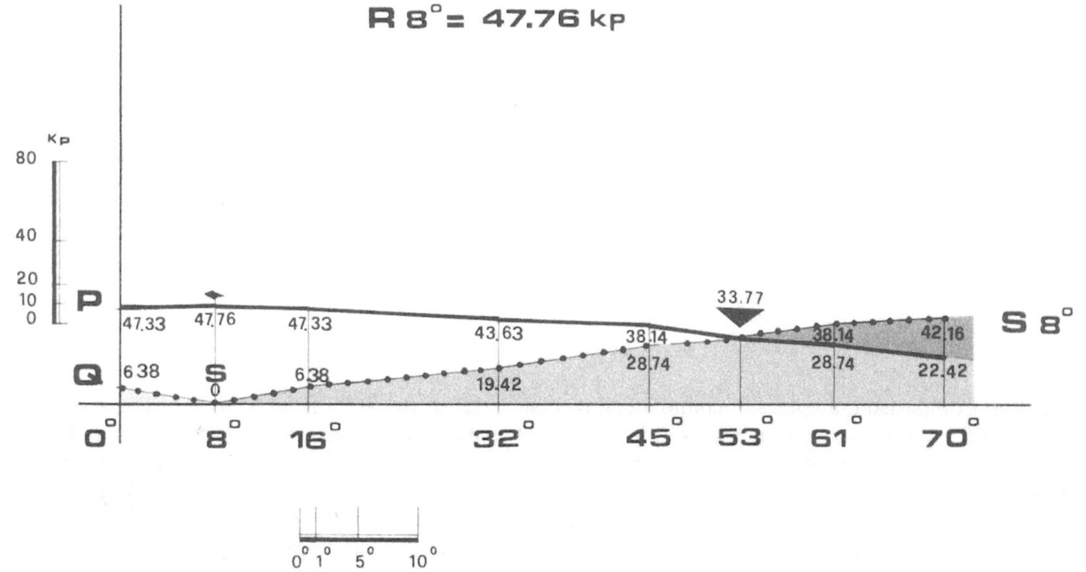

and P_R are greater in magnitude than in the normal hip (Fig. 26), whose neck-shaft angle is about 130°.

Anteversion of about 12° in the neck helps, with the pull of gluteus maximus, iliopsoas, the external rotators, and the adductors, to counteract the inward torsional stress in the upper part of the femur which is produced by the body weight of a flexed hip. When climbing a slope, negotiating stairs, or arising from a chair, the internal torque sustained by the proximal femur is significant (Fig. 27a, b). Theoretically, increased anteversion would appear to be more favorable because it converts torque to compression, but it would uncover the superomedial part of the head in erect posture.

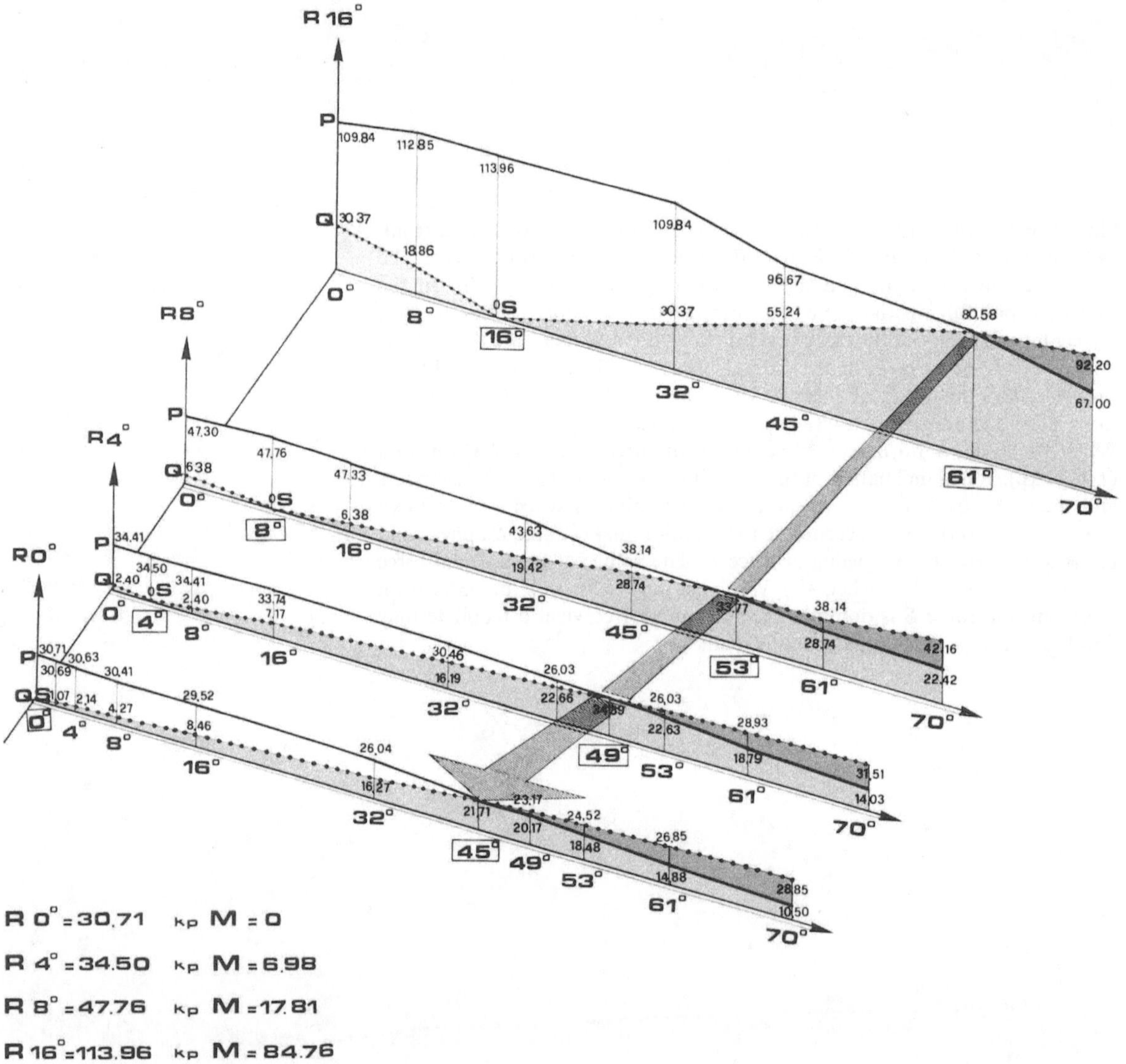

Fig. 20a. Comparison of effects of craniolateral inclination of WBS and trunk shift on reactive hip forces and the appearance of osteophytes. The diagram shows (1. different inclinations to the vertical of force *R* (16°, 8°, 4°, and 0°) and the corresponding values of forces *P*, *Q*, and *S*; (2. modifications in magnitude of force *P*, progressive disappearance of force *Q*, and appearance of force *S*, according to the inclination from the horizontal of the WBS from 0° to 70°. The arrow in the graph indicates the degree of inclination of the WBS to the horizontal in which the magnitudes of force *P* and force *S* correspond. In conclusion, the verticalization of force *R* and obliquity of the WBS enhance the disappearance of force *Q* and appearance of force *S*: in other words, the acceleration of osteophyte formation

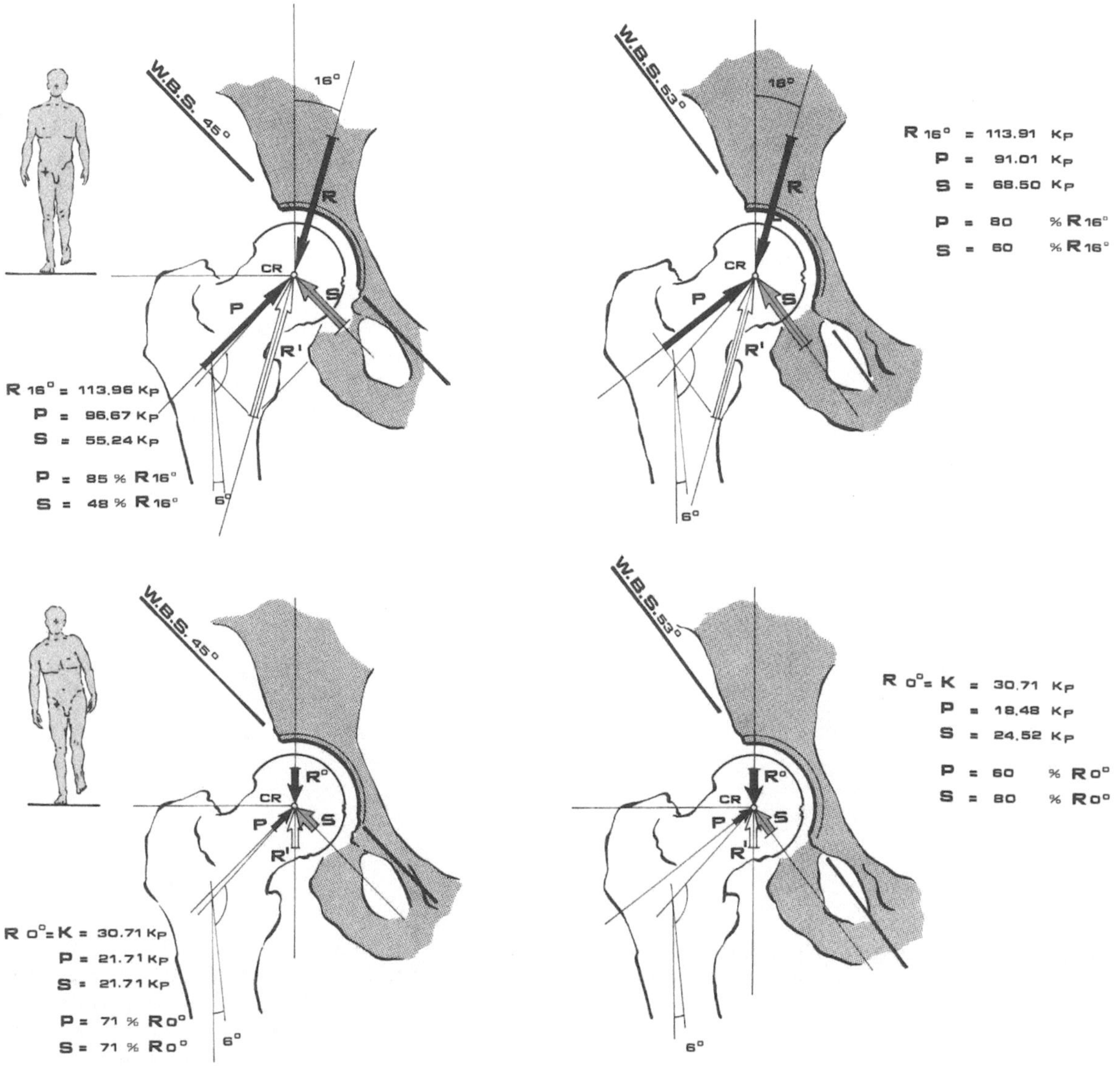

Fig. 20a (continued)

Fig. 20b. The force alteration of trunk shift (antalgic ▷ gait). For this example the anatomical WBS is craniolaterally inclined 32°. The trunk shift from *R* 16° to *R* 8° decreases the overall magnitude of all forces: (compare with case Fig. 19) *R* 16° (113.96 kp) to *R* 8° (47.76 kp), *P* 16° (109.84 kp) to *P* 8° (43.63 kp) and *S* 16° (30.37 kp) to *S* 8° (19.42 kp). However, force *S*, due to directional orientation parallel with the WBS, increases its relative percentage from 26% of *R* 16° to 44% of *R* 8°.

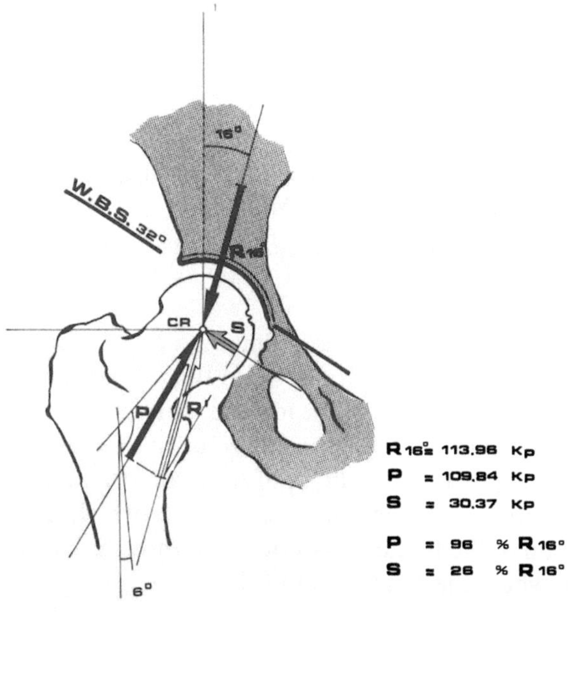

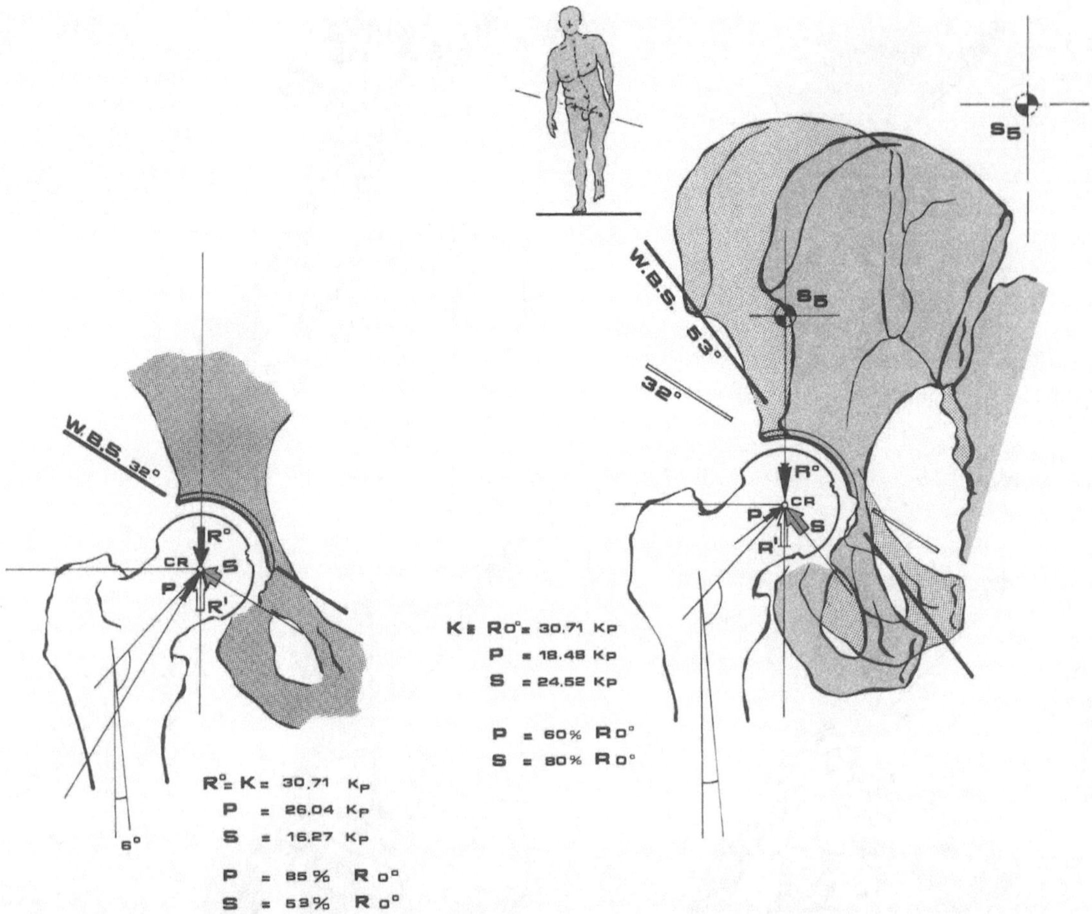

Fig. 20c. The force alteration of Trendelenburg gait. For this example the anatomical WBS is cranilaterally inclined 32°. In Trendelenburg gait there is trunk shift (*R* 16° to *R* 0°) and dynamic pelvic tilt, increasing the actual WBS to 53°. Despite reduction in the force *P* magnitude from 26.04 kp to 18.48 kp by the Trendelenburg gait, the force *S* magnitude increases from 16.27 kp to 24.52 kp, increasing in its relative percentage from 53% of *R* 0° before pelvic tilt to 80% of *R* 0° with pelvic tilt. The latter effect is due in great part to the directional orientation of force *S* parallel to the actual WBS, which results in maximal force dissipation into soft tissues

Selection of Treatment According to biomechanics in the Different Geometrical Combinations

Having dealt with the biomechanical meaning of abnormal direction in the WBS, shape variations in the femoral head, and different neck-shaft angles, let us now consider the forces in action when one or more of these abnormalities occurs, analyzing first the cases in which the head of the femur is spherical and then the cases in which the head is elliptical.

Spherical Femoral Head

With Horizontal WBS

A horizontal WBS means perfect concordance between (a) the forces $P_R (P_M + K)$ and P and (b) the forces $Q_R (Q_M)$ and Q (Fig. 28).

Fig. 22. Craniomedial inclination of the WBS predisposing to protrusio acetabuli. Congenital coxa profunda with deepened socket and normal joint space (*center*) must be distinguished from the coxa equatorialis seen when *Q* forces cause posteromedial depression of the head due to loss of joint space (*left*). Both conditions can result in protrusio OA (*right*) ▷

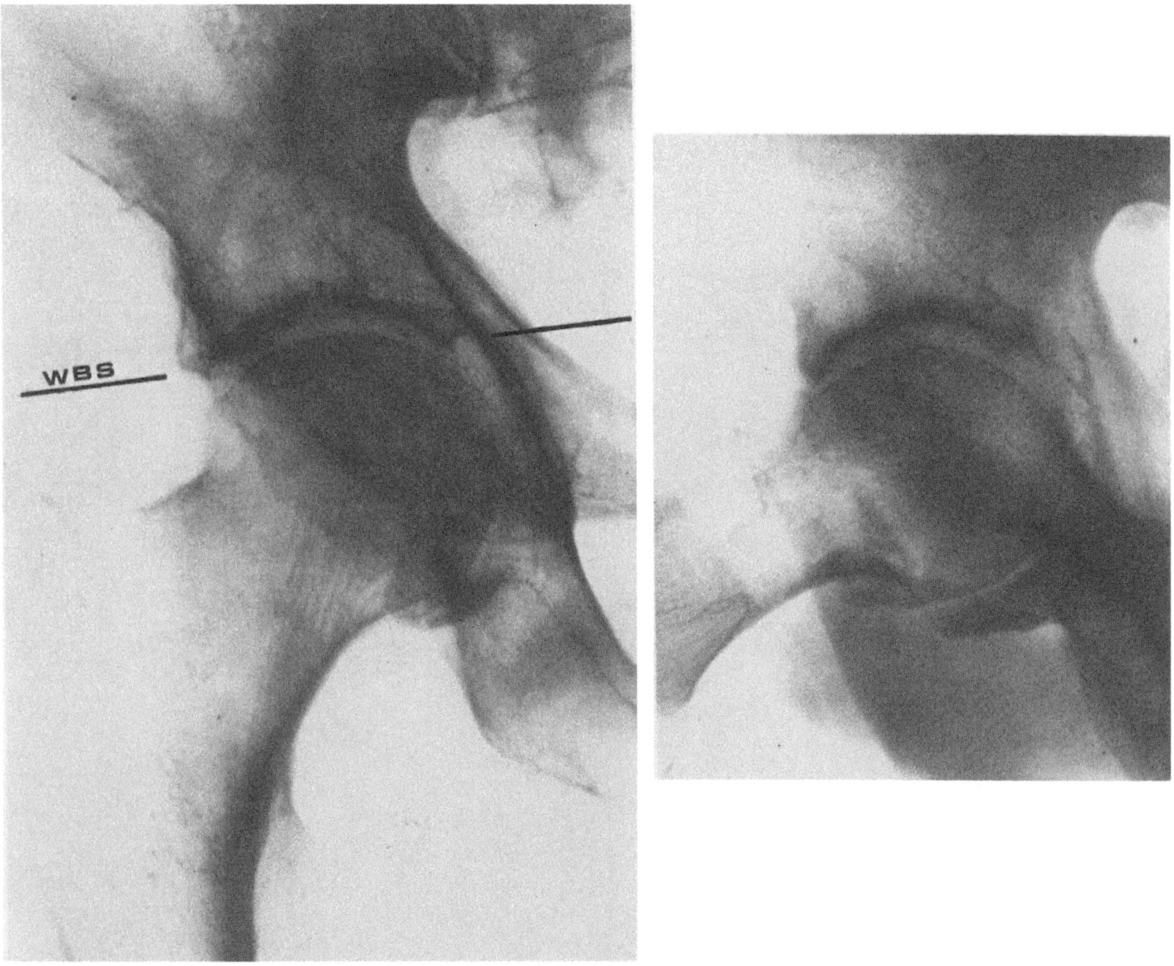

a b

Fig. 21 a, b. OA in the hip with craniomedial inclination of the WBS. On the AP view (**a**) the joint space is preserved under the sourcil, but in the axial view (**b**) the posteromedial joint collapse is revealed. Note that the head is angled posteriorly on axial view

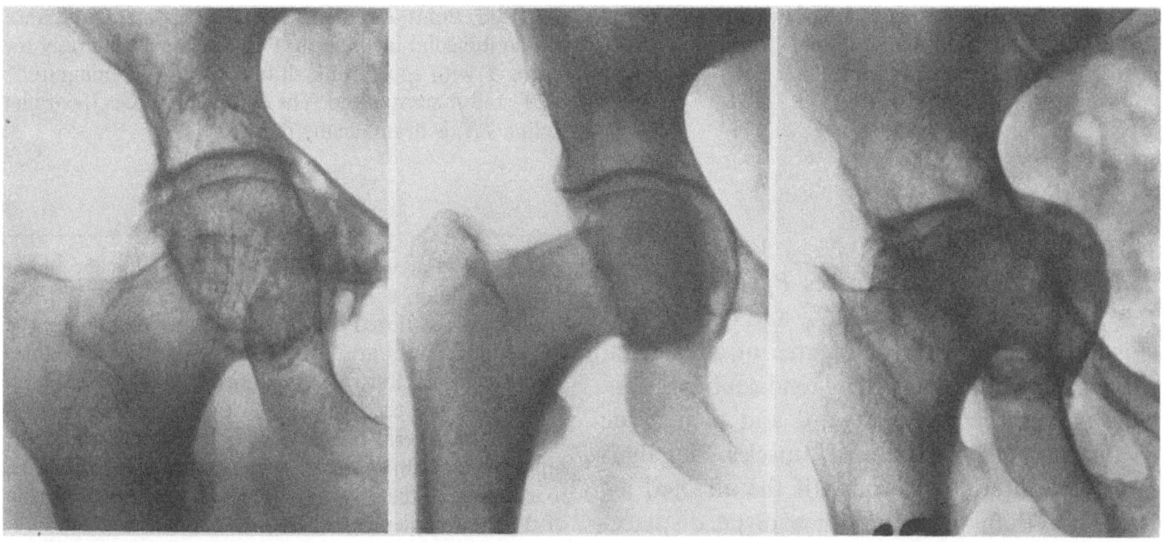

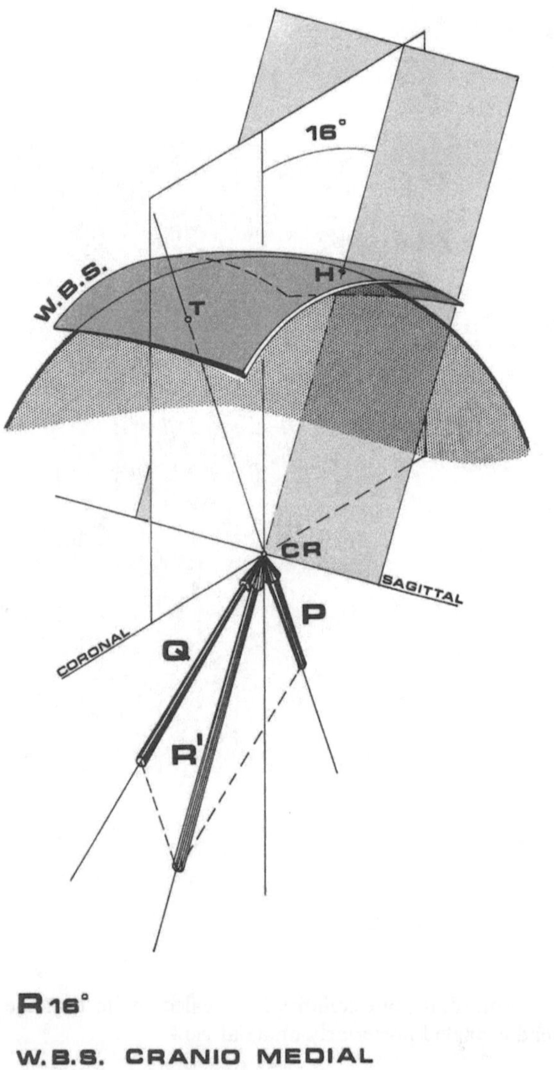

Fig. 23. Three-dimensional diagram of the right hip with craniomedial inclination of the WBS and no pain. Point T, as an extension of force P, translates laterally as the WBS inclines craniomedially. Point H remains with R_1 at 16°. Force Q is parallel to line $\overrightarrow{TH}$

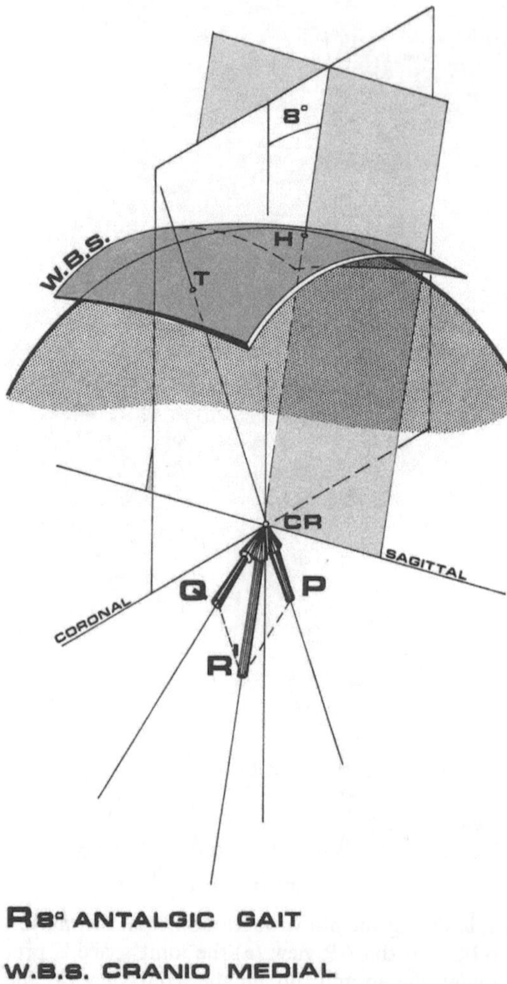

Fig. 24. Three-dimensional diagram of the right hip in antalgic gait of R 8° and craniomedial inclination of the WBS. Point T remains lateral with force P because of craniomedial inclination. Point H moves laterally towards T with each trunk shift to R 8°. The magnitude of R_1 and P are reduced. The damaging force Q, parallel to line $\overrightarrow{TH}$, is dramatically reduced

Varus Neck-Shaft Angle: Coxa Vara. In coxa vara, the magnitude of forces $P_R(K+P_M)$ and P is reduced, that of forces Q_M and Q increased (Fig. 29). The greater the degree of coxa vara, the more significant is the Trendelenburg sign. This makes the gait awkward and tiring, due to the impact on the spinal muscles. A valgus intertrochanteric osteotomy (if the affected leg is shorter than the other) or a distal displace-

Fig. 27a, b. Forces in the proximal femur on the flexed ▷ hip under load. a A dynamic vertical load (P_R), when applied to the flexed hip, creates large internal torque force along a lever arm from CR to the top of the diaphysis. The insert illustrates how torsion of the diaphyseal cylinder occurs, theoretically twisting lines of force from B to B_1. b Several powerful muscles tighten about the hip when the subject rises from a chair or climbing stairs, to counteract the internal torsional load. Anteversion of the neck implements this antitorsional effect

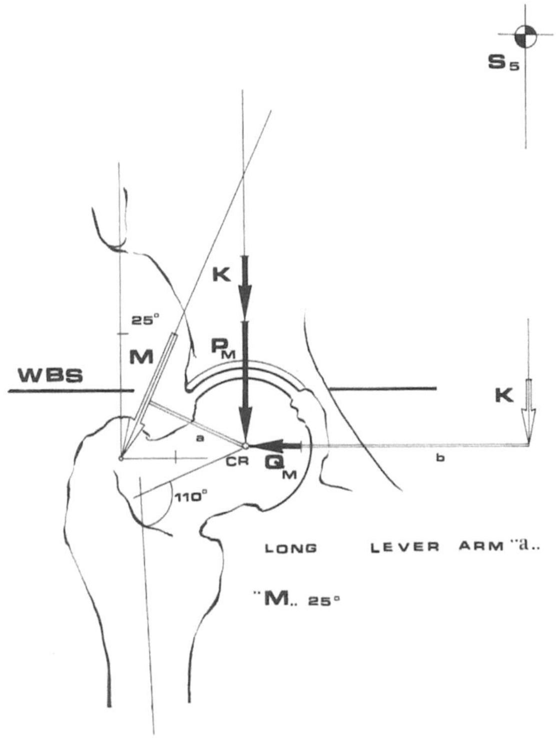

Fig. 25. Effect of cranial position of greater trochanter in coxa vara. The elevated position of the greater trochanter increases lever arm *a* and makes the direction of the abductors *M* more horizontal. The vertical component of *M*, P_M, is reduced by both phenomena

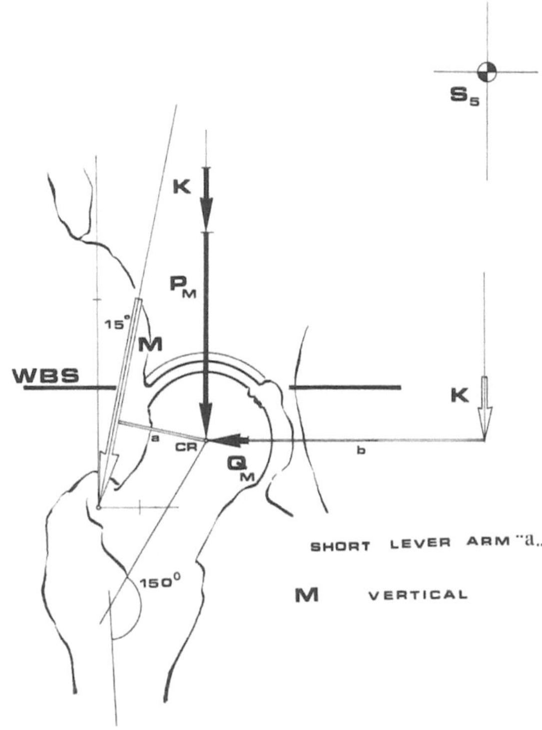

Fig. 26. Effect of caudal position of the greater trochanter in coxa valga. The caudal position of the greater trochanter decreases lever arm *a* and makes the direction of the abductors *M* more vertical. The vertical component of *M*, P_M, is increased by both phenomena

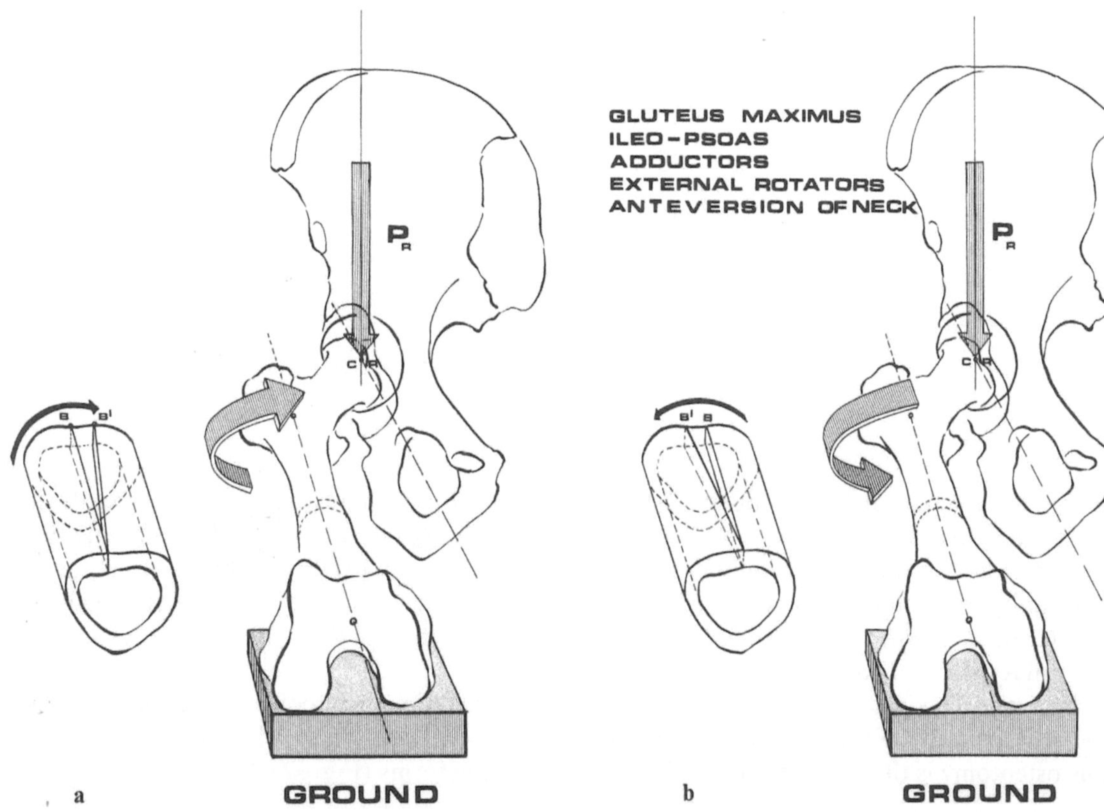

a b

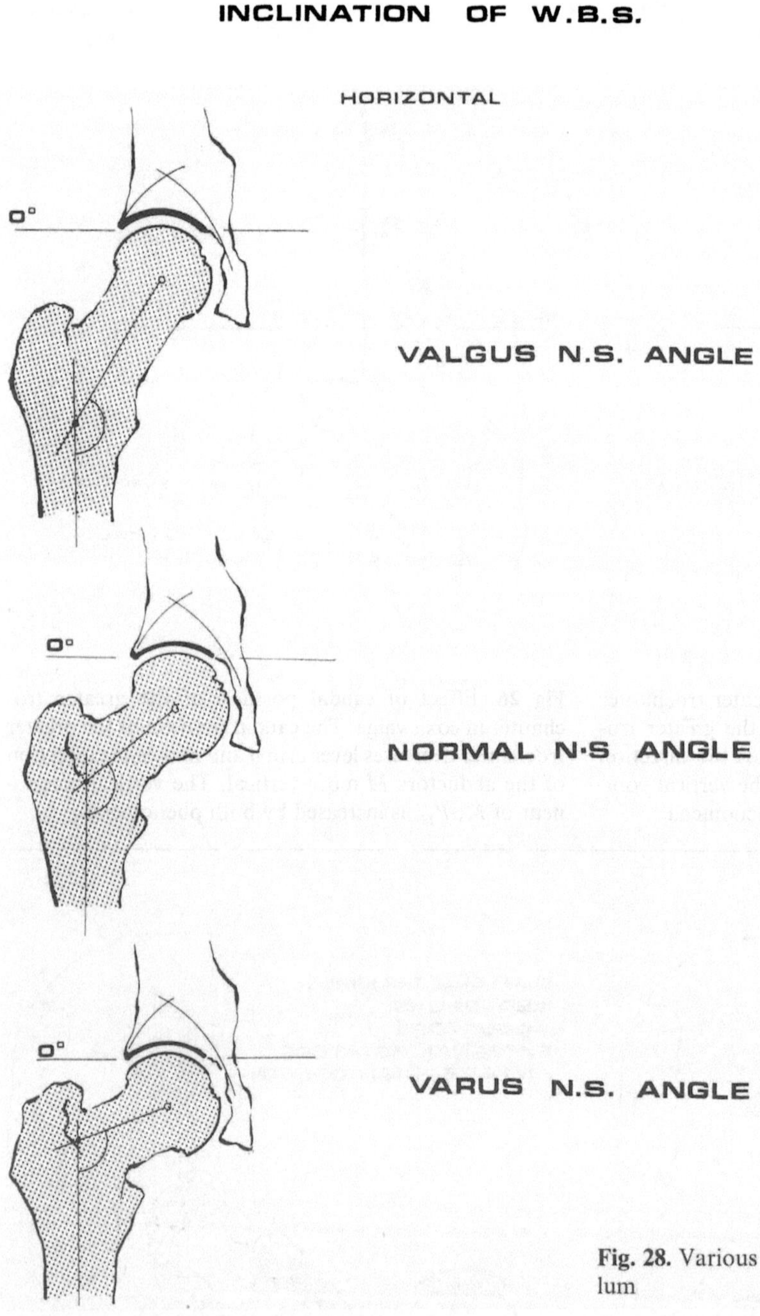

Fig. 28. Various neck-shaft angles with normal acetabulum

ment of the greater trochanter alone (if there is no limb length discrepancy) corrects the pathological gait and restores the magnitudes of the vertical and horizontal forces to physiological values. Coxa vara, while beneficial for the joint, is harmful for the neck, because it increases flexion stress and can produce a fatigue fracture of the neck (Fig. 30). Even in such a condition, valgus osteotomy is the treatment of choice.

Normal Neck-Shaft Angle. The forces acting vertically, P_R and P, and the forces acting horizontally, Q_M and Q, have physiological magnitudes (Fig. 31). In spite of the geometrical normality, the hip may be affected by OA in three ways:

- Altered bone metabolism (osteopenia): when the bone cannot stand a normal load, the joint deforms (Fig. 32).

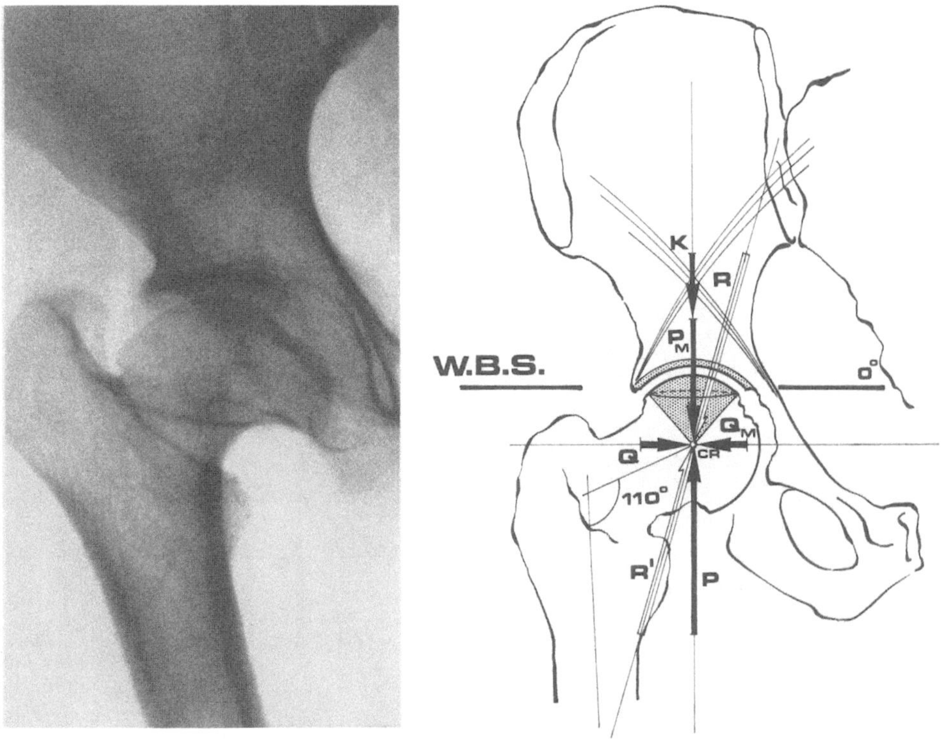

Fig. 29. Example of coxa vara, spherical head and horizontal WBS. The radiograph illustrates a typical case and the diagram depicts the forces acting. Note that force P_M is very low

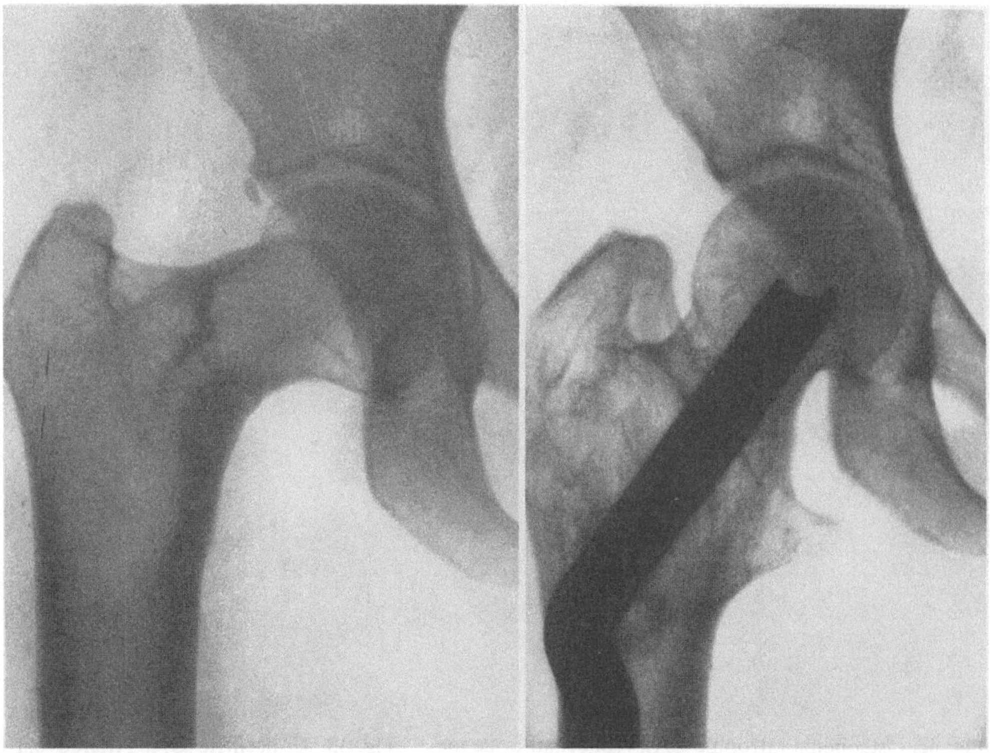

Fig. 30. Fatigue fracture from coxa vara. Coxa vara shields the joint from stress by diminishing force P_M, but exposes the neck to increased bending stress, in this case resulting in a fatigue fracture medially. Treatment involves 35° valgus osteotomy to overcome the deficiency in bone alignment

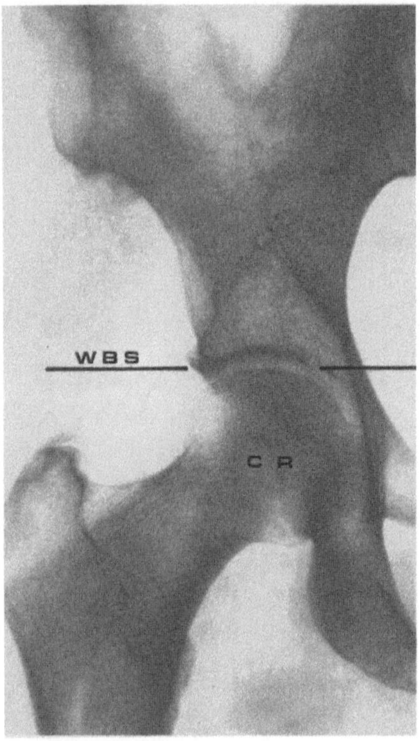

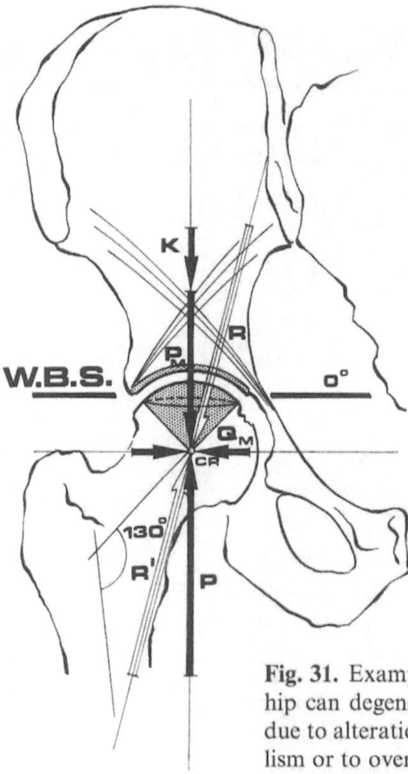

Fig. 31. Example of normal hip. The normal hip can degenerate, despite normal structure, due to alterations in bone or cartilage metabolism or to overuse

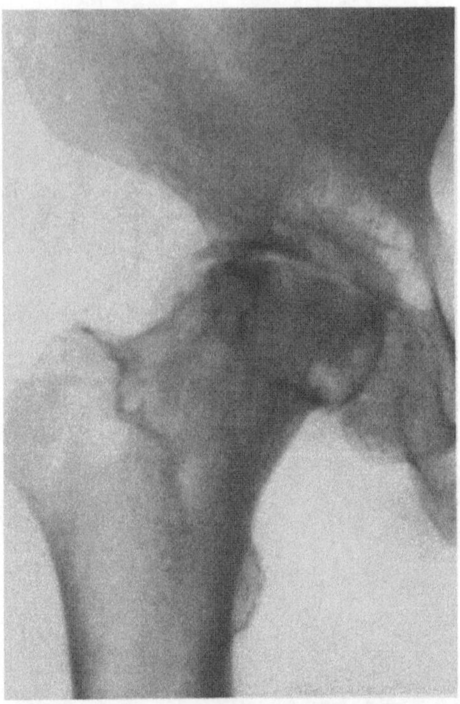

Fig. 32. Osteopenia (atrophic OA). Abnormal bone metabolism leads to intrinsic weakening and structural collapse in an anatomically normal hip. Osteophytes are usually absent

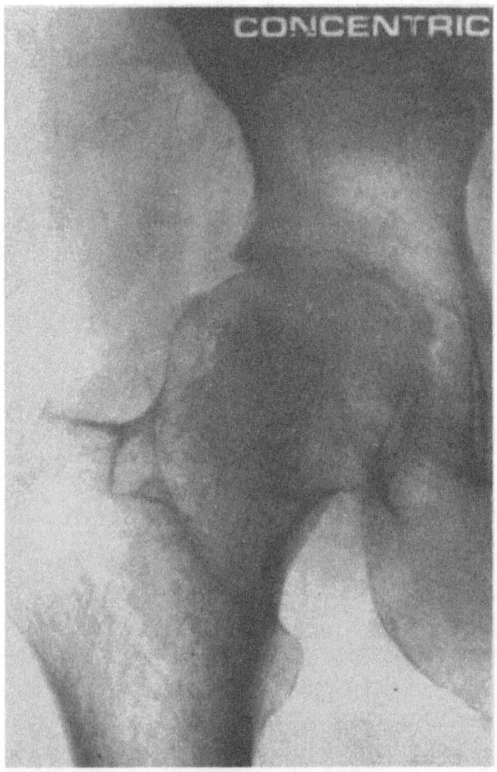

Fig. 33. Concentric OA. Altered cartilage metabolism with global disappearance of joint space will also lead to OA despite normal structure. Because motion is present, this must be distinguished from chondrolysis

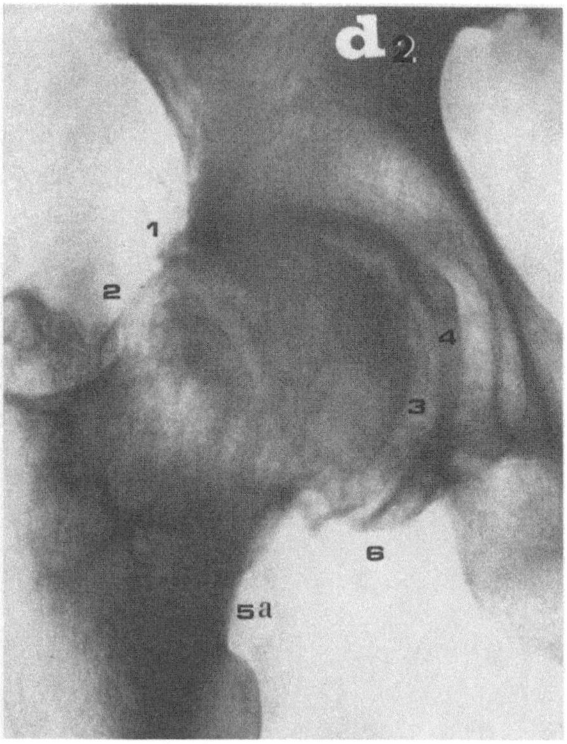

Fig. 34. Overuse OA (type d) [6]. Normal anatomy and normal metabolism can be overwhelmed by overstress, such as in professional athletes or chronically obese subjects. The result is frequently hypertrophic OA with exuberant osteophyte formation. This hip illustrates six types of osteophyte: *1* roof; *2* superior cervical; *3* capital drop; *4* curtain; *5a* inferior cervical (*5b* elephant trunk not present); *6* floor osteophyte

- Altered cartilage metabolism can make the joint space disappear in spite of a spherical head (concentric OA (Fig. 33).
- Overstress from repetitive high dynamic force, e.g., in certain athletic pursuits or in chronic obesity [6], wears out the joint (Fig. 34).

In atrophic OA, no osteotomy is advised. In concentric OA or in overuse, varus osteotomy may be indicated (Fig. 35).

Valgus Neck-Shaft Angle: Coxa Valga. In coxa valga, forces P_R and P increase in magnitude and forces Q_R and Q decrease (Fig. 36). Forces P_R and P are responsible for the destruction of the cartilage on the weight-bearing part of the head and on the acetabular WBS (Fig. 37).

A consequent therapy is therefore varus osteotomy, which shifts the greater trochanter cranialward, making the lever arm a longer and the direction of the abductor muscles (M) more horizontal, thereby reducing the magnitude of forces M and P_M and therefore of reaction force P, allowing regeneration of the joint space (Figs. 35–38).

With Abnormal Direction of WBS

Abnormal direction of the WBS, whether combined with varus, normal, or valgus femoral

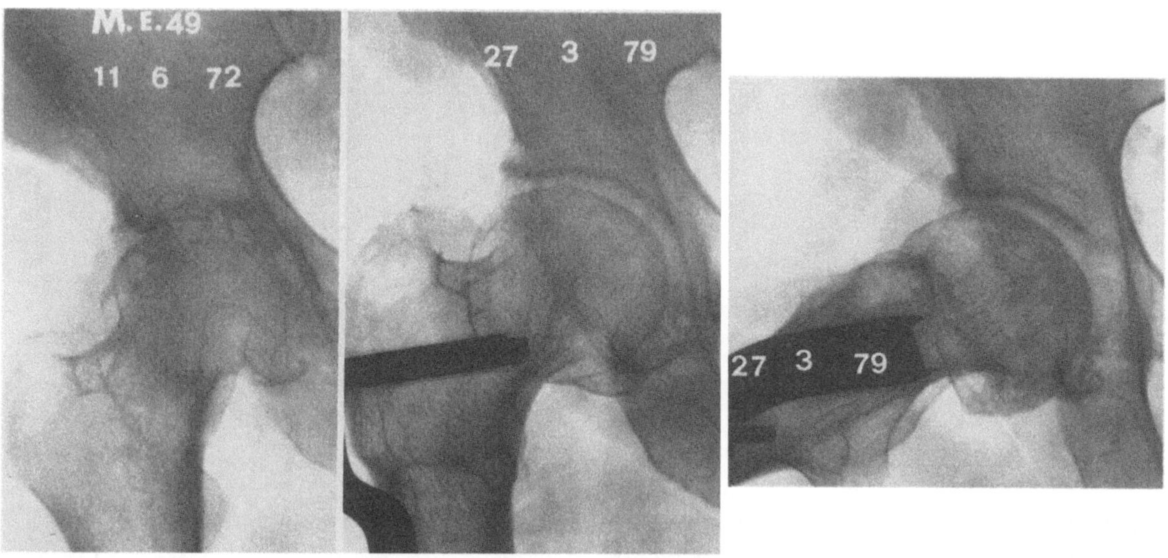

Fig. 35. Varus osteotomy for concentric OA. Seven years following varus osteotomy the joint space has been restored

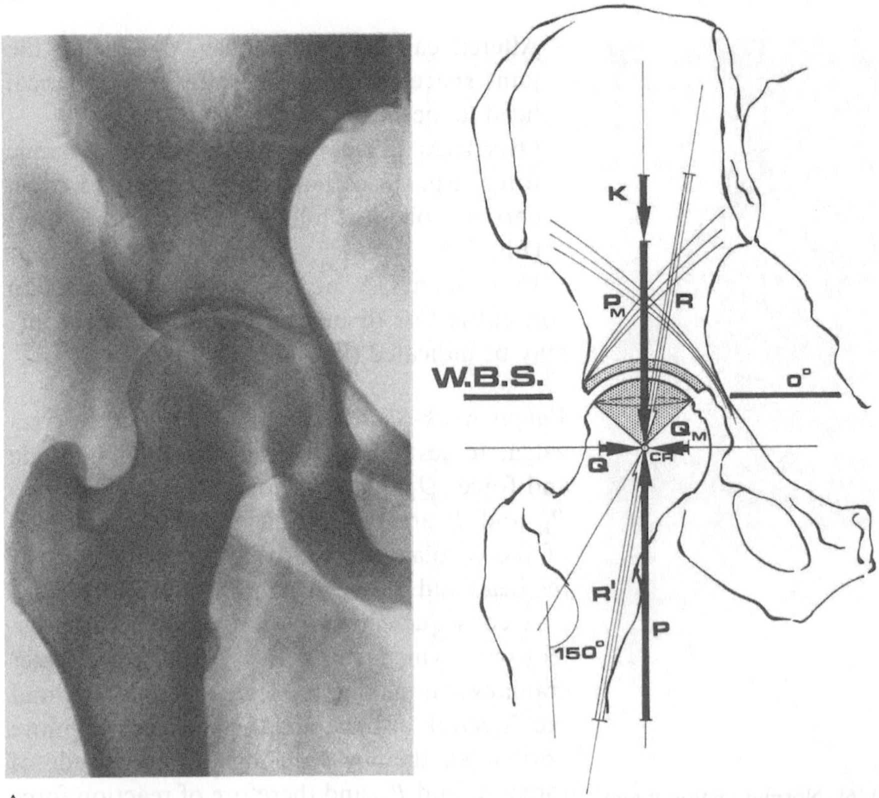

△

Fig. 36. Example of coxa valga, spherical head, and horizontal WBS. The radiograph illustrates a typical case and the diagram depicts the forces acting. The cephalad position of the greater trochanter is responsible for an increase in force P_M

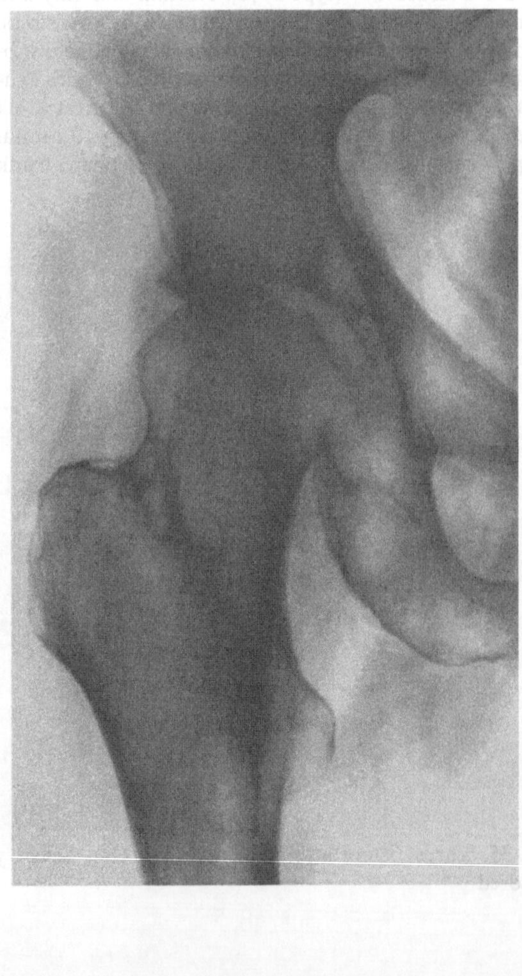

▷

Fig. 37. Joint degeneration caused by coxa valga. The normal horizontal WBS and spherical head are vulnerable to the increased *P* forces of coxa valga, resulting in loss of joint space under the sourcil

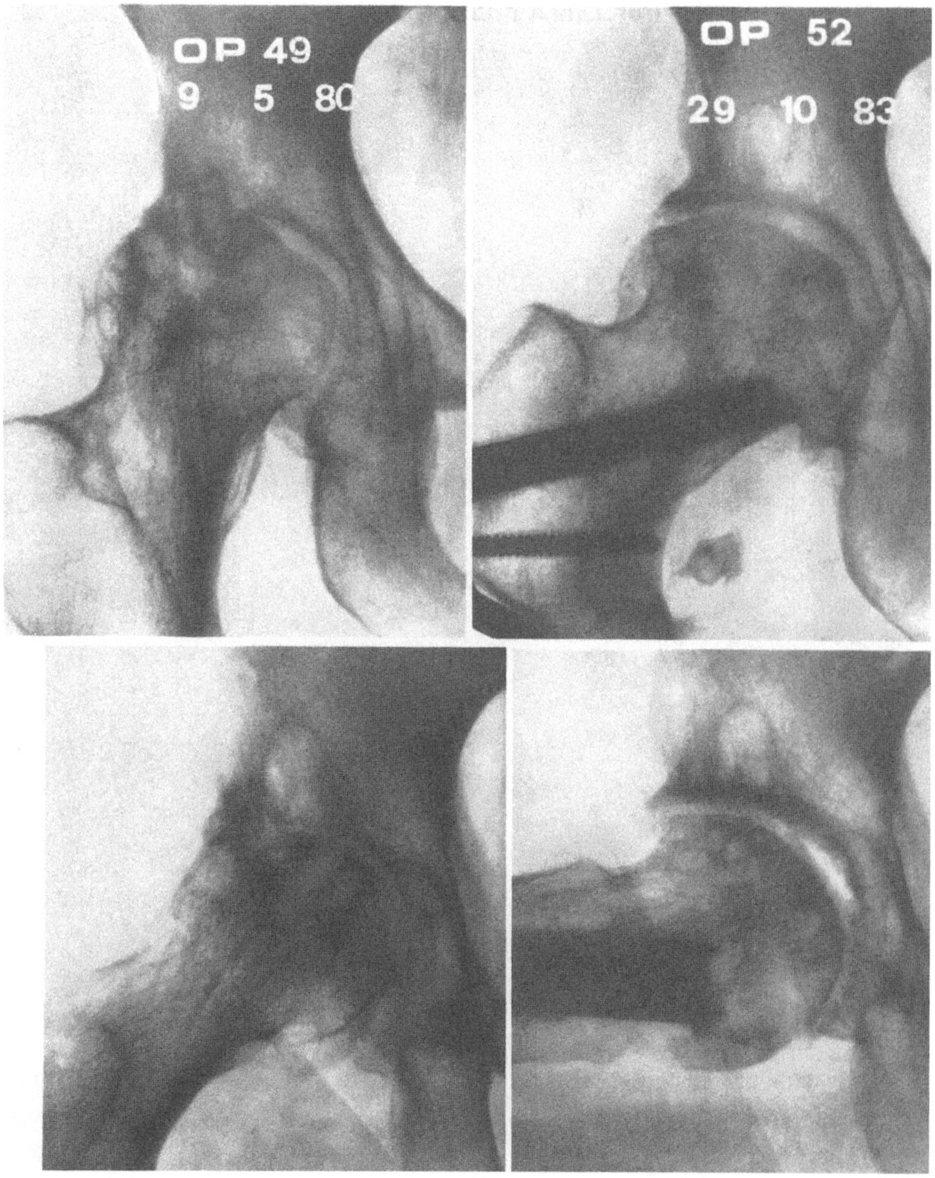

Fig. 38. Treatment of coxa valga. In this case joint space regeneration and disappearance of pain are seen 3 years after reduction of P forces by varus osteotomy

neck, poses a rather complicated problem whose solution requires an understanding of the pathological direction of the forces in action. Once the answer is found, an operation may be planned and performed with the aim of reducing the abnormal magnitude of forces and correcting their altered directions.

Craniolaterally Inclined WBS. As already described, a craniolateral inclination of the WBS (Fig. 10a–d) produces a discrepancy between the component forces of R and the component forces of R_1. The shearing component of R_1 (force Q) decreases and cannot counteract force Q_M. The femoral head glides anterocraniolaterally out of the acetabulum. Force P progressively increases up to the point of reversal and then decreases, when the shearing force S appears. It is worth repeating that in cases of craniolateral inclination of the WBS the femoral head glides not only craniolaterally, but also anteriorly (Fig. 72). Based upon this fact, when an

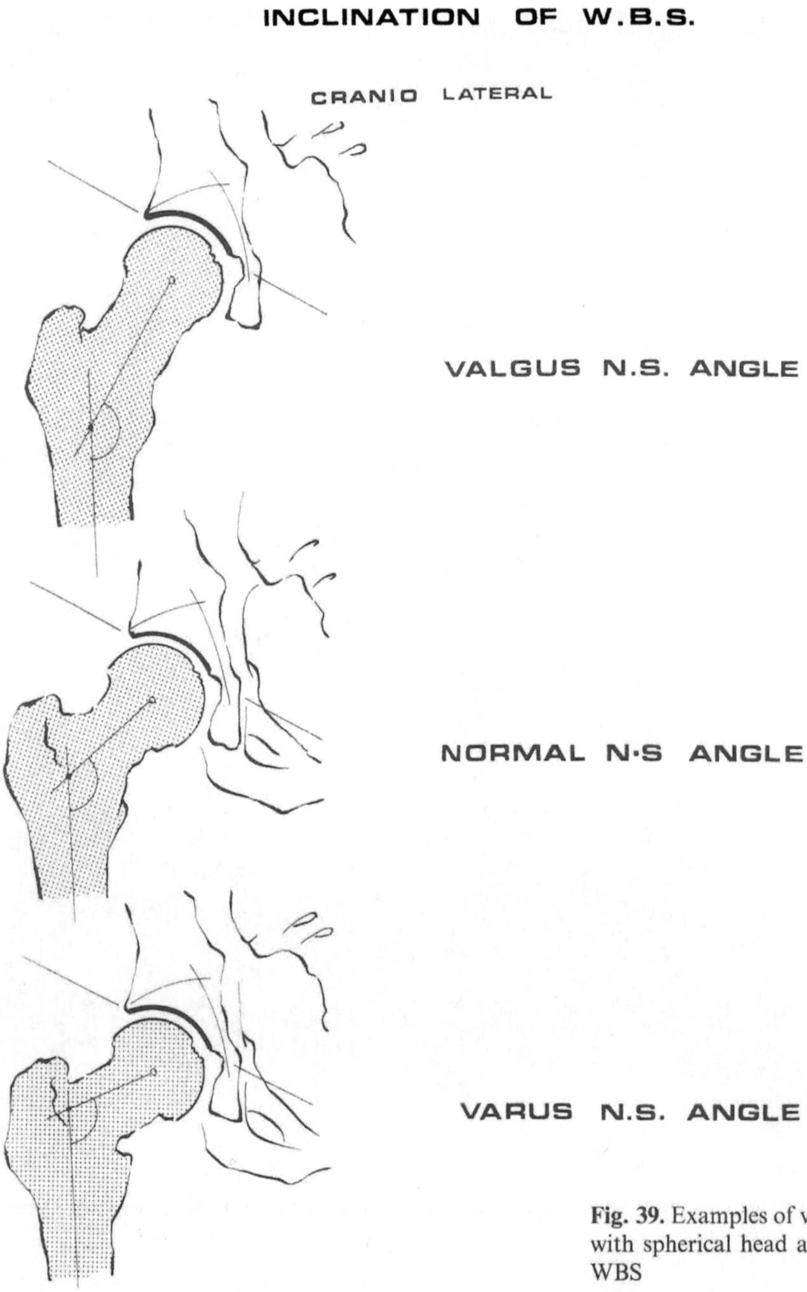

Fig. 39. Examples of various neck-shaft angles combined with spherical head and craniolateral inclination of the WBS

intertrochanteric osteotomy has to be performed, the position of the head must be corrected both in the coronal plane (varus + valgus) and in the sagittal plane (by means of an extension).

In the case of a *varus* neck (coxa vara; Fig. 40) there is a Trendelenburg gait. A valgus-extension intertrochanteric osteotomy is advised in order to eliminate the Trendelenburg gait and correct the tendency of the head to subluxate anteriorly (Fig. 41). When the inclination of the WBS exceeds 15°–20°, it is also necessary to add pelvic osteotomy, acetabuloplasty (Fig. 42), or a shelf. The common goal is to make the WBS horizontal and redirect the component forces of R_1. Force P becomes vertical (cranially directed), force S disappears, and the horizontal (medially directed) force Q reappears.

Where the neck-shaft angle is *normal* (Fig. 43), it is necessary, when the inclination

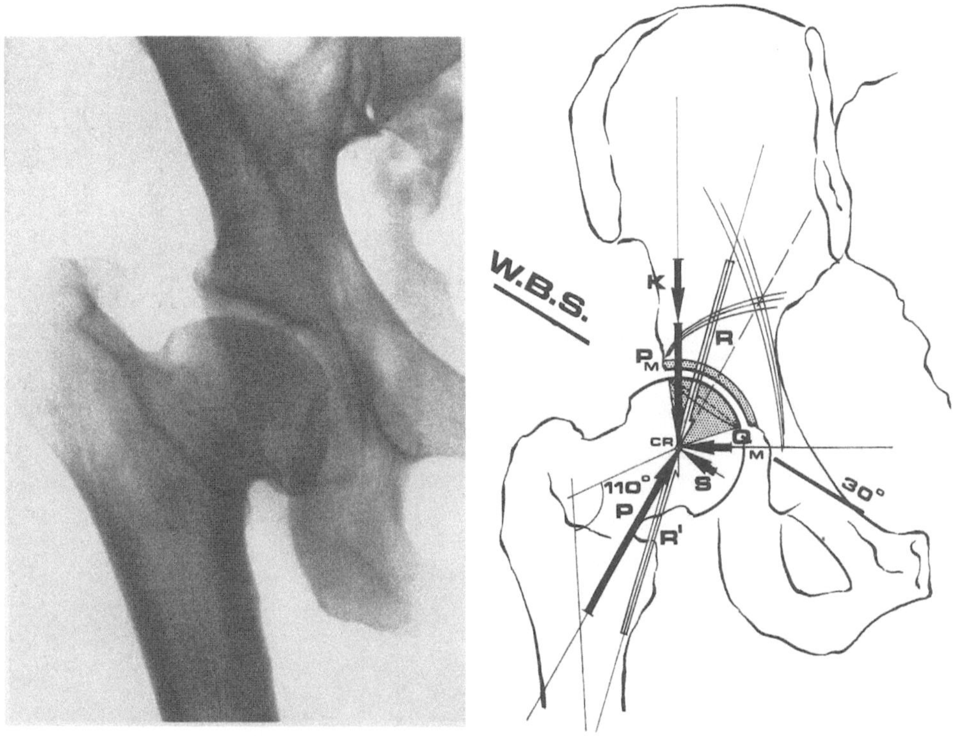

Fig. 40. Example of coxa vara, spherical head and craniolateral inclination of the WBS. The hip seen in the radiograph is prone to subluxate anteriorly because of combined S and Q_M forces. The patient usually presents with a Trendelenburg gait, but pain is absent. Valgus-extension osteotomy corrects the tendency to late subluxation and Trendelenburg gait

of the WBS exceed 15°–20°, to perform pelvic osteotomy, acetabuloplasty (Fig. 44), or shelf-plasty.

In cases where the neck-shaft angle is *valgus* (coxa-valga; Fig. 45) and the inclination of the WBS exceeds 15°–20°, the deformities in both pelvis and femoral neck are to be corrected. The valgus must be reduced by varus-extension intertrochanteric osteotomy. After the operation the neck-shaft angle must be in the range of 120°–125° and the WBS must be horizontal (Fig. 46). In patients of over 35–40 years of age, it is wise to postpone the pelvic osteotomy to a second stage (10–12 months after the intertrochanteric osteotomy). In fact the Trendelenburg gait, in many instances resulting from slight varus, evokes the roof osteophyte on the anterolateral edge of the acetabulum, spontaneously correcting the pathological inclination of the WBS (Fig. 47).

The following results are obtained with the above-mentioned operations:

- The pelvic operations create a horizontal WBS, making the components of force $R(P_R, Q_R)$ and force $R_1(P, Q)$ equal in magnitude and opposite in direction. At the same time, the area of contact between the acetabulum and the femoral head increases.
- Varus intertrochanteric osteotomy reduces the magnitudes of forces P_R and P and the extension component relocates the anteriorly subluxated femoral head into the acetabulum.
- In adult patients the roof osteophyte which frequently forms after varus-extension osteotomy, due to a transient Trendelenburg gait, has the same effect as pelvic osteotomy or shelf-plasty.

Craniomedially Inclined WBS. When the WBS is inclined craniomedially (Fig. 48), force Q is always dominant over force Q_M, whatever the neck-shaft angle, and progressively displaces the femoral head posteromedially against the fundus acetabuli.

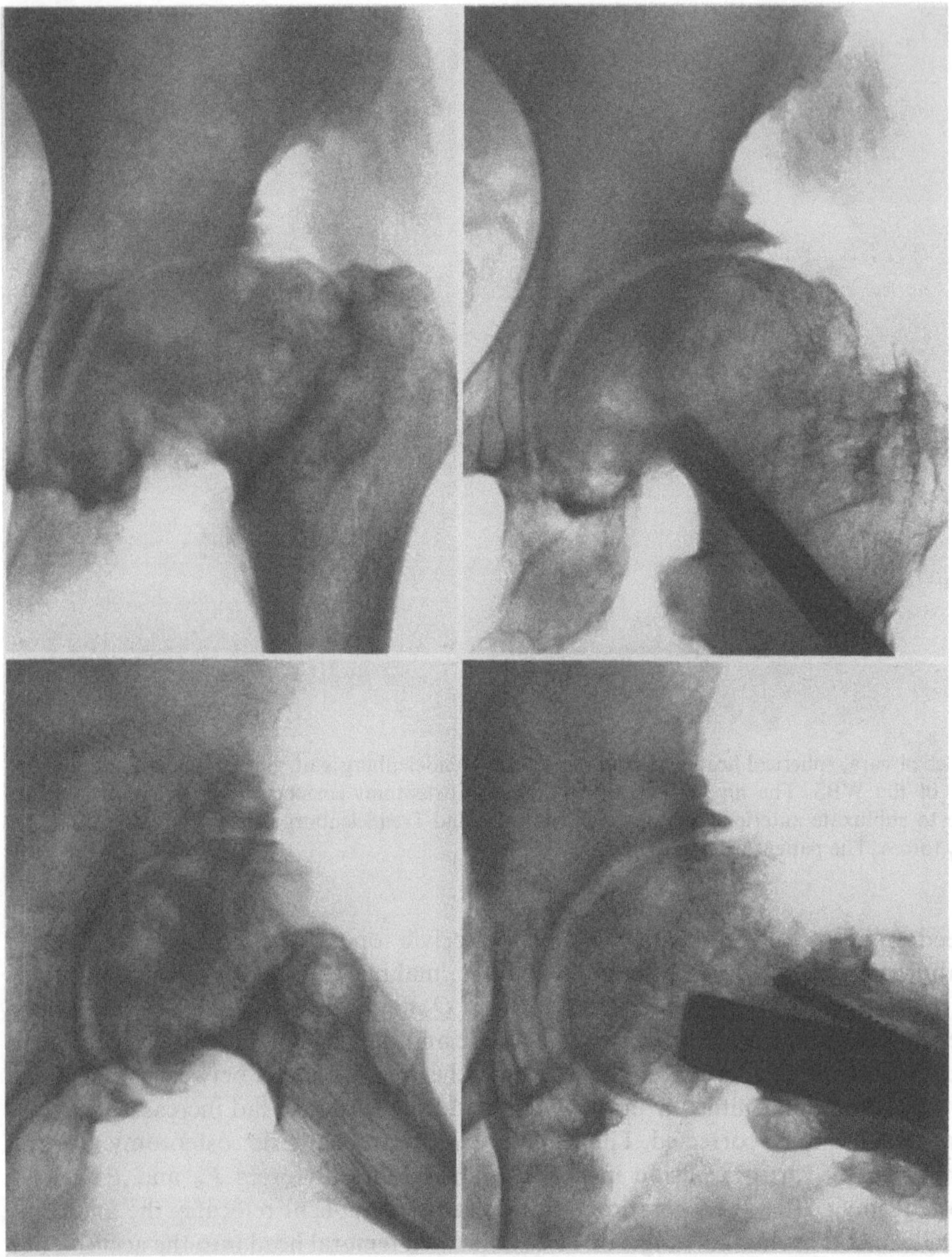

Fig. 41. Coxa vara and craniolateral inclination of the WBS. Severe OA in this 45-year-old patient is corrected by valgus-extension osteotomy. Note that the stimulation of a roof osteophyte has helped restore normal joint forces by creating a horizontal WBS. Joint space is restored as seen in this 5-year follow-up

The cartilage covering the posteromedial or equatorial part of the head wears out against the lamina quadrilatera. In the long run, this pathological situation produces the medial type of OA, coxa equatorialis, coxa profunda, or protrusio acetabuli. The joint cartilages of the upper part of the femoral head and of the corresponding acetabulum are preserved by the reduced compressive force *P*.

The neck-shaft angle may be *varus* (Fig. 49) or *normal* (Fig. 50). So far, I have not found a craniomedially inclined WBS combined with a valgus neck (Fig. 51), although such a combination could exist. Since a valgus osteotomy

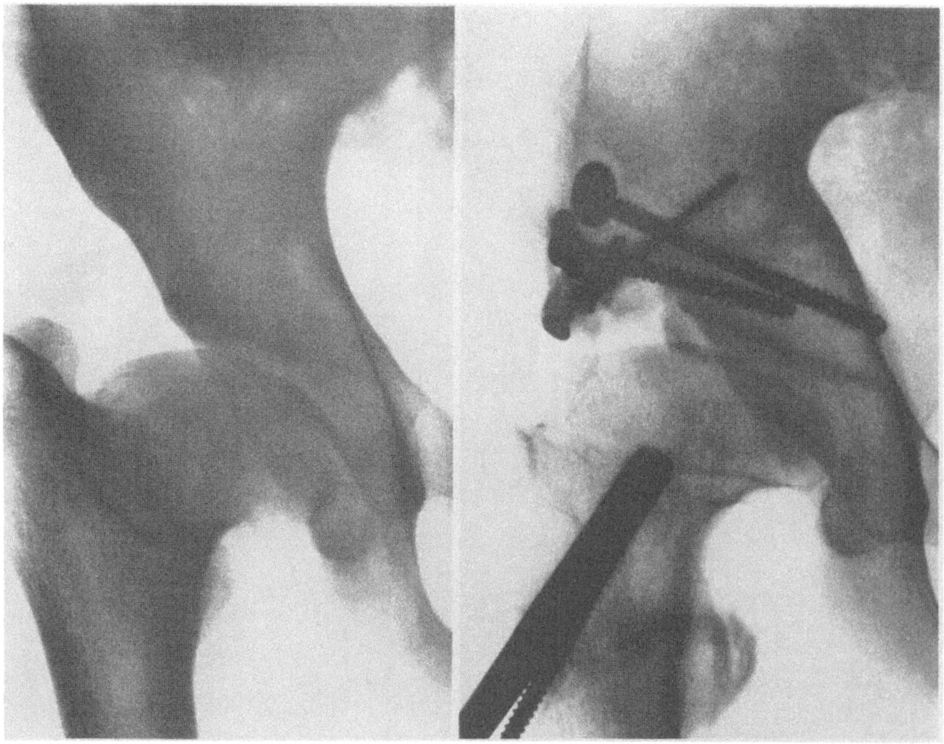

Fig. 42. Combined femoral and pelvic osteotomies. This 16-year-old patient had a Trendelenburg gait but no pain. The coxa vara and craniolateral inclination with a spherical head required a Chiari pelvic osteotomy augmented by a shelf buttress because of uncovering after the valgus-extension osteotomy of the femur. The patient was too young to form spontaneously a roof osteophyte.

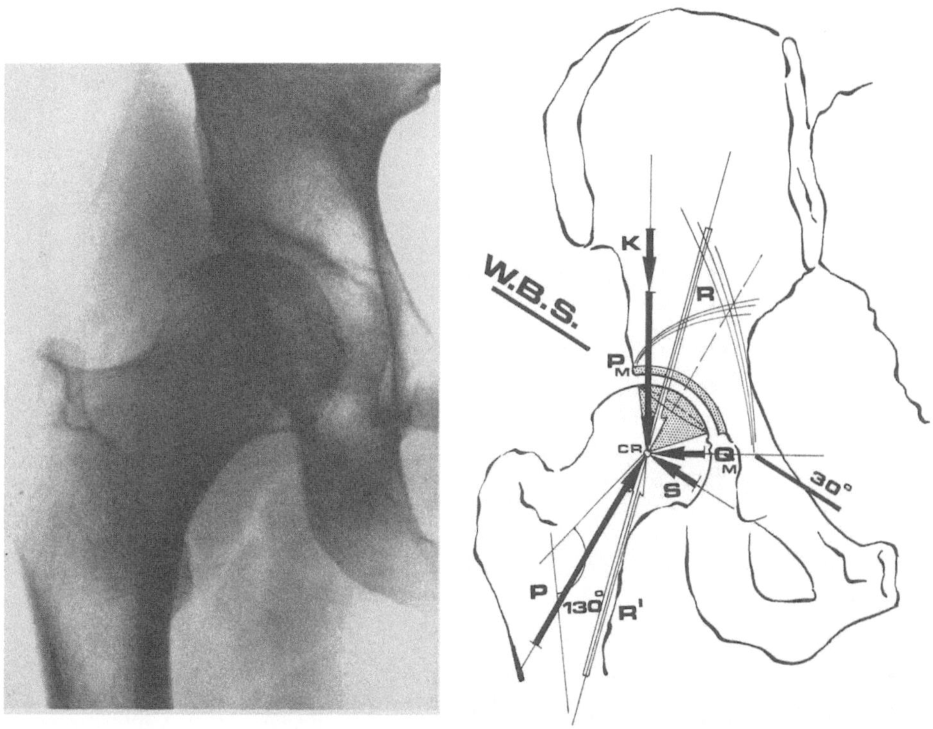

Fig. 43. Example of normal neck-shaft angle, spherical head, and craniolateral inclination of the WBS. Forces Q_M and S produce anterocraniolateral subluxation

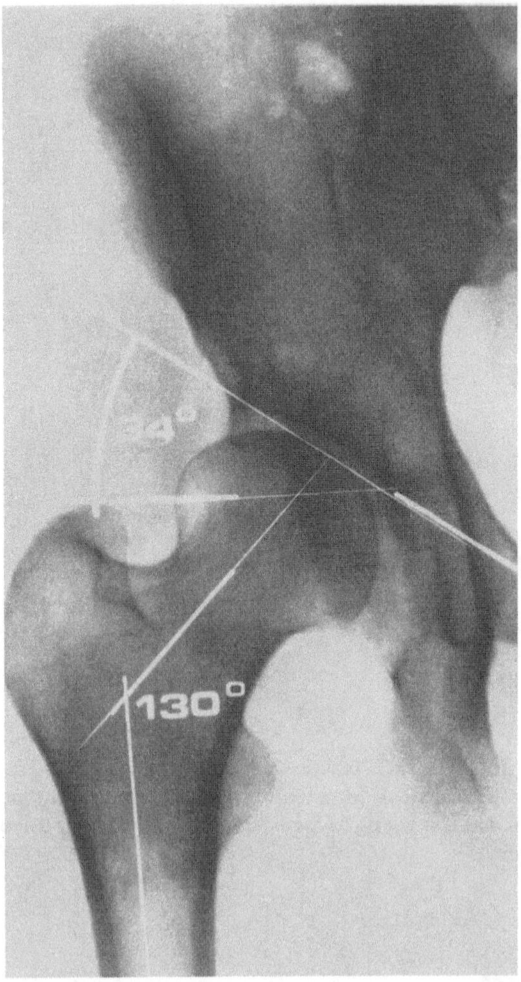

Fig. 44. The radiograph illustrates a typical case suitable for acetabuloplasty according to Wagner

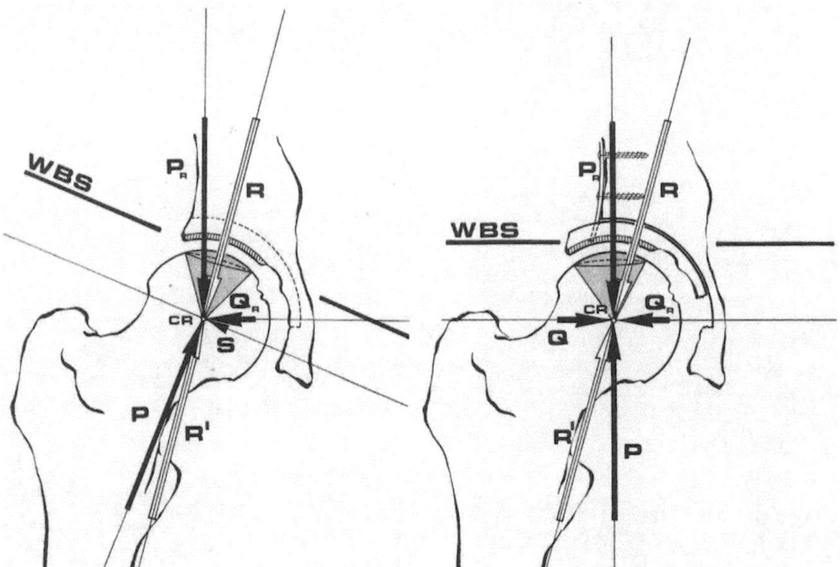

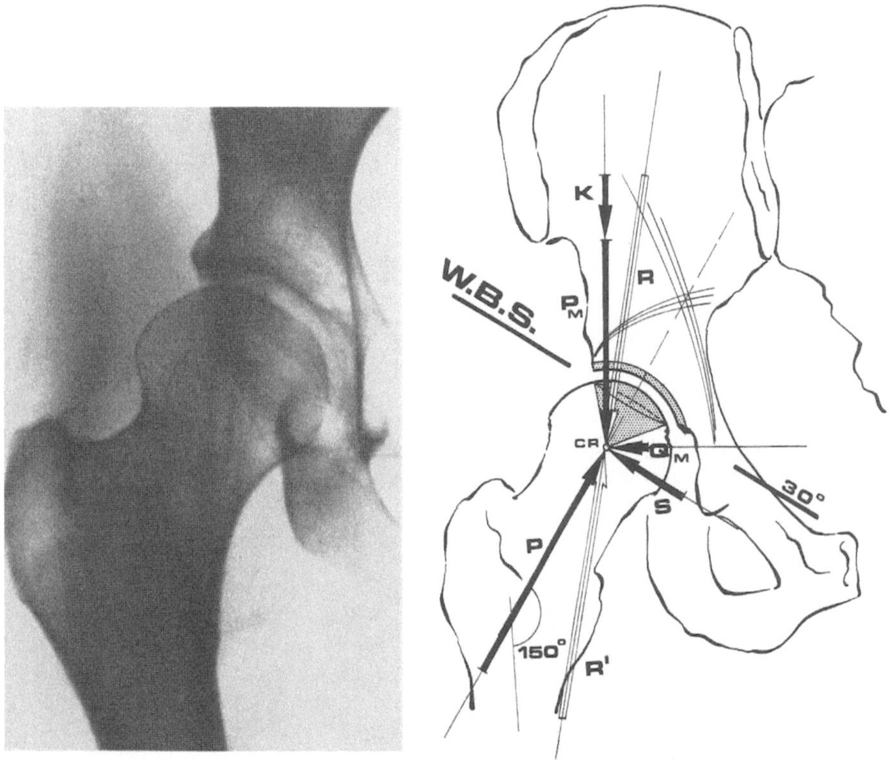

Fig. 45. Example of coxa valga, spherical head, and craniolateral inclination of the WBS. This patient is at high risk for early OA because of high *P* forces and high shear forces (S and Q_M)

gives favorable results when the WBS is craniomedially inclined, it is possible that primary valgus eliminates any ill effects of such WBS inclination.

In cases of coxa equatorialis congenital coxa profunda, the femoral head maintains a spherical shape; in cases of protrusio acetabuli, the head becomes conical. The consequent therapy in the presence of a spherical head is valgus osteotomy of 35°–40°, combined with flexion osteotomy of 20°–30° to recenter the posteromedially migrated head into the acetabulum. This operation must be performed *only* when the head is spherical; there is no indication in protrusio acetabuli. The flexion osteotomy is performed only when passive flexion exceeds 45° and no flexion contracture is present.

The greater trochanter has to be displaced laterally and cranially to increase the lever arm of the abductors and to obtain a modest Trendelenburg gait (Fig. 52). The slight contralateral tilt in monopodal stance obtained by the Trendelenburg gait makes the WBS horizontal. In order to avoid any lengthening of the limb, a cylinder 1.5–2 cm long must be removed from the shaft.

With Elliptical Femoral Head

An elliptical femoral head is always combined with a WBS craniolaterally inclined WBS and tends to glide anterocraniolaterally. The amount of anterocraniolateral displacement is not constant, but depends on the initial degree of inclination of the WBS and on the time elapsing before treatment (Fig. 53). The head may be:

- Completely dislocated.
- Highly subluxated (reseated into a false acetabulum at the level of the upper brim of the original acetabulum). A horizontal line tangent to the apex of the head would cross the sacro-iliac joint.

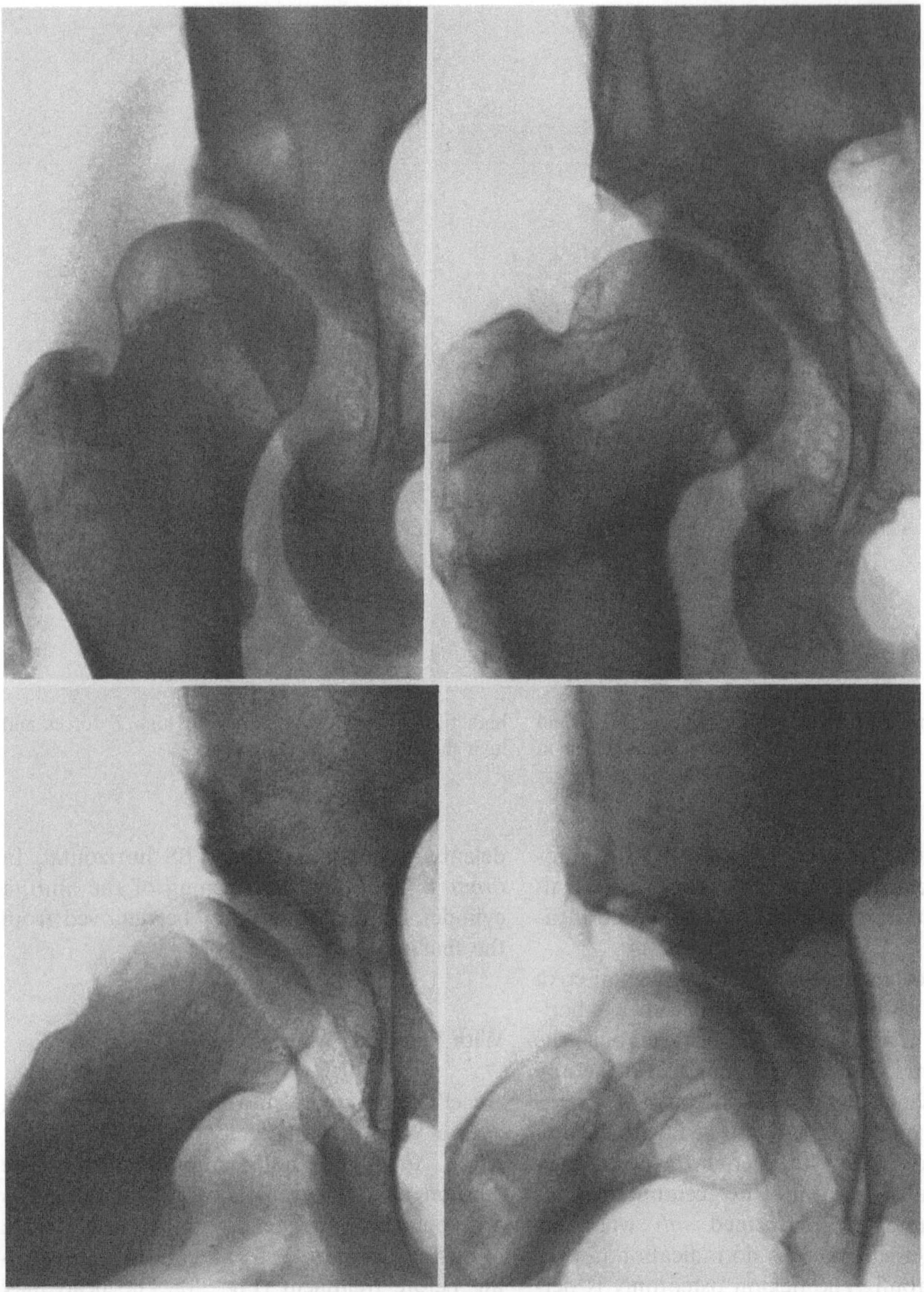

Fig. 46. Coxa valga and craniolateral inclination of the WBS in a young patient. Varus-extension osteotomy and Chiari pelvic osteotomy were performed in this 17-year-old patient in 1979. The plate had been removed by the time of this follow-up radiograph in 1982

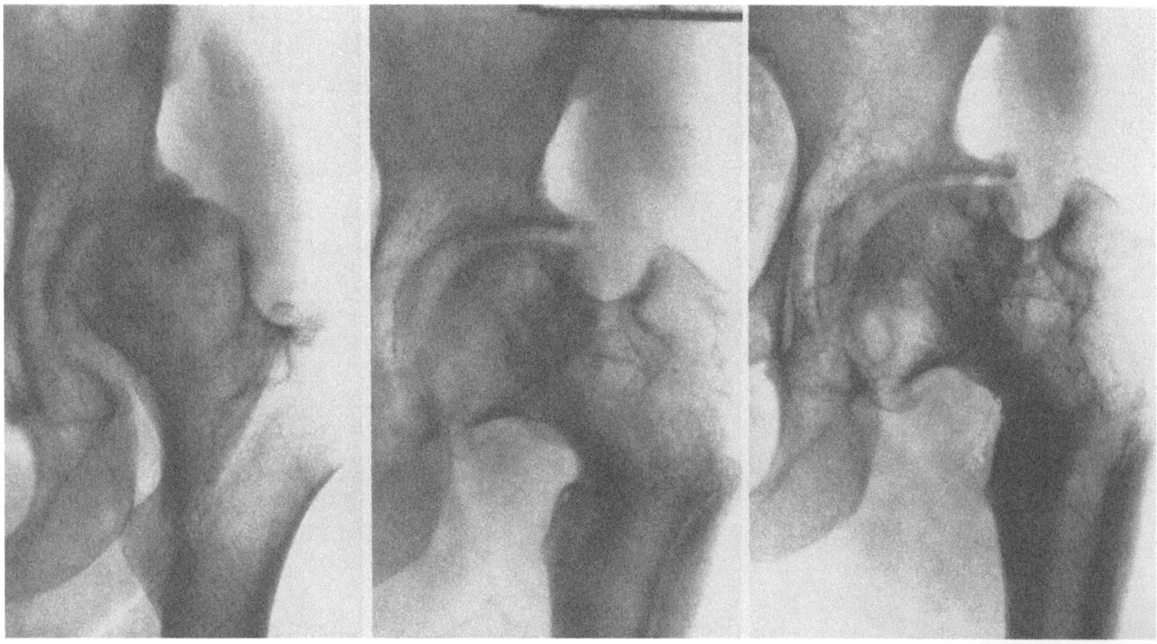

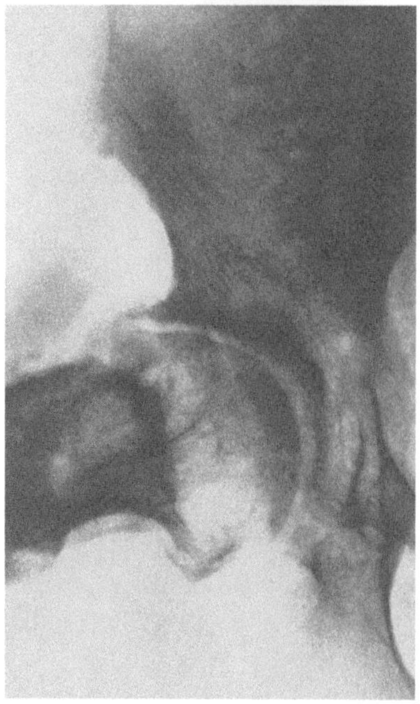

Fig. 47. Coxa valga and craniolateral inclination of the WBS in an older patient. Varus-extension osteotomy alone was enough in this 55-year-old lady, as the temperary Trendelenburg gait stimulated formation of the roof osteophyte. Postoperative radiographs demonstrate 7- and 10-year follow-ups

- Only in part anterocraniolaterally subluxed. A horizontal line traced at a tangent to the top of the head would run caudal to the sacro-iliac joint.
- Uncovered anterocraniolaterally, but still in the acetabulum.

Treatment must redirect the pathological forces, correct the obliquity of the WBS, decrease the magnitude of forces, and increase the area of the WBS. The neck-shaft angle plays no role in the choice of operation.

I believe that no osteotomy is advisable in case of complete dislocation. The Schanz osteotomy results in an ugly and tiring gait.

In high subluxation, valgus-extension intertrochanteric osteotomy is indicated (Fig. 54). Pain disappears, but Trendelenburg gait is not improved. The distal lateral displacement of the

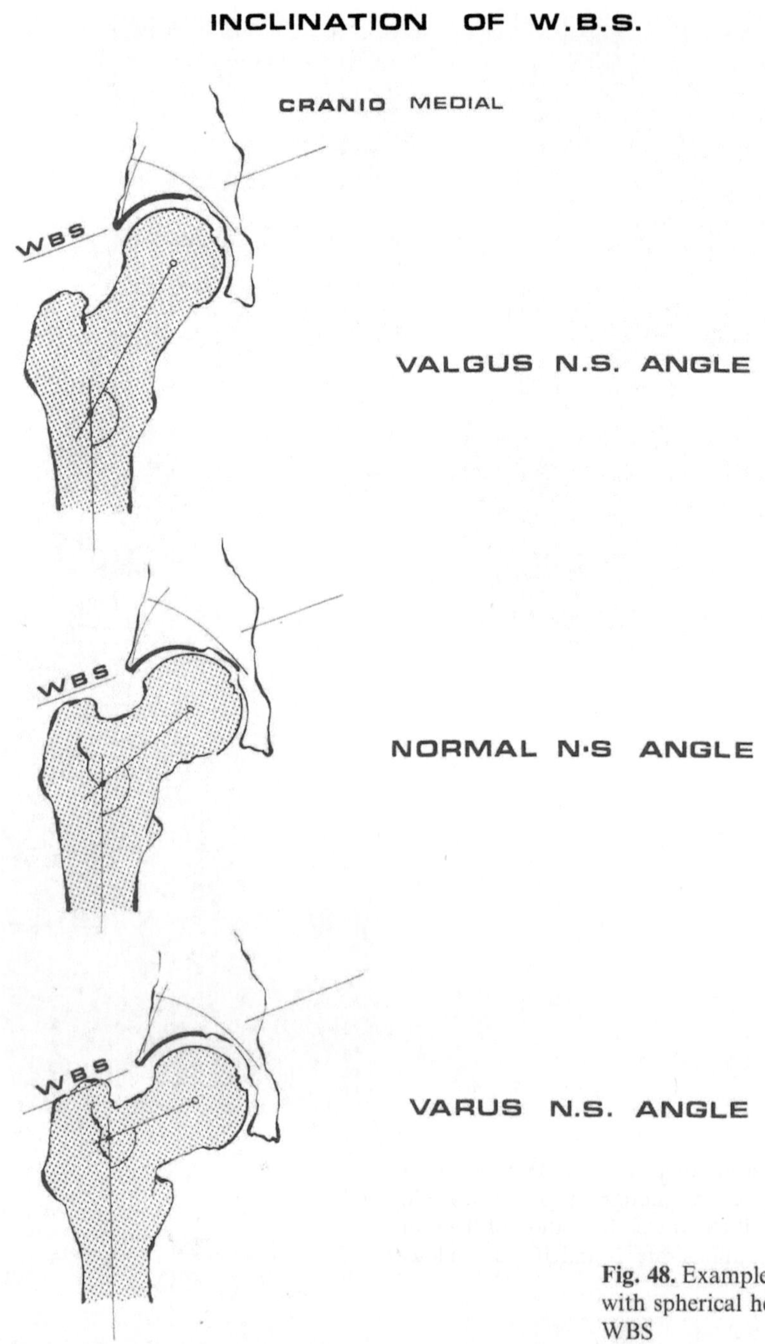

Fig. 48. Examples of various neck-shaft angles combined with spherical head and craniomedial inclination of the WBS

shaft lengthens the limb by only 1 cm. It is not possible to perform a pelvic osteotomy to cover the femoral head, because the head is too highly positioned. The pelvic osteotomy line would end up at the level of the sacrum.

In partial subluxation, valgus-extension intertrochanteric osteotomy is the operation of choice (Figs. 55, 56). If this uncovers too much of the head, pelvic osteotomy must be performed if feasible. It increases the contact surface in the joint and corrects the lateral inclination of the WBS (Fig. 57).

I have found that despite horizontal correction of the WBS, a pelvic osteotomy results in

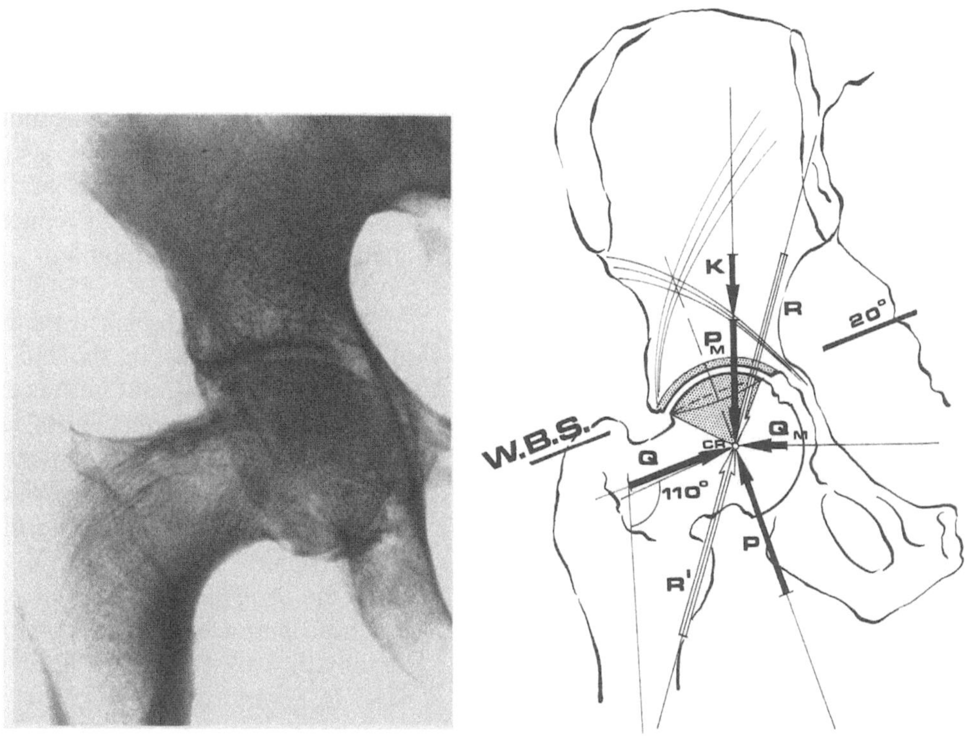

Fig. 49. Example of coxa vara, spherical head and craniomedial inclination of the WBS. This combination is common. Note the dominance of force Q over Q_R tending toward posteromedial migration

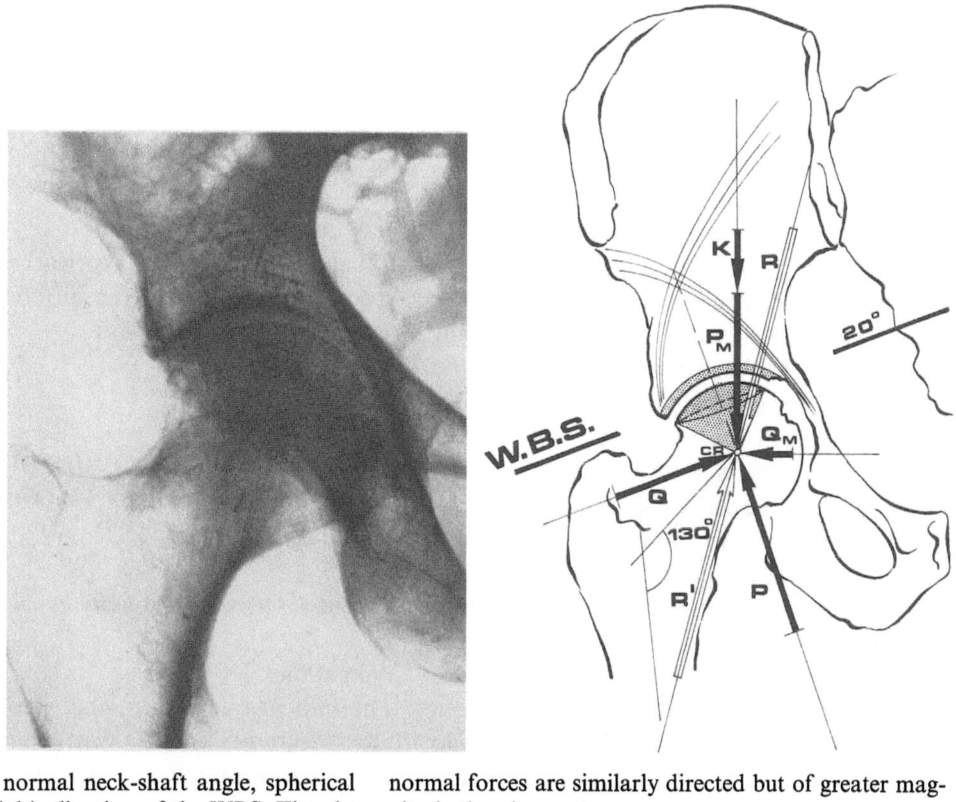

Fig. 50. Example of normal neck-shaft angle, spherical head and craniomedial inclination of the WBS. The abnormal forces are similarly directed but of greater magnitude than in coxa vara

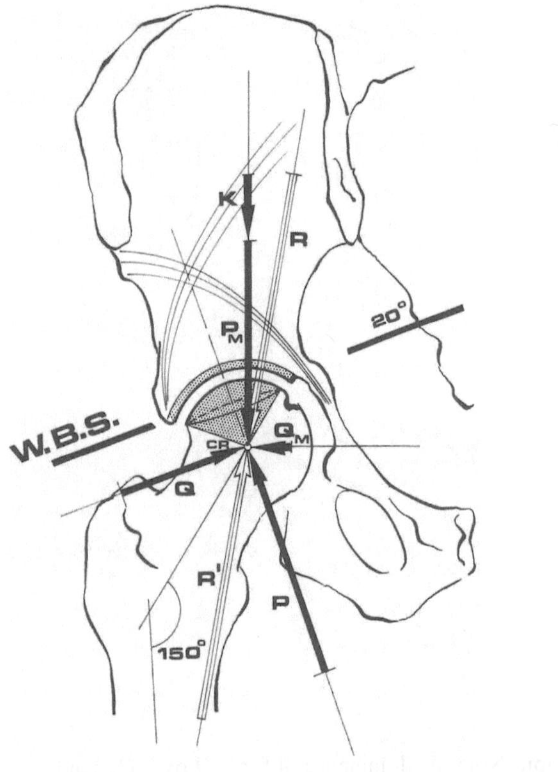

Fig. 51. Diagram of coxa valga, spherical head and craniomedial inclination of the WBS. I have so far found no corresponding X-ray

a permanent Trendelenburg gait in 65% of cases. In 35% of cases it disappears 18–24 months after operation.

The valgus osteotomy realizes a temporary medial shifting of the center of rotation. In fact the capital drop and the curtain osteophyte (double fundus acetabuli) act as a fulcrum for this movement. The lever arm *b* of the weight of the body (*K*) is shortened, and at the same time the lever arm *a* of the abductors is increased. As a result the magnitudes of the abductor force *M* and its vertical component P_M are reduced. The extreme downward pull in the craniolateral part of the capsule evokes a new roof osteophyte or increases the size of a roof osteophyte already present. This neoformation, like a spontaneous shelf, realizes horizontal correction of the WBS (Figs. 57–58).

The extension component of the operation, reduces the anteriorly subluxated femoral head into the acetabulum and creates a wider head-acetabulum contact. Clinically, before the operation, the anteriorly subluxated head may be palpated in the lateral portion of the groin. During the operation, it may be seen extruding from the anterior edge of the acetabulum when the anterior aspect of the capsule is opened longitudinally along the direction of the connective fibers. Flexion of the tigh reduces the subluxated head into the acetabulum.

So far we have discussed the indications for different operations in the hip, according to morphological type, but not taken into account the biological reaction, which depends on the vascularization of the components: bone, synovial membrane, and capsule. We divide biological reactions into atrophic, normotrophic, and hypertrophic.

In the *atrophic* type, the bone trabeculae of the head and acetabulum tend to collapse. Osteophytes are scarce, the head diminished in size. In *normotrophic* OA, areas of eburnation and bone cysts are present in both head and acetabulum. In *hypertrophic* OA, the head is deformed and crowned by an exuberant growth of osteophytes. Huge osteophytes develop all around the edges of the acetabulum.

An osteotomy must never be performed in elderly people, in presence of atrophic OA or in severe bilateral cases. Clinically the range of motion must exceed 45° of flexion in anesthetized patient, otherwise in 80% cases the joint may end up with a fusion.

Table 1 shows a classification of OA that takes into account all the different components we have mentioned so far.

Technical Considerations of Valgus-Extension and Varus Osteotomies

Valgus-Extension Osteomy

Indications

The indications for valgus osteotomy (Table 5) are as follows:

- Valgus alone: coxa vara with a short limb (Fig. 68).

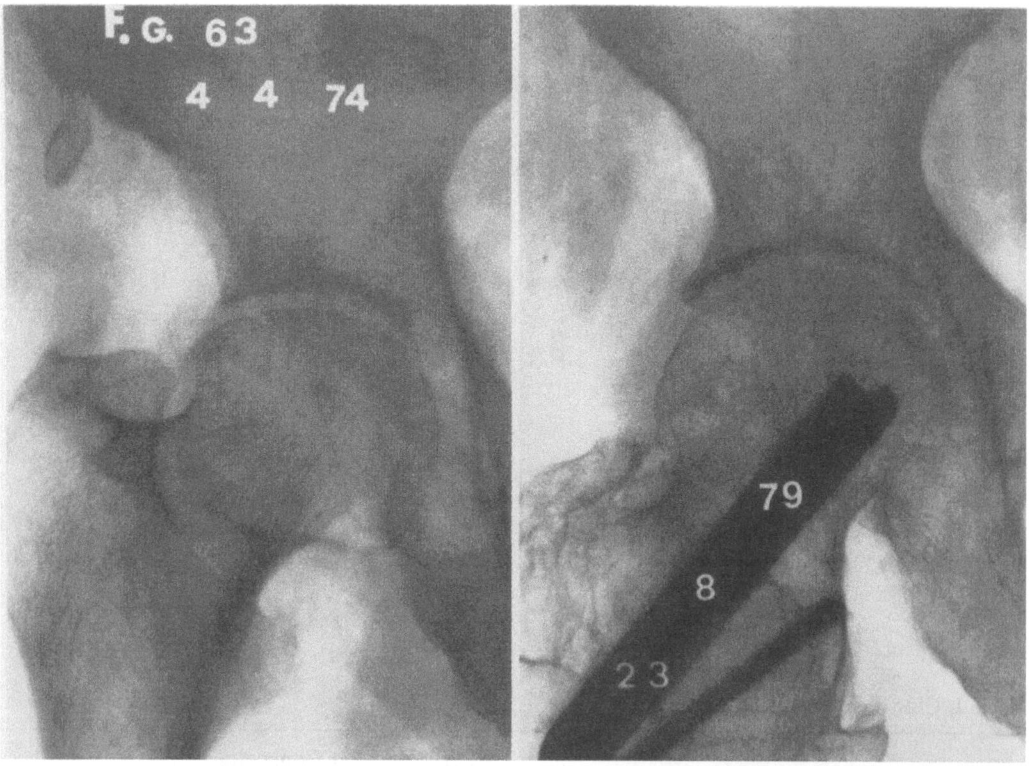

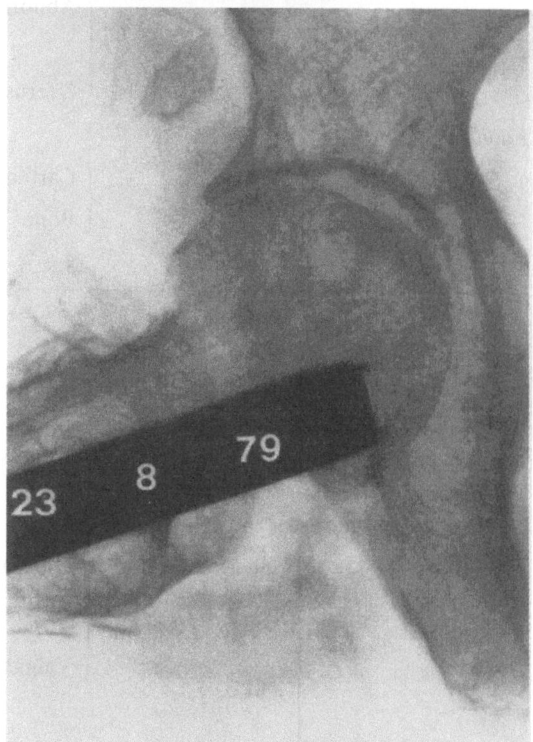

Fig. 52. Craniomedial WBS treated by pure valgus osteotomy. Five-year follow-up after surgery in a 63-year-old patient. Note elevation of greater trochanter and joint space regeneration. In medial OA of the hip, valgus osteotomy (35°–40°) recenters the femoral head in the acetabulum, shifting it laterally from the fundus acetabuli to the WBS

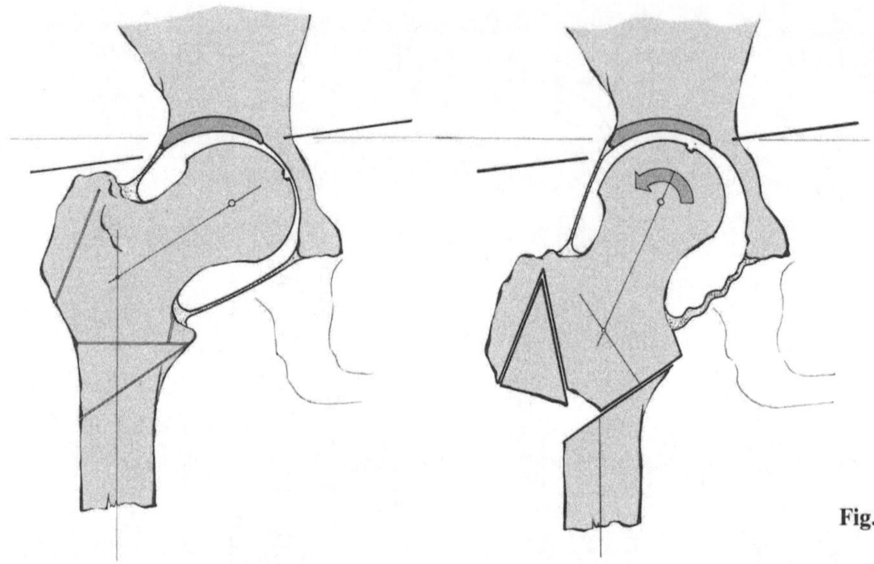

Fig. 52 (continued)

Table 1. Classification of OA of the hip

Etiology	Mechanical	Abnormal Geometry	Congenital	
			Acquired	
		Overuse	High dynamic force	
			Overweight	
	Metabolic	Cartilage		
		Bone	Osteoporosis	
			Osteomalacia	
	Combined			
Biological reaction	Atrophic			
	Normotrophic			
	Hypertrophic			
Morphology	Spherical head	Varus NSA	Inclination WBS	CL
				H
				CM
		Normal NSA	Inclination WBS	CL
				H
				CM
		Valgus NSA	Inclination WBS	CL
				H
				CM
	Elliptical head	NSA plays no role	WBS always CL	Iliac dislocation
				High subluxation
				Subluxation
				Uncovering

NSA, neck-shaft angle; WBS, weight-bearings surface; CL, craniolateral; H, horizontal; CM, craniomedial

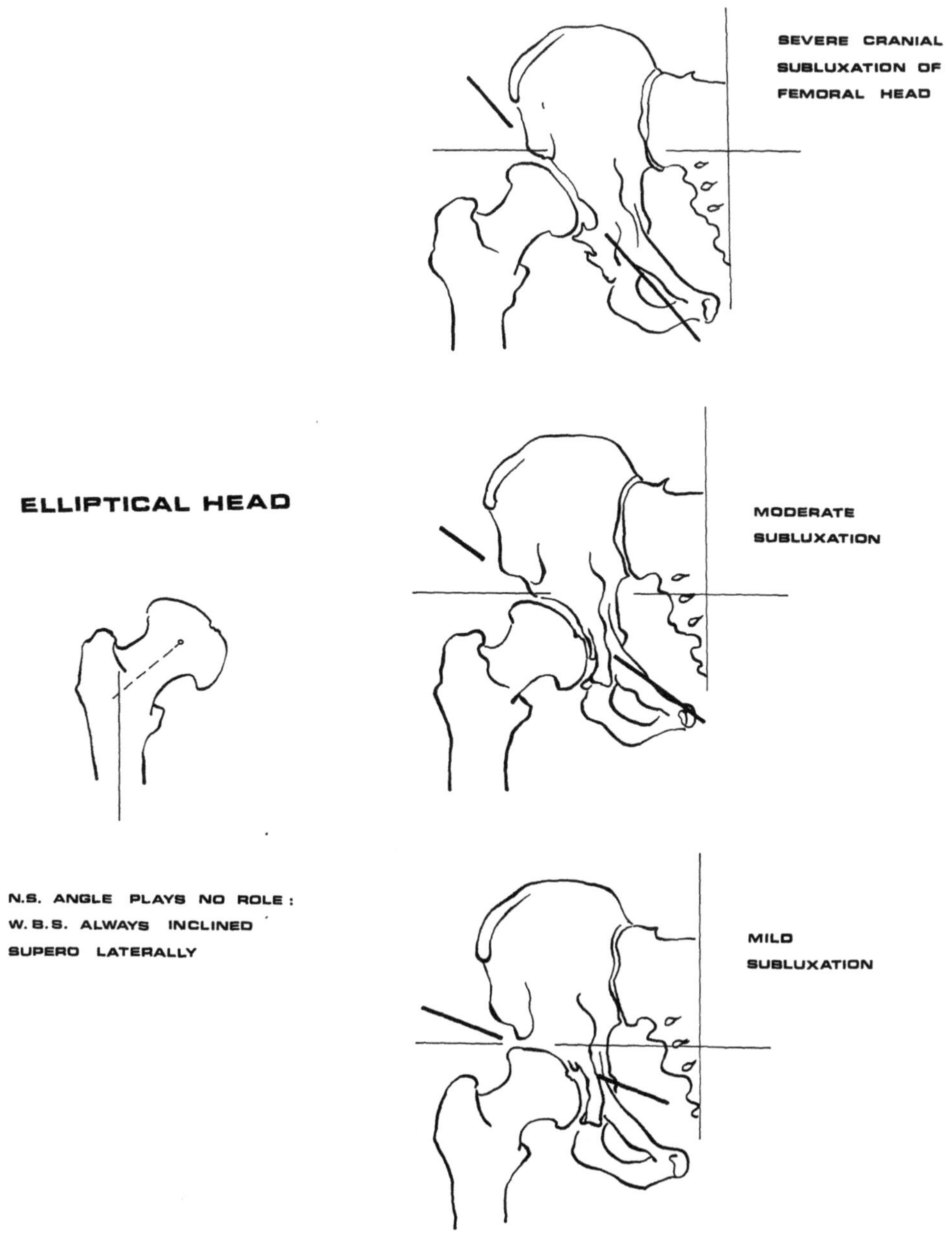

Fig. 53. Elliptical head and craniolateral inclination of WBS. The neck-shaft angle does not affect the choice of treatment. The problem is subluxation of the femoral head. Early valgus-extension osteotomy is essential to prevent dislocation. A high subluxation will respond, but this osteotomy is contraindicated if dislocation is complete

- Valgus-extension: femoral head elliptical (due to formation of the capital drop and antero-craniolateral flattening), as seen in types b, c, and d_2. An extension component must always be, included when the WBS is craniolaterally inclined. In most cases the degree of extension exceeds the degree of valgus.
- Valgus-flexion: medial osteoarthritis (coxa equatorialis or coxa profunda) where the WBS is craniomedially inclined (Fig. 71).

Aims in Craniolateral Osteoarthritis

Since the pathological process has eliminated force Q and created force S, pushing the head

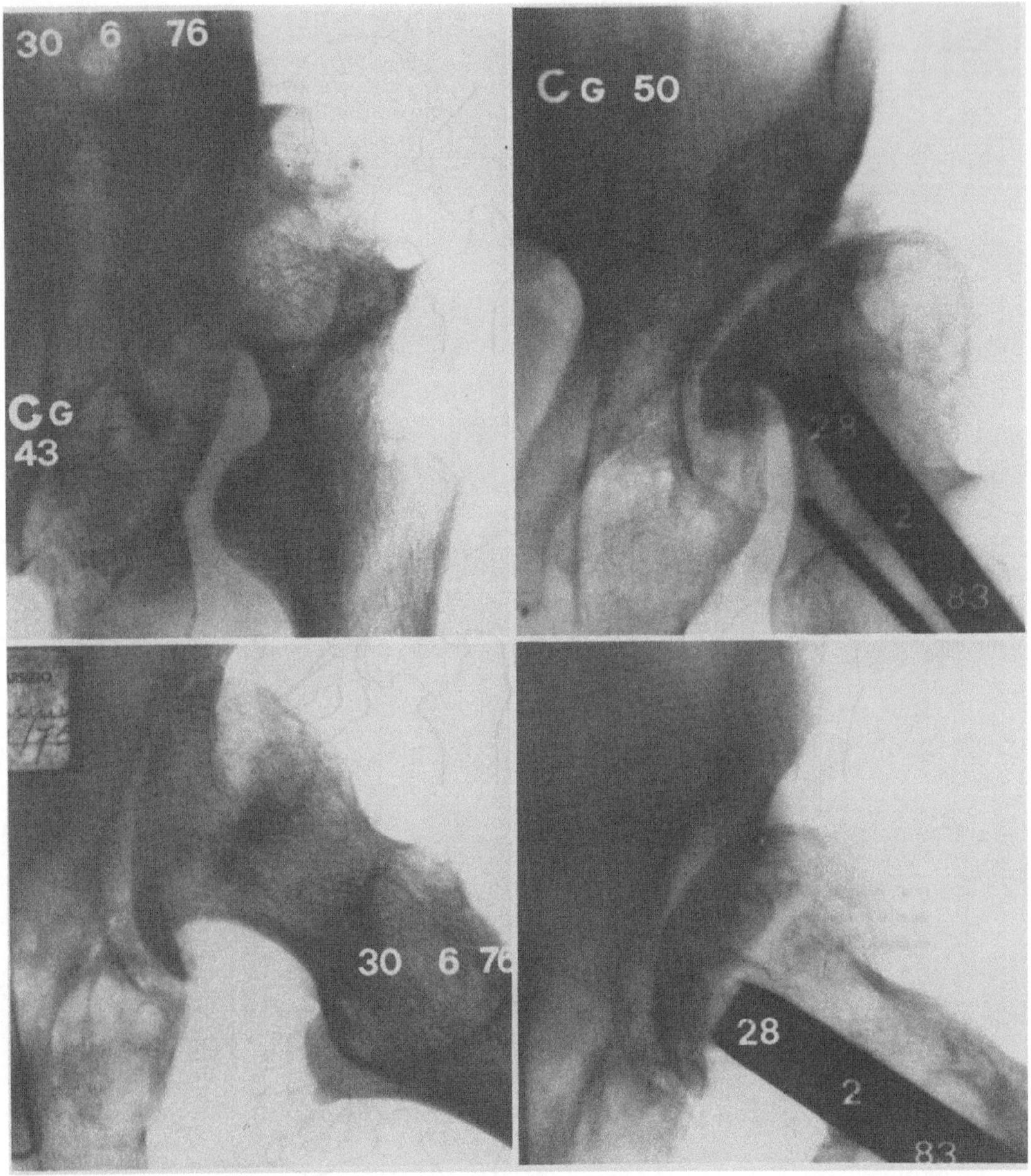

Fig. 54. Example of valgus-extension osteotomy in elliptical head, craniolateral inclination of the WBS, and high subluxation. Despite persistent Trendelenburg gait and shortening, pain is relieved. The joint space has reappeared. Note the 7-year follow-up

out of the acetabulum, created pain for the patient and forced him to walk unnaturally, our treatment must:

1. Eliminate force *S* and restore force *Q*
2. Reduce force *R* at least temporarily while the joint heals
3. Reduce the unit pressure in the head by restoring joint space and increasing the WBS
4. Encourage the growth of osteophytes
5. Exploit the hydraulic mechanism
6. Avoid valgus in the knee

The essence of valgus extension osteotomy is very simple. If the pathological forces can be removed from the joint, the bone will be able to heal itself, and in time, with the growth of osteophytes, will form a new joint. We achieve this by turning the head so that the capital drop and tent osteophytes come into contact in such

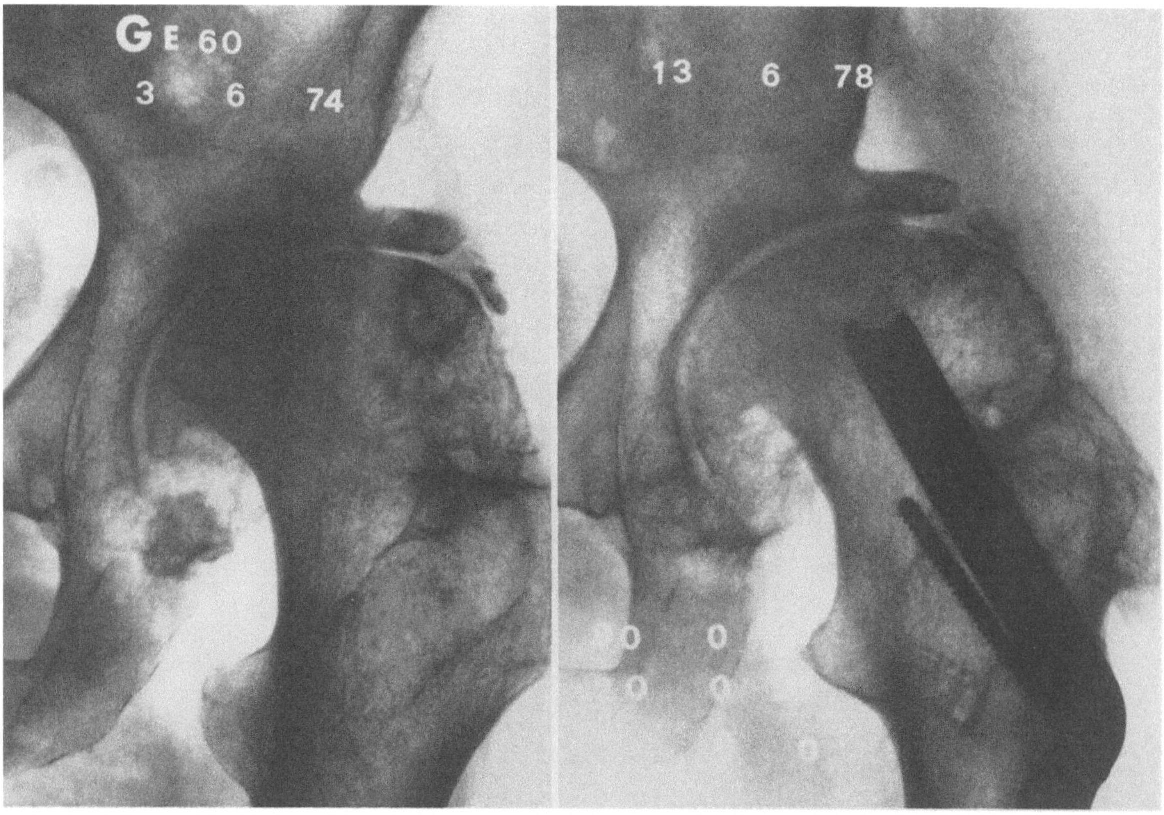

Fig. 55. Mild subluxation, elliptical head. Joint pain is relieved and anterior subluxation is corrected by valgus-extension osteotomy

a way as to provide a fulcrum of movement, which will be painless since osteophytes are not innervated (Fig. 69).

The advantages are clear (Fig. 58). CR_1 is transferred from the painful anterocraniolateral area (1) to the painless fulcrum on the curtain osteophyte (2). The lever arm a_1 of M_1 about CR_1 is increased, and the lever arm b_1 of K is decreased.

As a result, $M_1 \cdot \frac{(K \cdot b_1)}{a_1}$ is diminished along with its resultant force R. The weight-bearing joint space has widened considerably and the capsule fills with fluid. As the joint is compressed cyclically, this fluid "massages" the bone and joint back to life, encouraging it to regain its healthy shape and distribute the resultant force R over more of the WBS. The displacement of the head has stretched the joint capsule and its synovial membrane. As time goes on, these undergo bone metaplasia and form an osteophyte, which makes the WBS more horizontal and makes force S disappear. Gradually, the fulcrum becomes molded (Fig. 59) and less important. The superior parts of the head then take over their original function and CR_1 is relocated at the center of the new head. The diameter of the new head is grater than that of the old one, meaning that it is subject to less unit pressure (stress) and is more competent to carry out its function because of less strain.

Operating Technique

The patient lies supine on an ordinary operating table. The limb is left free, not placed in traction. When the patient has been anesthetized, the limb is cautiously flexed, abducted, and adducted. The passive movements are generally much greater than the active movements. Lack of 45° flexion or 15° adduction is a contraindication to osteotomy.

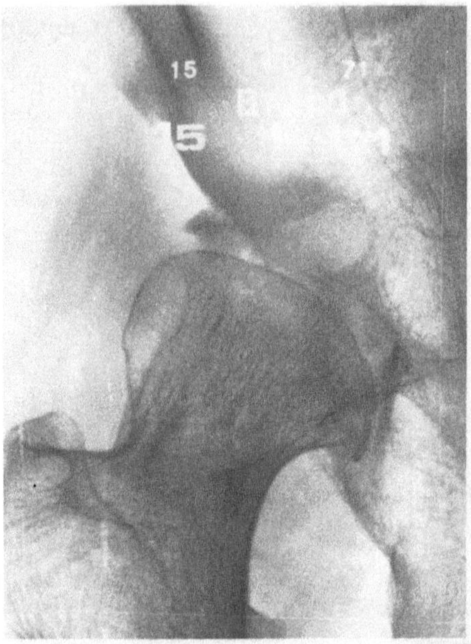

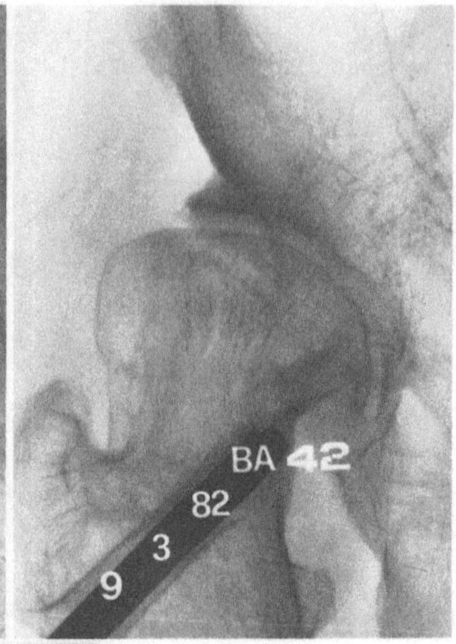

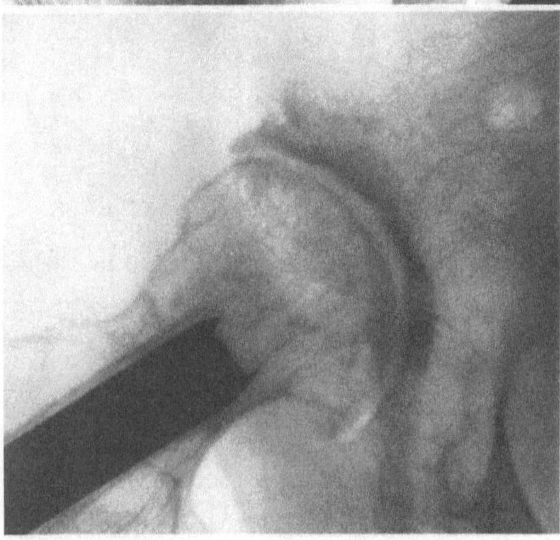

Fig. 56. Eleven-year follow-up of valgus-extension osteotomy in a 31-year-old patient

The area to be disinfected extends from a level five fingers above the navel to the toes of the affected limb. The operative area, which is protected by a plastic sheet, stretches along the laterosuperior surface of the thigh from the distal third to about 2 cm above the iliac crest.

The approach employed is the Watson-Jones. The incision is straight for 20 cm along the lateral surface of the thigh and then curves toward the anterosuperior iliac spine for about 10 cm from the inferior margin of the greater trochanter, taking on the shape of a hockey stick.

The fascia lata is incised in line with the skin incision. The dissection extends close to the greater trochanter between the tensor of the fascia lata and the anterior fibers of the gluteus medius. The nerve and artery of the tensor of the fascia lata are left intact.

The vastus lateralis muscle is detached from the lateral intermuscular septum and is divided in its proximal part, leaving a tract of about 2 cm of its tendon attached to the inferior margin of the greater trochanter. The perforating veins and arteries are ligated with absorbable suture material. The anteromedial and superior surfaces of the joint capsule are exposed by use of three Hohmann retractors, the lower one placed around the inferior surface of the capsule, the middle one hooked around the anterior rim of the acetabulum, and the superior one

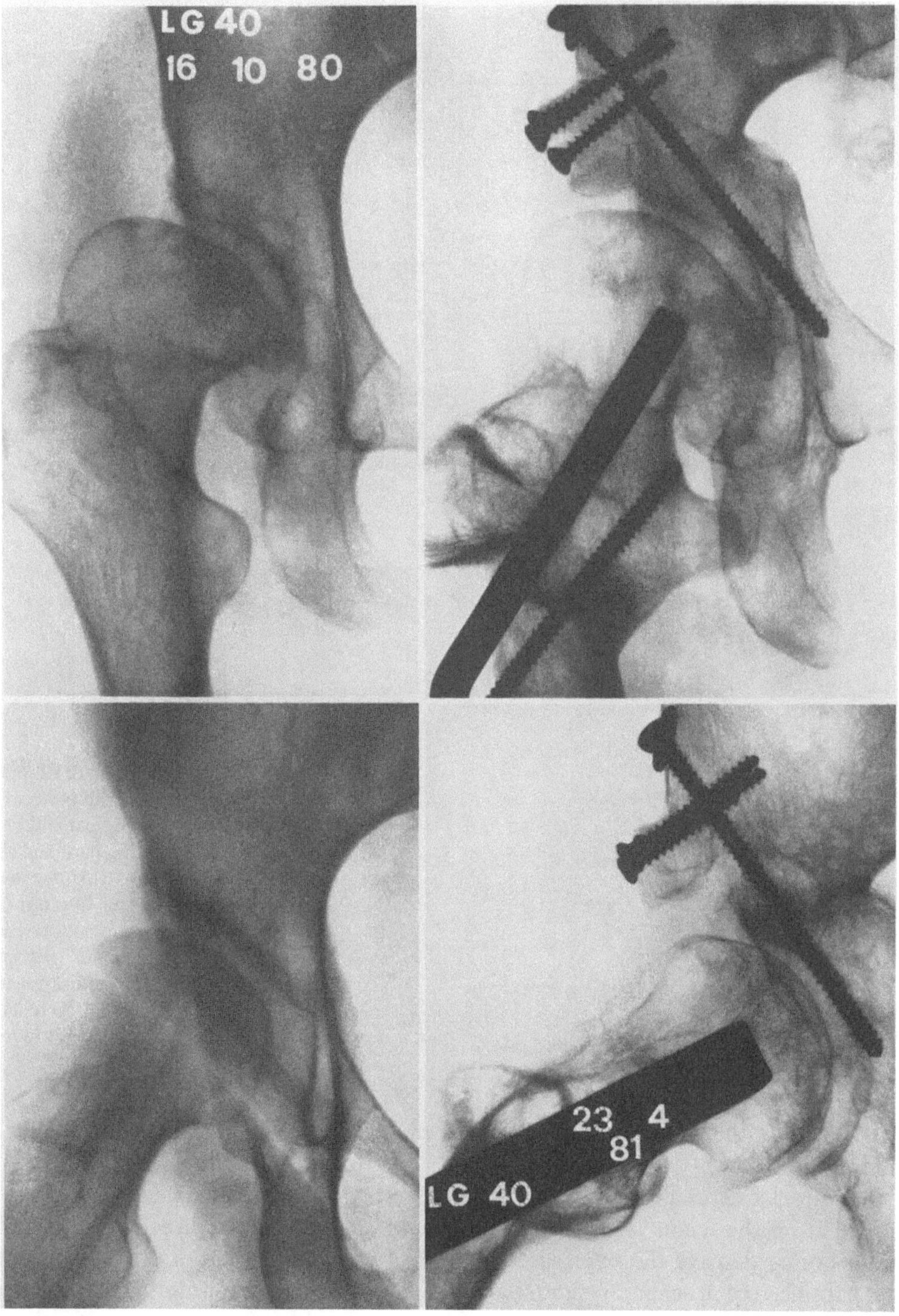

Fig. 57. When valgus-extension osteotomy uncovers the head laterally, pelvic osteotomy should be utilized in the younger patient, since a roof osteophyte will not form until much later

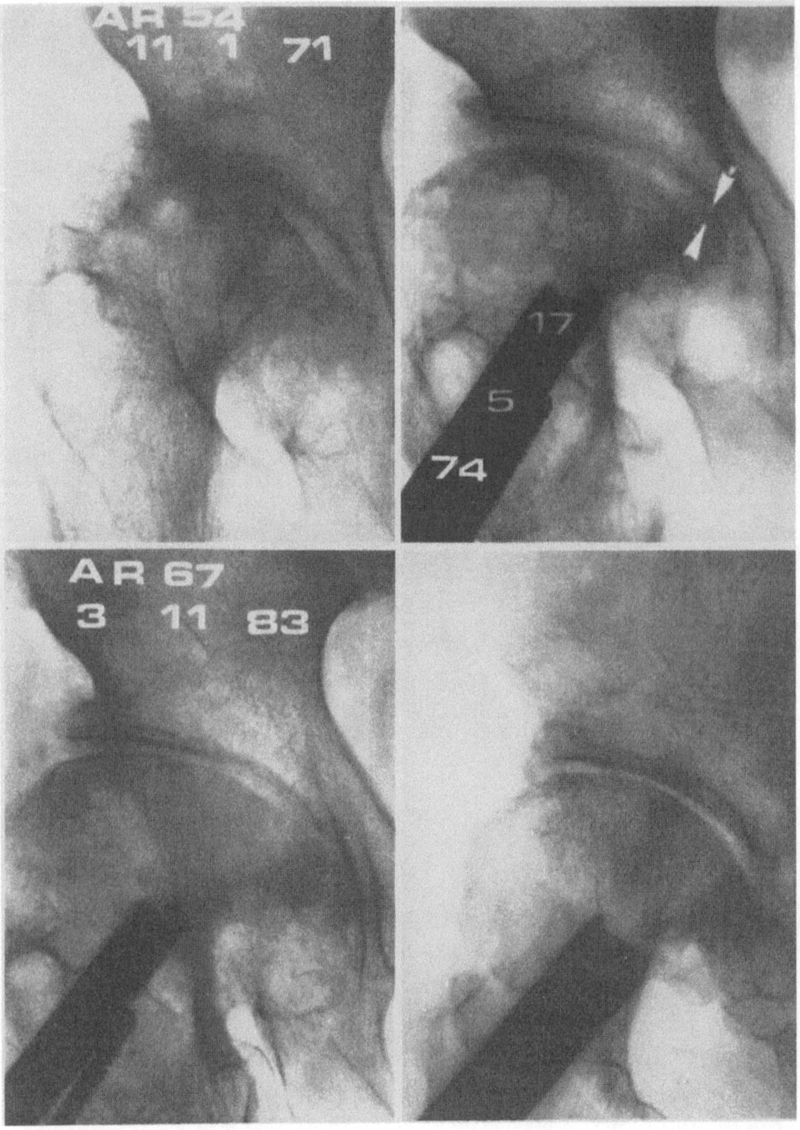

Fig. 58. Elliptical head and anterocraniolateral subluxation. This 54-year-old patient had debilitating pain and shortening. Valgus-extension osteotomy created a new fulcrum CR_1 at the point of contact between capital drop and curtain osteophytes (*arrows*). Pain disappeared as force reorientation fostered joint regeneration. Follow-up is at 12 years

passed above the superior surface of the capsule.

The greater trochanter is then partially detached from the femur using an osteotome. In order not to damage the inferolateral fibers of the capsule, the trochanter should remain attached to the femoral neck by its proximal part, which acts as a hinge. The inferolateral fibers of the capsule, when placed under traction by frontal rotation in valgus of the femoral head, provoke the formation of the roof osteophyte. The anterior and posterior fibers of the gluteus medius must remain intact. In this way a pocket is created where a bone transplant will be placed to lengthen the lever arm of the abductors muscles about *CR*.

The joint capsule is then cut longitudinally following the direction of its fibres and the Hohmann retractors previously inserted are placed in the same order, but inside the capsule. That is, the inferior retractor is placed in direct contact with the inferior surface of the femoral neck, the middle one overrides the limbus and the anterior rim of the acetabulum, and the superior one is in contact with the superior surface of the femoral neck. This last retractor should not be pushed too far dorsally lest damage to the posterosuperior artery of the femoral head occur.

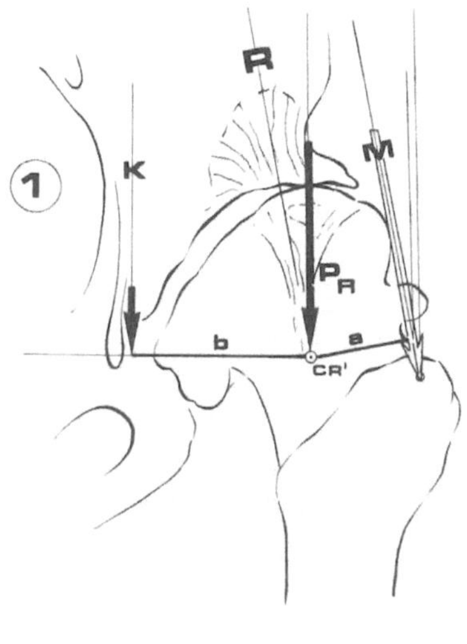

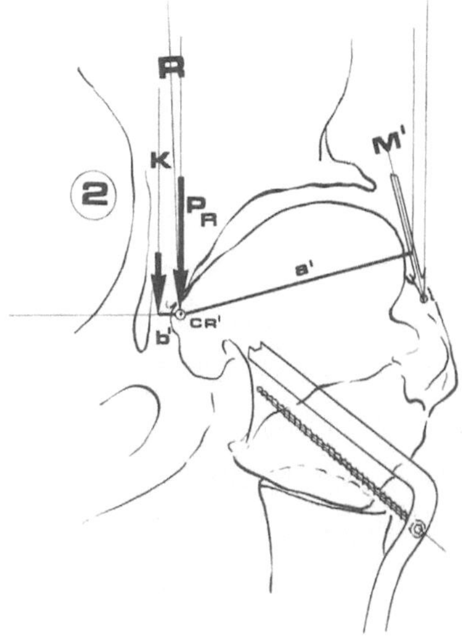

$$M \cdot a = K \cdot b$$

$$M = \frac{K \cdot b}{a}$$

$$M' = \frac{K \cdot b'}{a'}$$

$$b > b' \qquad a < a'$$

$$M' < M$$

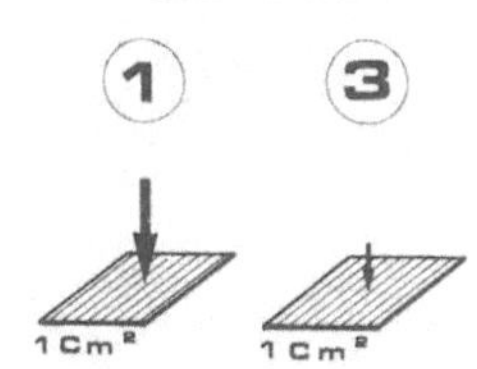

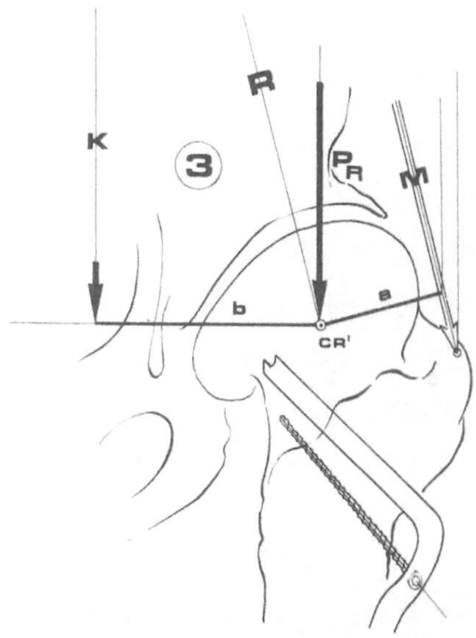

Fig. 58 (continued)

Arthrotomy facilitates the operation in four ways. It allows:

- Calculation of the degree of anterior subluxation of the femoral head and determination of the exact amount of extension to be carried out.
- Visual control as the seating chisel is introduced. The channel for the blade plate in the neck and head of the femur is thus safely prepared, obviating X-ray control.
- Exact calculation of blade length.
- Contouring of the capital drop or elephant trunk osteophyte when too large to fit into the acetabulum with valgus rotation.

If the femoral head is subluxed anteriorly, which frequently happens, the femur is flexed until the head is completely covered by the acetabulum. The angle between the axis of the shaft of the femur and the plane of the operating table is the angle of extension to be performed (usually 30° or more). The preparatory chisel is inserted in the neck and head of the femur with the blade vertical. The angle which the chisel should form with the axis of the shaft of the femur, is the supplementary angle of the plate (e.g., with a plate of 130°, this would be 50°) to which is added the necessary angle of valgus (Fig. 60) and the necessary angle of correction

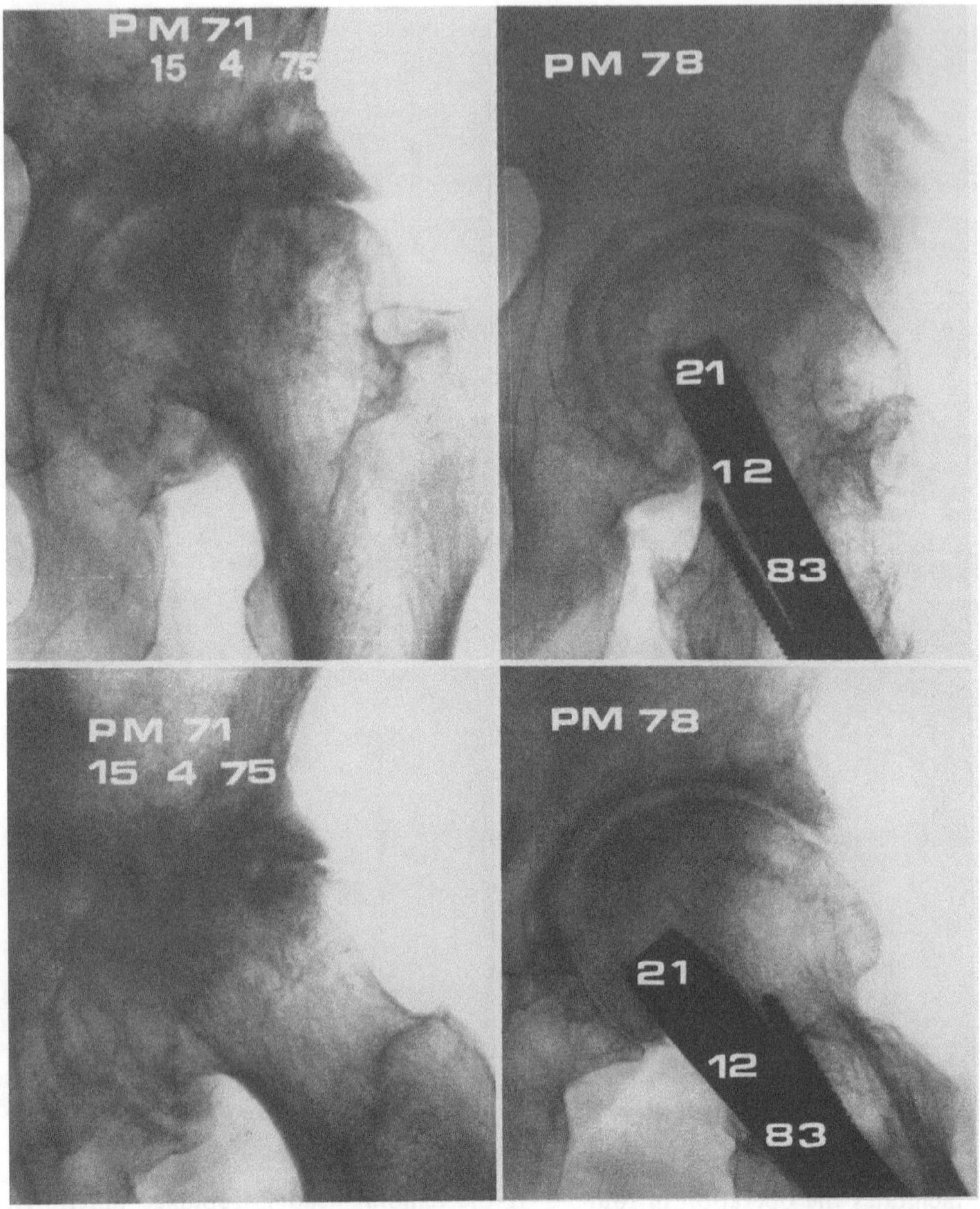

Fig. 59. Valgus-extension osteotomy in this 71-year-old patient not only restored joint space and relieved pain, but, as shown, the capital drop has remodelled

when there is associated extension (see table, Fig. 61). The depth to which the blade of the preparatory chisel is to be introduced, may be read on the shaft of the chisel itself.

The preparatory chisel must be introduced with regard for all three planes: (a) the sagittal plane for extension, (b) the coronal plane for the valgus, and (c) the horizontal plane for any pathological ante- or retroversion of the head. If rotation of the hip is inadequate this is compensated by rotation of the shaft until the patella points anteriorly.

When the preparatory chisel has been introduced, the oscillating saw is used to resect a bone wedge based posteriorly and laterally corresponding to the degree of extension and valgus desired. The wedge is removed in one piece.

The proximal line of section is perpendicular to the axis of the shaft of the femur and is 2–2.5 cm distal to the point of insertion of the

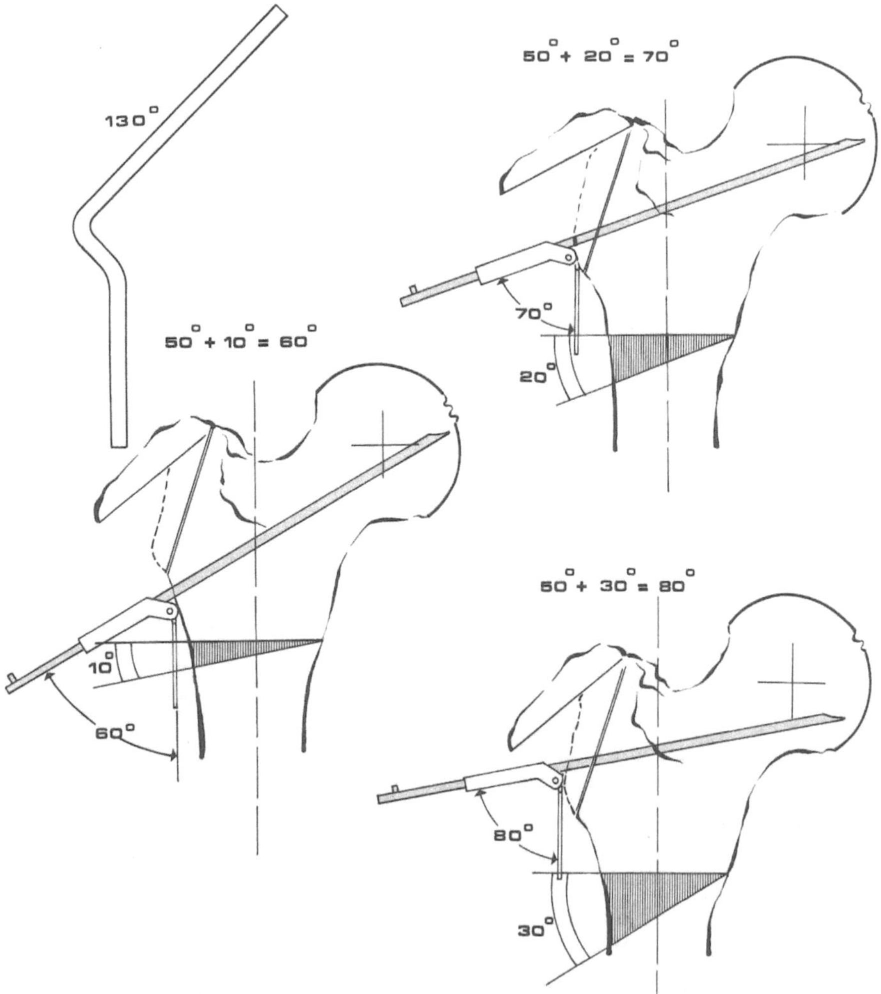

Fig. 60 ANGLE CHISEL-SHAFT = SUPPLEMENTARY ANGLE + ANGLE OF WEDGE TO REMOVE OF ANGLED PLATE 130°

seating chisel, which chisel serves temporarily to maneuver the proximal fragment of the femur. Following the proximal osteotomy, the limb is rotated in order to direct the patella anteriorly and a second osteotomy is carried out with the proper degree of obliquity to create valgus and extension.

If a piece of lesser trochanter remains connected to the proximal portion of the femur, it should be removed to avoid it impinging against the inferior margin of the acetabulum when the head of the femur is rotated into valgus. Any portion of the lesser trochanter which remains part of the shaft of the femur is left intact, as it will serve to increase the contact surface of the osteotomy, adding support to the proximal portion when it is under pressure.

The fibers of the tendon of the iliopsoas are separated from the lesser trochanter and the proximal fibers of the pectineus insertion from the medial surface of the shaft. Detaching these muscles from the distal fragment permits both permanent reduction of joint pressure and lateralization of the femoral shaft.

The amount of lateral displacement produced in the shaft depends upon the shape of the knee. If the patient has a varus knee, we usually displace not at all or very little (0.5–1 cm). If the patient has a valgus knee we displace 2.5 cm or more. In the presence of a normal knee we displace about 2 cm [6].

The preparatory chisel is extracted and the blade of the angled plate is introduced. The blade should be longer than the measurement

HOW EXTENSION AFFECTS THE SHAFT-NECK ANGLE

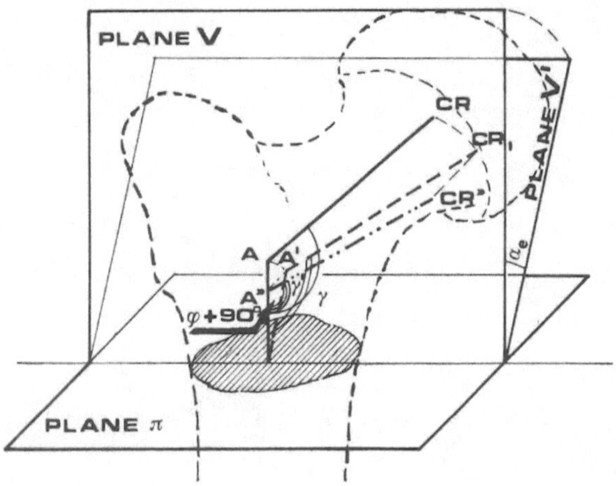

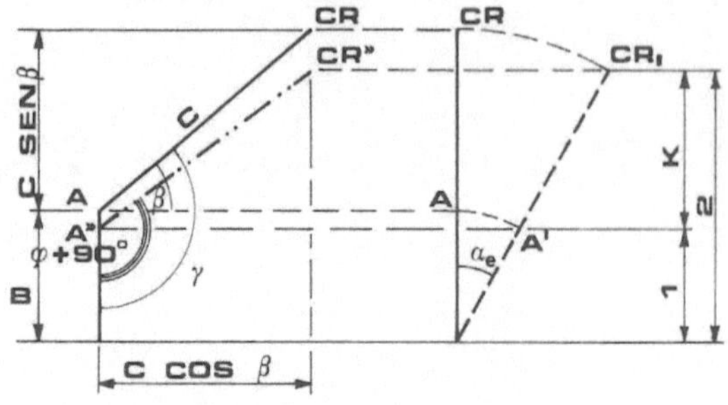

α_e = ANGLE OF EXTENSION

$\beta = \gamma - 90°$

$K = 2 - 1$

$1 = B \cos \alpha_e$

$2 = (B + C \operatorname{sen} \beta) \cos \alpha_e$

$K = (B + C \operatorname{sen} \beta) \cos \alpha_e - B \cos \alpha_e$

$K = C \operatorname{sen} \beta \cos \alpha_e$

$$\operatorname{tg} \varphi = \operatorname{tg} \beta \cos \alpha_e$$

$$\operatorname{tg} \varphi = \frac{C \operatorname{sen} \beta \cos \alpha_e}{C \cos \beta}$$

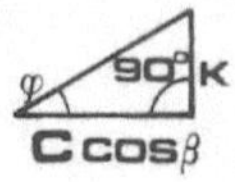

$$\operatorname{tg} \varphi = \frac{K}{C \cos \beta}$$

STARTING VALUE OF SHAFT-NECK ANGLE	FINAL VALUES OF SHAFT-NECK ANGLE (φ+90°) AFTER EXTENSION										
0°	10°	15°	20°	25°	30°	40°	50°	60°	70°	80°	90°
160°	159°43'	159°21'	158°50'	158°07'	157°12'	154°35'	150°29'	143°57'	133°13'	115°30'	90°
150°	149°37'	149°08'	148°26'	147°30'	146°19'	143°	138°04'	130°54'	120°39'	106°45'	90°
140°	139°34'	139°01'	138°14'	137°13'	135°54'	132°24'	127°27'	120°47'	112°11'	101°41'	90°
130°	129°34'	129°01'	128°15'	127°15'	126°	122°44'	118°20'	112°46'	106°	98°17'	90°
120°	119°37'	119°09'	118°29'	117°37'	116°34'	113°51'	110°21'	106°06'	101°10'	95°43'	90°
110°	109°48'	109°22'	108°53'	108°15'	107°30'	105°35'	103°10'	100°19'	97°06'	93°37'	90°
100°	99°51'	99°40'	99°24'	99°05'	98°41'	97°41'	96°28'	95°02'	93°27'	91°45'	90°

Fig. 61

read on the chisel (usually 1.5–2 cm), so that the shaft can move laterally abutting the side plate.

The space which forms between the elbow of the plate and the two femoral portions, metaphysis and diaphysis, is filled with bone fragments taken from the removed proximal segment of the lesser trochanter and from the bone wedge.

Should it be necessary to shorten the femur, a bone cylinder corresponding to the shortening desired is taken from the shaft and placed medially to the elbow of the plate. The angled plate is fixed to the proximal portion of the femur by means of a long cortical screw, which passes through the hole in the elbow of the plate, through the bone wedge, and grips the calcar femoris. The purchase obtained by this screw blocks backout of the blade from the neck when the osteotomy is compressed. The femoral shaft is adapted, reduced, and temporarily held to the plate with two Verbrügge clamps. The patella should face anteriorly in rotational alignment.

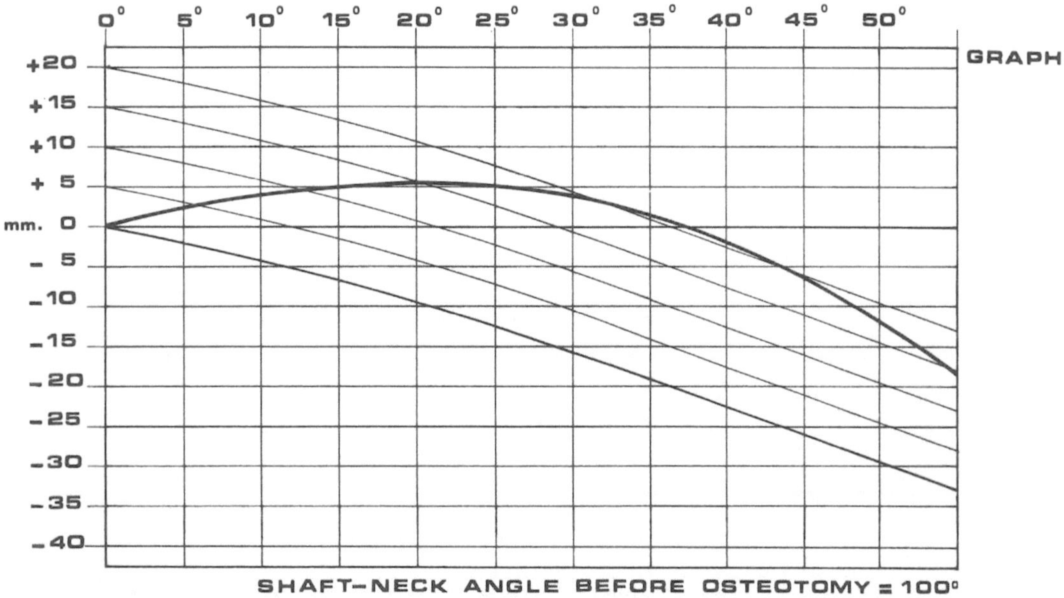

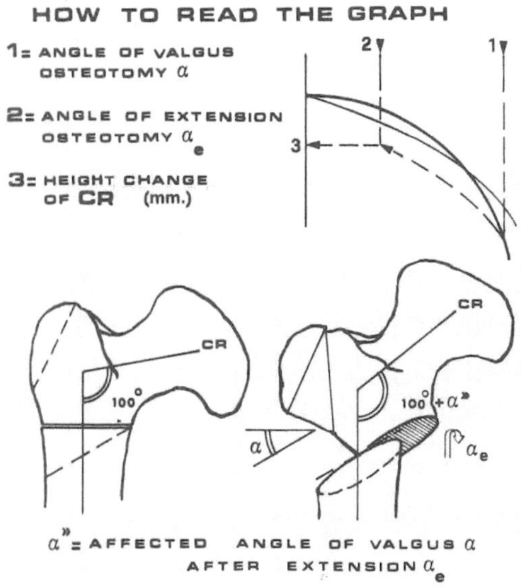

1/2 SHAFT DISPLACEMENT

TABLE

$\gamma = 100°$		ANGLE OF EXTENSION OSTEOTOMY						
		0°	10°	15°	20°	30°	40°	50°
ANGLE OF VALGUS OSTEOTOMY	0°	0.00	– 4.34	– 6.87	– 9.61	–15.63	–22.22	– 29.19
	10°	+ 8.30	+ 3.96	+ 1.43	– 1.31	– 7.33	–13.92	– 20.89
	15°	+11.87	+ 7.53	+ 5.00	+ 2.26	– 3.76	–10.35	– 17.32
	20°	+14.93	+10.59	+ 8.04	+ 5.32	– 0.70	– 7.29	– 14.26
	30°	+19.25	+14.91	+12.38	+ 9.64	+ 3.62	– 2.97	– 9.94
	40°	+20.49	+16.15	+13.62	+10.88	+ 4.86	– 1.73	– 8.70
	50°	+17.49	+13.15	+10.62	+ 7.88	+ 1.86	– 4.73	– 11.70

Fig. 62

A compression device is fixed to the distal part of the femur. After compression of the surfaces of the osteotomy and fixation of the plate to the shaft with cortical screws, the device is removed (Fig. 70).

The capsule is resutured. The bone wedge previously taken out is now placed in the artificial pocket created under the greater trochanter. The wedge does not need to be fixed with screws or wire; gentle impaction suffices.

Tables (Figs. 62–65) allow us to judge the alteration in length of the limb after such an osteotomy according to the CCD angle of the femur before the operation and the degree of valgus-extension osteotomy. To obtain the maximum lengthening of the limb (approximately 1.5 cm), the bone wedge should not be removed when carrying out a valgus-extension osteotomy.

Two sets of suction tubes are inserted; one leaves the wound at its distal extremity with the perforated sections lying along the medial side of the osteotomy line, the other at the proximal extremity with the perforated sections lying on

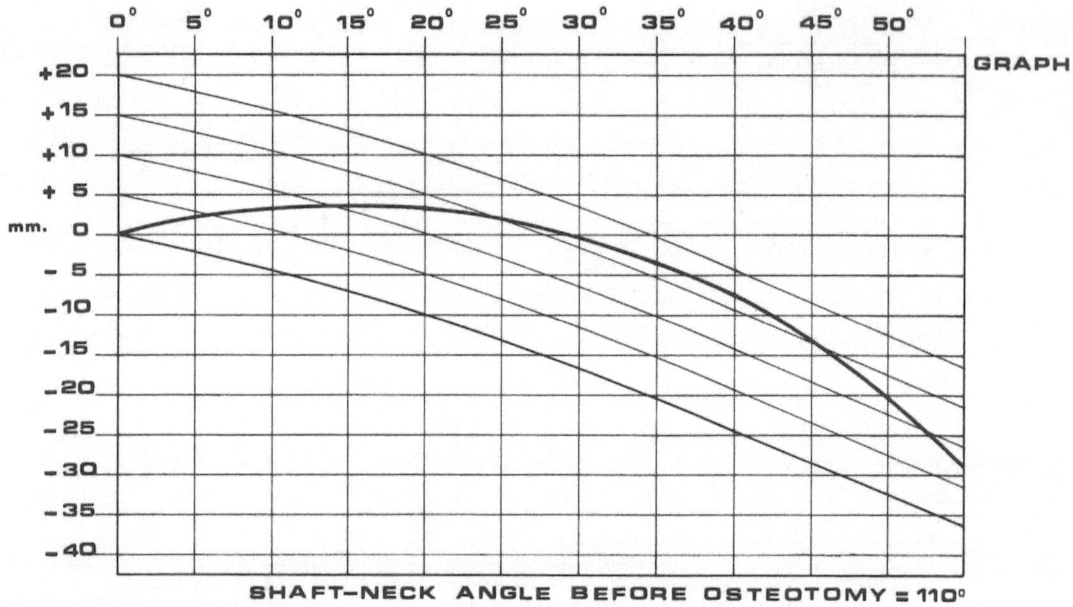

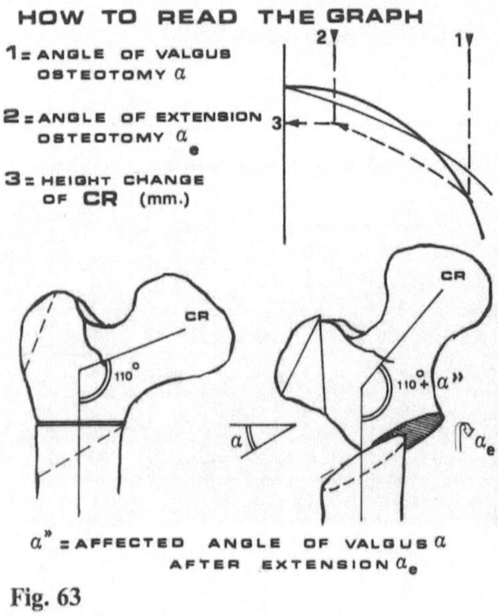

1/2 SHAFT DISPLACEMENT

TABLE

γ=110°		ANGLE OF EXTENSION OSTEOTOMY						
		0°	10°	15°	20°	30°	40°	50°
ANGLE OF VALGUS OSTEOTOMY	0°	0.00	– 4.48	– 7.19	–10.17	–16.87	–24.39	–32.50
	10°	+ 7.73	+ 3.25	+ 0.54	– 2.44	– 9.14	–16.66	–24.77
	15°	+10.91	+ 6.43	+ 3.72	+ 0.74	– 5.96	–13.48	–21.59
	20°	+13.53	+ 9.05	+ 6.34	+ 3.36	– 3.34	–10.86	–18.97
	30°	+16.77	+12.29	+ 9.58	+ 6.60	– 0.10	– 7.62	–15.73
	40°	+16.73	+12.25	+ 9.54	+ 6.20	– 0.14	– 7.66	–15.77
	50°	+12.28	+ 7.80	+ 5.09	+ 2.11	– 4.59	–12.11	–20.22

Fig. 63

the intermuscular septum between the shaft and the vastus lateralis. The vastus lateralis muscle is stitched to the lateral intermuscular septum and proximally to the portion left attached to the inferior margin of the greater trochanter. Deep closure with an absorbable material (e.g., Dexon) reduces the late foreign body reaction seen with nonabsorbable sutures. A third set of suction tubes is inserted between the vastus lateralis and the fascia lata and leaves the wound distally. The fascia lata and skin are closed in layers, and finally a compressive dressing is applied.

Postoperative Management

We leave the six suction drains in place for 48 h. We do not use anticoagulants or antibiotics on a prophylactic basis. The patients is encouraged to perform chin-up exercises with the trapeze in bed the day after the operation, and after 5 days he may walk with two crutches.

When he walks, he must set one foot directly in front of the other. In this way he stretches the ligamentum teres and the craniolateral zone of the joint capsule. He is encouraged to exercise the limb and the body as much as possible, with partial weight-bearing for about 6 months using

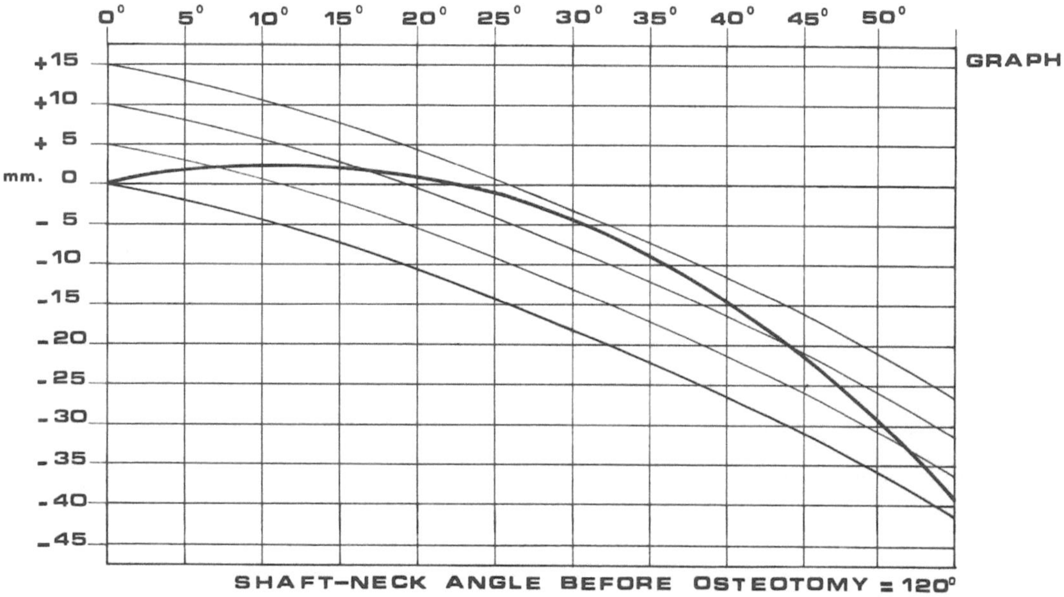

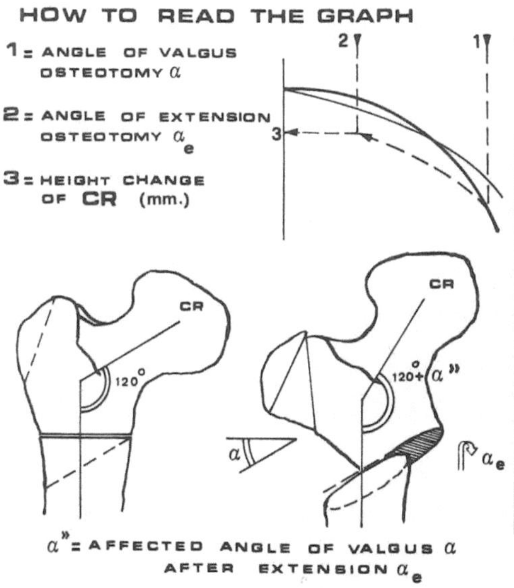

1/2 SHAFT DISPLACEMENT

TABLE

γ = 120°		ANGLE OF EXTENSION OSTEOTOMY						
		0°	10°	15°	20°	30°	40°	50°
ANGLE OF VALGUS OSTEOTOMY	0°	0.00	– 4.62	– 7.48	–10.69	–18.03	–26.42	–35.61
	10°	+ 6.89	+ 2.27	– 0.59	– 3.80	–11.14	–19.53	–28.72
	15°	+ 9.56	+ 4.94	+ 2.08	– 1.13	– 8.47	–16.86	–26.05
	20°	+11.62	+ 7.00	+ 4.14	+ 0.93	– 6.40	–14.80	–23.99
	30°	+13.58	+ 8.96	+ 6.10	+ 2.89	– 4.45	–12.84	–22.03
	40°	+12.09	+ 7.47	+ 4.61	+ 1.40	– 5.94	–14.33	–23.52
	50°	+ 6.07	+ 1.45	– 1.41	– 4.62	–11.96	– 20.35	–29.54

Fig. 64

two crutches. Sometimes may use one crutch for an additional 2 or 3 months.

Varus Osteotomy

Indications

The indications for varus osteotomy (Table 3) are as follows:

1. Coxa valga with spherical head combined with a WBS from 0° to craniolateral inclination of 15°–20°. In younger patients (under 35 years) varus osteotomy must be combined with a pelvic osteotomy or acetabuloplasty. When the WBS is craniolaterally inclined, extension must be combined with varus.
2. Concentric osteoarthritis.
3. Overuse osteoarthritis during the early phase, when the head is still spherical and the floor osteophyte has not yet fused with the curtain osteophyte.

Aims

Since the pathological process has damaged the bone and cartilage of the weight-bearing sector

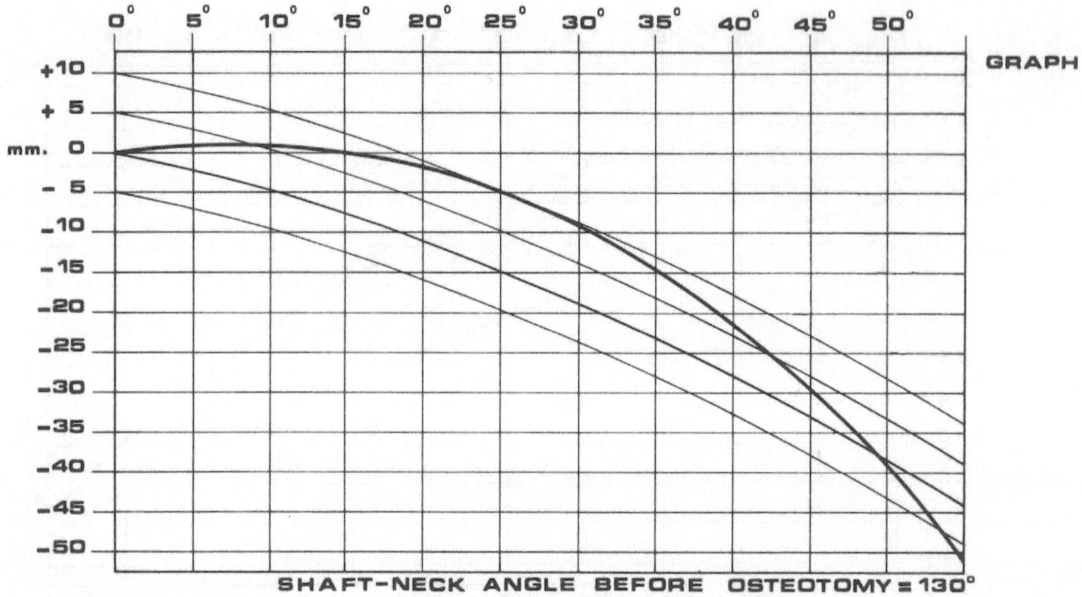

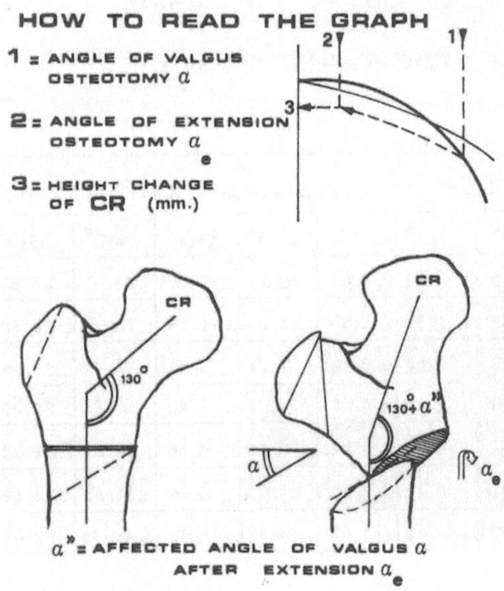

1/2 SHAFT DISPLACEMENT

TABLE

γ = 130°		ANGLE OF EXTENSION OSTEOTOMY						
		0°	10°	15°	20°	30°	40°	50°
ANGLE OF VALGUS OSTEOTOMY	0°	0.00	– 4.74	– 7.75	–11.16	–19.09	–28.26	–38.41
	10°	+ 5.82	+ 1.08	– 1.93	– 5.34	– 13.27	–22.44	–32.59
	15°	+ 7.87	+ 3.13	+ 0.12	– 3.29	– 11.22	–20.39	–30.54
	20°	+ 9.26	+ 4.52	+ 1.51	– 1.90	– 9.83	–19.00	–29.15
	30°	+ 9.78	+ 5.04	+ 2.03	– 1.38	– 9.31	–18.48	–28.63
	40°	+ 6.72	+ 1.98	– 1.03	– 4.44	– 12.37	–21.54	–31.69
	50°	– 0.95	– 5.69	– 8.70	– 12.11	– 20.05	–29.21	–39.36

Fig. 65

through an abnormally high compressive force $P_R(K+P_M)$, varus osteotomy aims to:

1. Reduce force P_M by increasing lever arm *a* of the abductors and by making their direction more horizontal (Fig. 66).
2. Exploit the biological response of patients over the age of 35 to create a roof osteophyte, thereby spontaneously correcting the abnormal inclination of WBS to 0° (horizontal). This is accomplished by a temporary Trendelenburg gait (Fig. 67).
3. Maintain the mechanical axis through the center of the knee, avoiding genu varus [see 6].

Technique

Preparation. The angle of varus can be found in the way described by Pauwels [24]. From an AP X-ray of the hip on which the axis of the shaft is dotted, an outline of the head, neck,

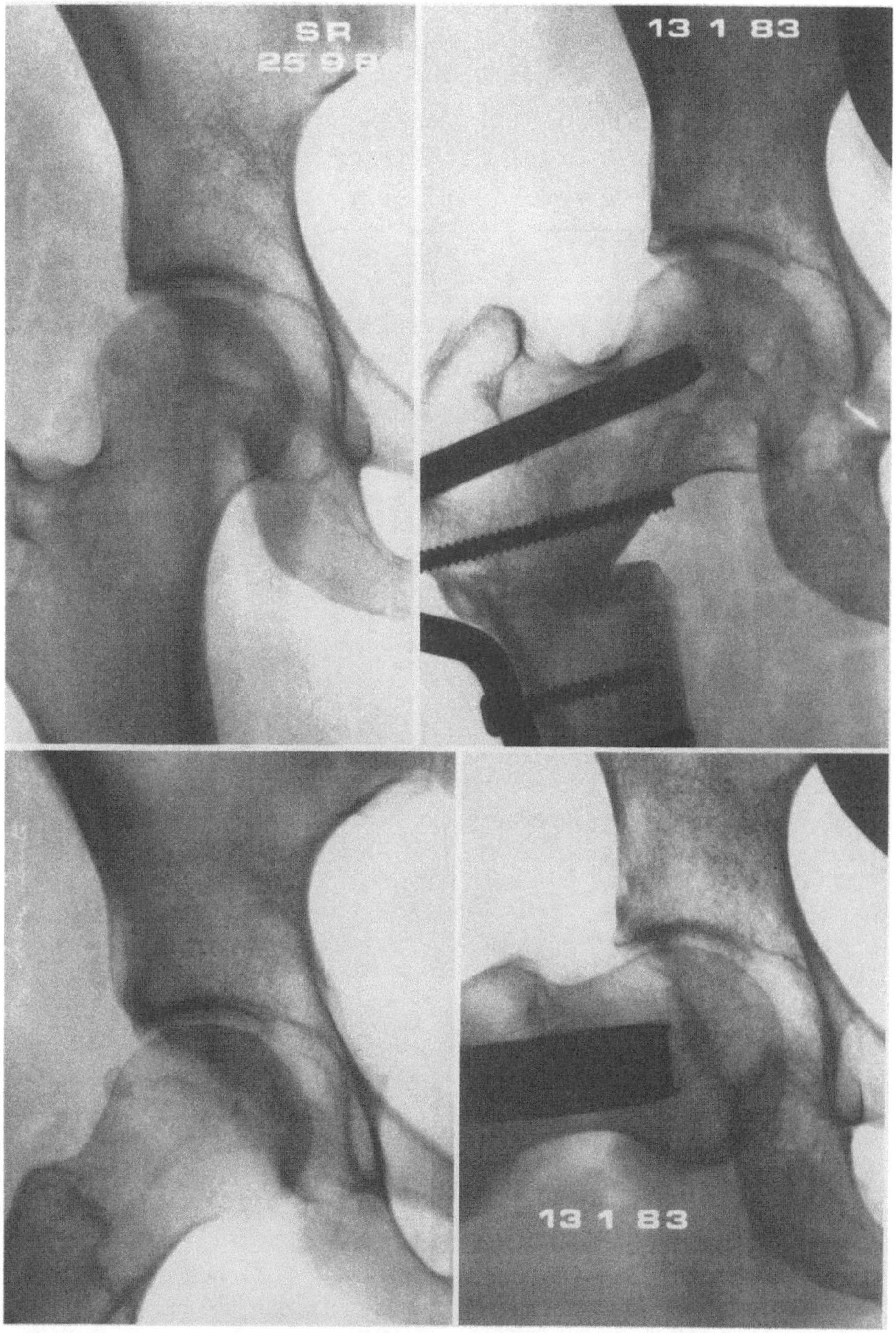

Fig. 66. Aims of varus osteotomy. In order to decrease P_M the greater trochanter is shifted cranially with the proximal fragment. Lever arm *a* increases in length and the direction of the abductors becomes more horizontal

metaphysis and part of the shaft of the femur is drawn on tracing paper, marking the axis of the shaft. The tracing of the head, superimposed on the original X-ray, is turned inwards in the socket until maximum concentric coverage of the head by the acetabulum is obtained. The angle between the axis of the shaft on the tracing paper and the axis of the shaft on the X-ray is determined: this is the angle of varus correction.

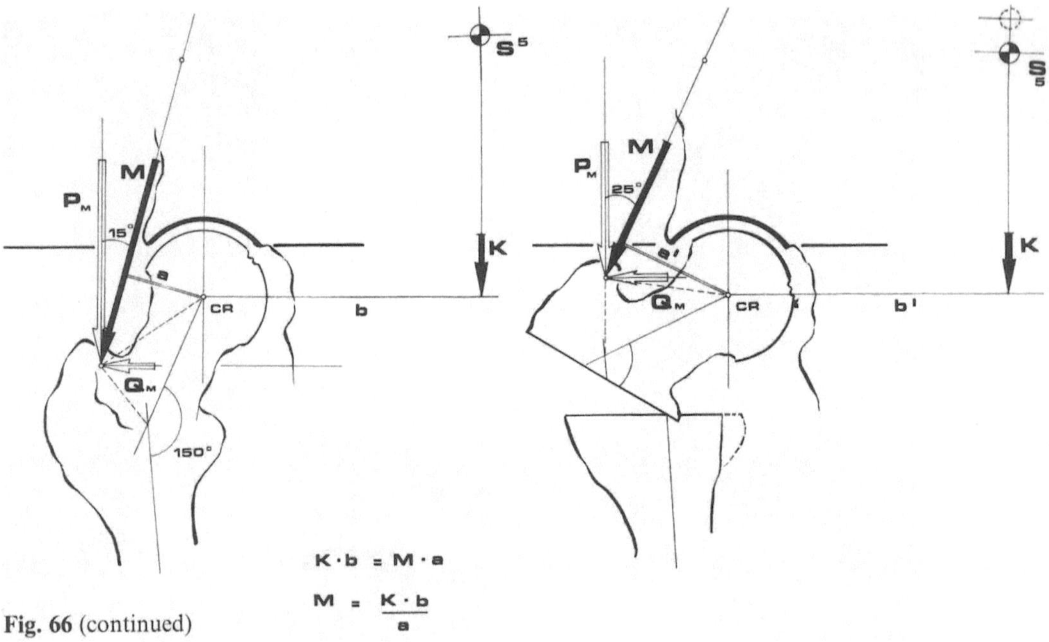

Fig. 66 (continued)

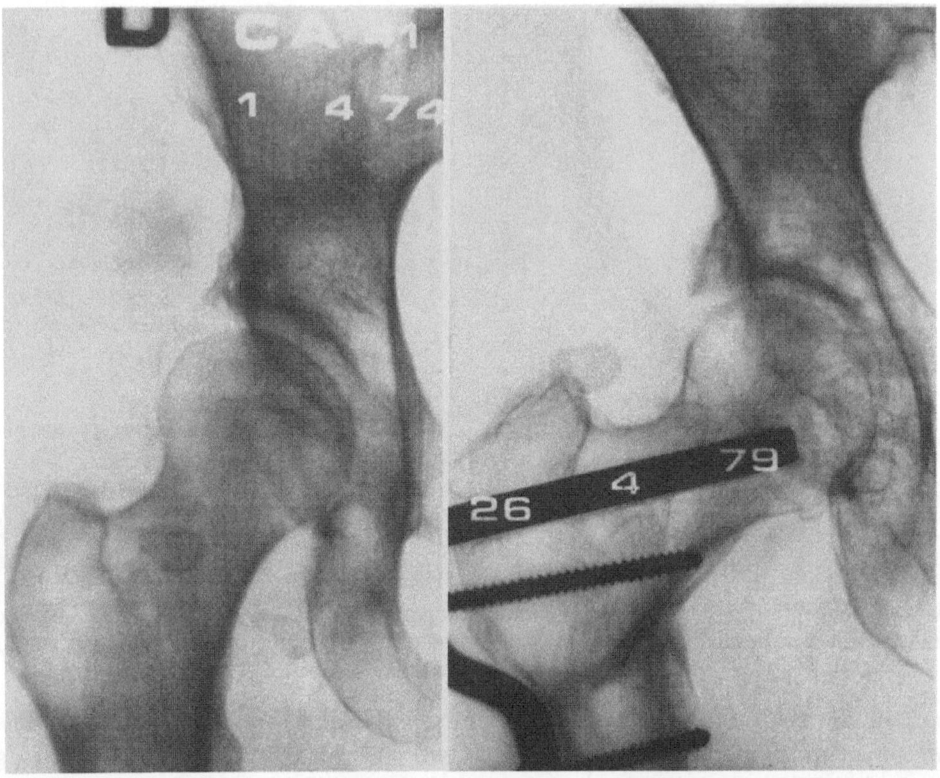

Fig. 67. C.A., aged 41. Varus osteotomy for coxa valga, spherical head and craniolateral inclination of the WBS. Compressive forces are diminished by cranial migration of the greater trochanter. An intermittent and transient Trendelenburg gait stimulates the roof osteophyte to horizontalize the WBS

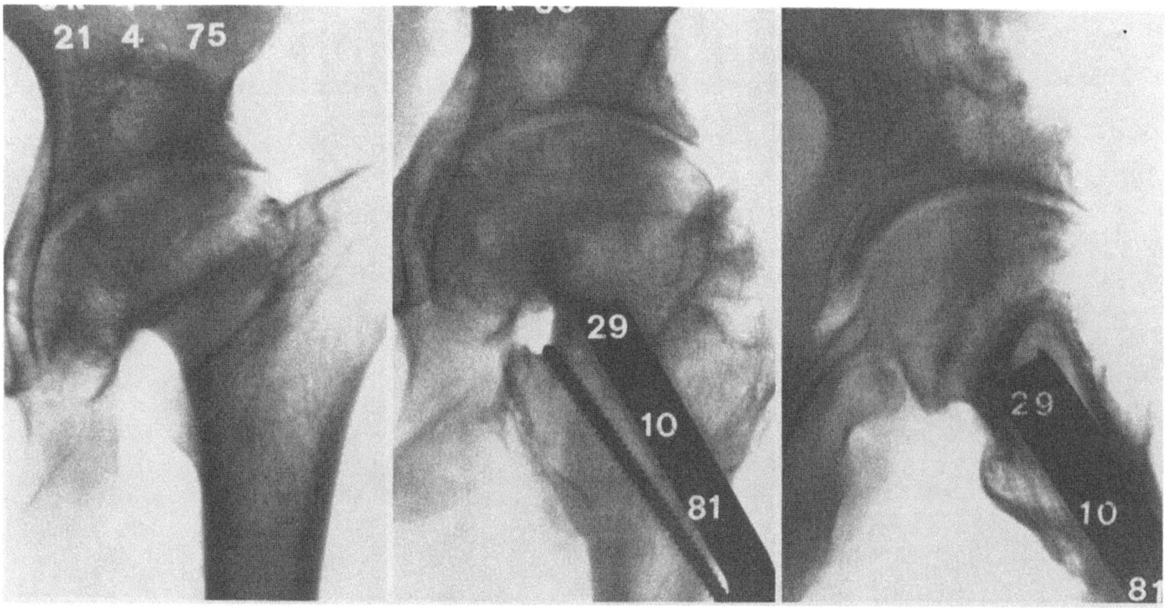

Fig. 68. G.R., aged 44. Valgus-extension osteotomy in coxa vara with elliptical head. The limb usually needs to be lengthened. The resting lenght of the abductors is reconstituted, eliminating the Trendelenburg gait, and the lateral capsule is placed under constant tension, stimulating a roof osteophyte to horizontalize the WBS

Varus osteotomy always shortens the femur. Figure 73 indicates the exact amount of shortening, which depends on whether no bone wedge or a bone wedge of full or half thickness is removed. When a bone wedge must be removed, it is advisable to cut it from the distal fragment, otherwise Adam's arch becomes weaked.

Operation. The patient lies supine on the operating table and the approach is similar to that already described for valgus osteotomy (i.e., Watson-Jones), including the opening of the capsule and the insertion of the Hohmann retractors. The seating chisel is inserted into the neck of the femur. The apex of the chisel must lie in the inferior quadrants of the femoral head, and the inclination of the chisel to the axis of the shaft of the femur depends upon the degree of varus to be realized.

The AO 90°-angled plate is, in the author's opinion, advisable. If a 90°-angled plate is utilized and a varus correction of 20° is necessary, the chisel preparing the blade channel must be introduced into the neck of the femur at an angle of 70° to the axis of the shaft.

On the frontal plane the angle between the chisel and the axis of the shaft of the femur must be 90° minus the angle of correction. Therefore:

To obtain a varus of 10°: $90° - 10° = 80°$
To obtain a varus of 20°: $90° - 20° = 70°$
To obtain a varus of 30°: $90° - 30° = 60°$
and so on (Fig. 74).

These two prerequisites make the choice of the point of entry of the seating chisel through the lateral cortex very simple; the more varus indicated, the lower the point of entry. The location of the lesser trochanter, the height of which varies according to the CCD angle, plays no role in determining the point of entrance.

Having chosen the exact point of entry on the lateral cortex, when the anterior quadrants of the head are uncovered we must flex the limb in order to relocate the head into the acetabulum. This procedure is easily controlled when the joint is opened anteriorly and the head inspected. The angle between the shaft of the femur and the table is the angle of extension required. The seating chisel is then inserted with blade perpendicular in the cortex, making the required angle with the shaft in the frontal plane (for varus of 20° the angle is 70°). The osteotomy cut is made 1.5 cm below the point of

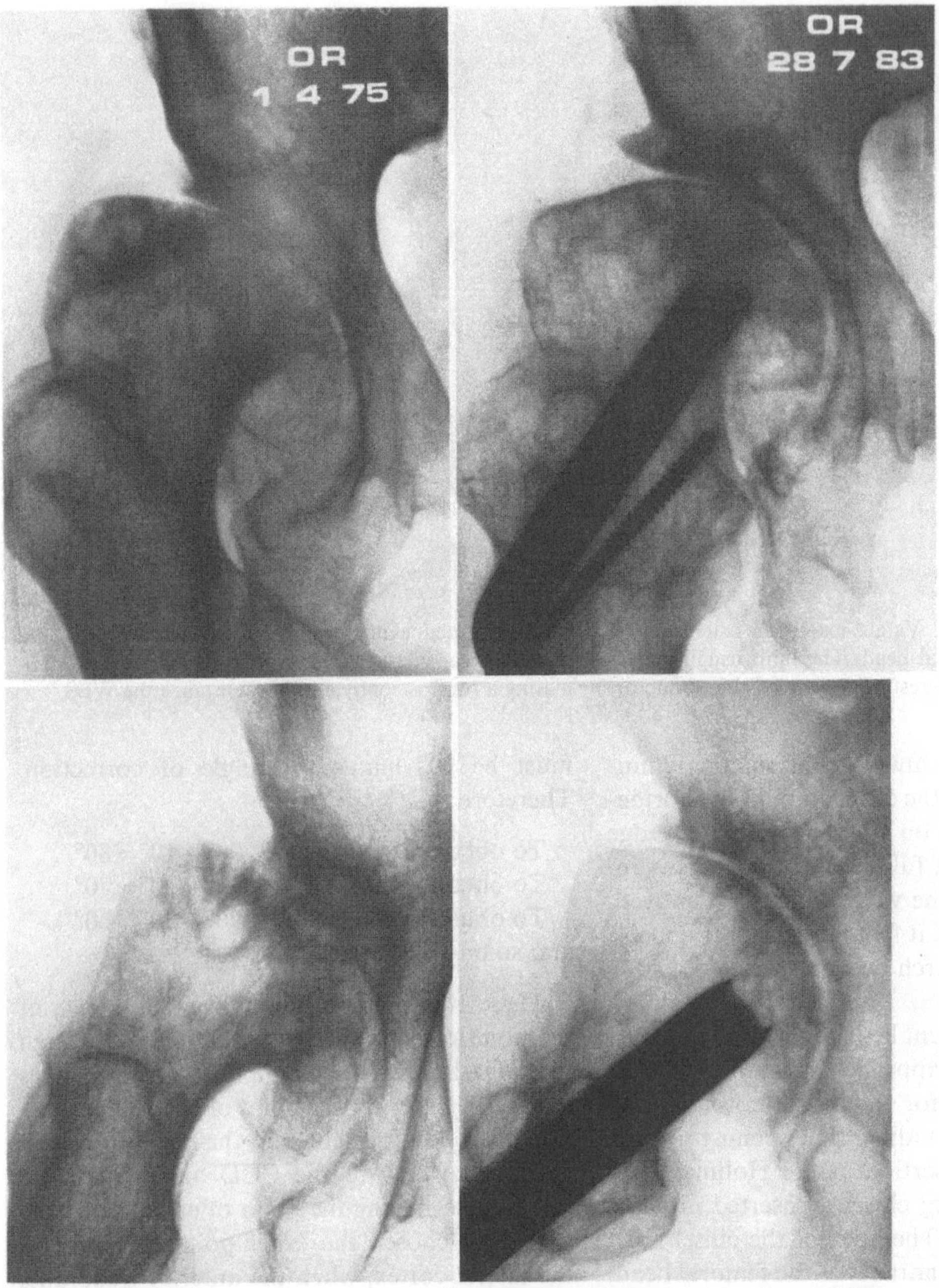

Fig. 69. O.R., aged 65. The radiographs demonstrate 8-year follow-up of valgus-extension osteotomy in mechanical craniolateral OA in a 65-year-old woman. The drawings illustrate the aim of this osteotomy: to realign the WBS to the horizontal by stimulating a roof osteophyte, decreasing the forces by temporarily medializing *CR* to CR_1, and transferring contact to the painless medial osteophytes. In time, cartilage regeneration increases the area of surface contact and *CR* returns to normal

entry in order to have enough cortical bone to apply compression later.

After the bone has been transected, the assistant adducts and externally rotates the limb and the surgeon, pulling a hook placed in the medullary canal of the shaft, exposes the lesser trochanter and cuts the iliopsoas tendon (to reduce the permanent compression). When the lesser trochanter is inserted on the distal fragment, part or all of it is sawn off and will serve as

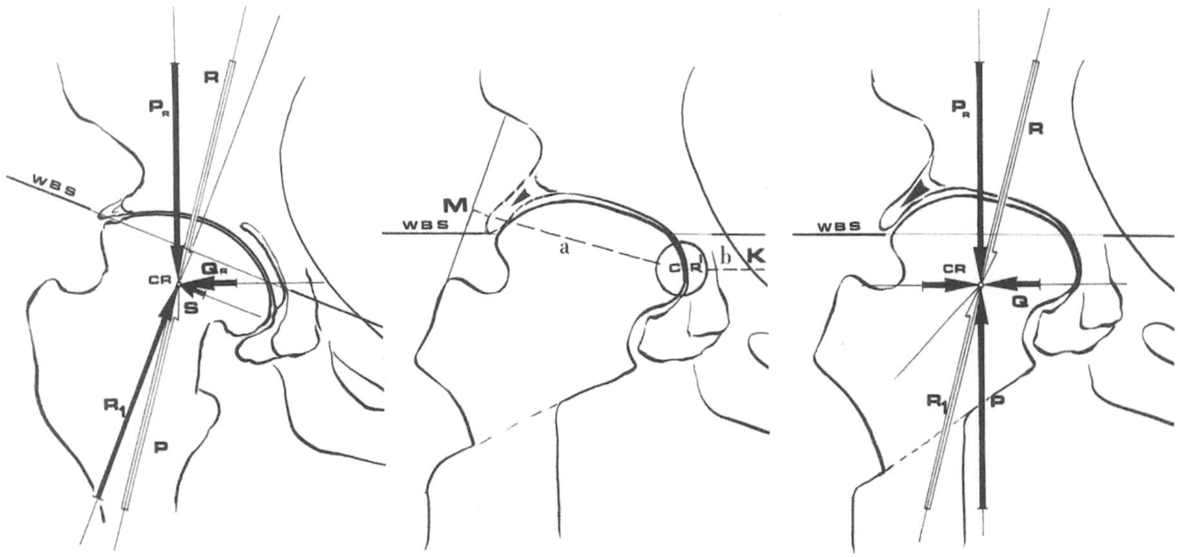

Fig. 69 (continued)

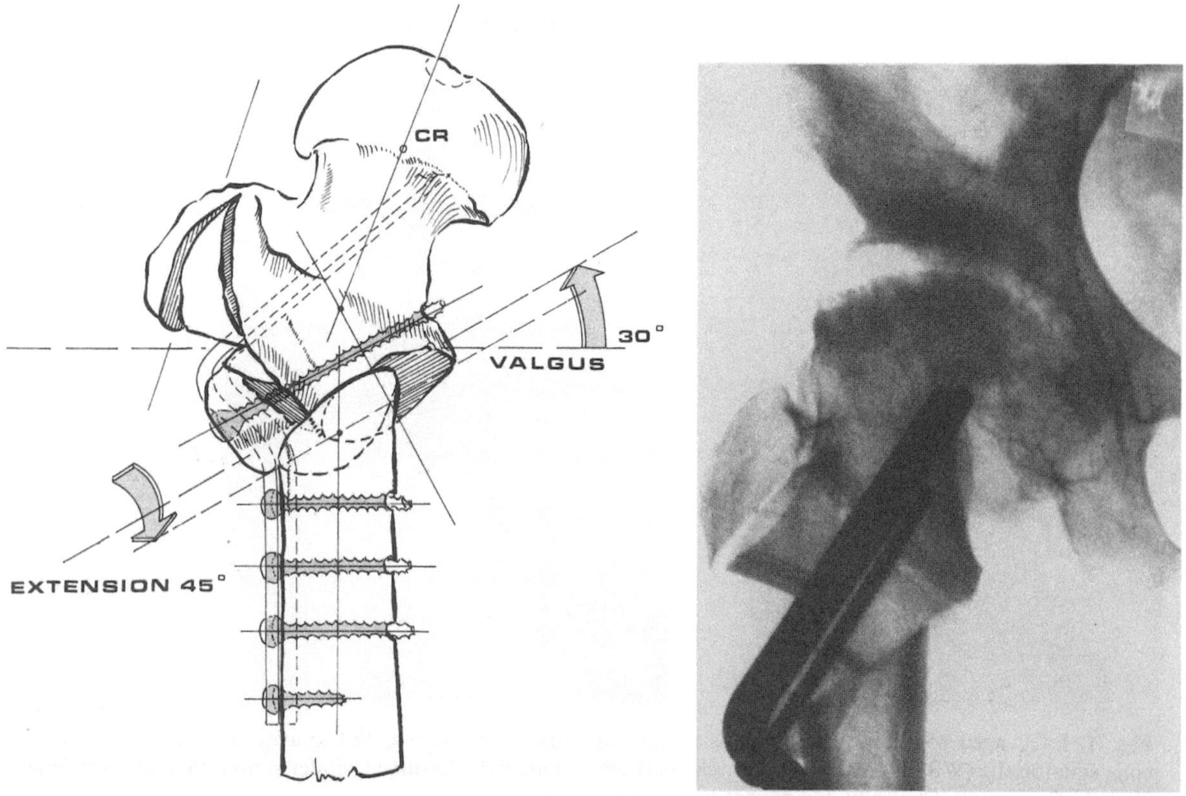

Fig. 70. Diagram of valgus-extension osteotomy. The proximal fragment is flexed and shifted into valgus. The distal fragment is returned to neutral, shifted laterally, and compressed with a 130° blade plate. Osteotomy of the greater trochanter leaves a cranially based hinge with anterior and posterior soft tissue pocket. Bone graft is inserted under the elbow and held by a long cortical screw across to the calcar

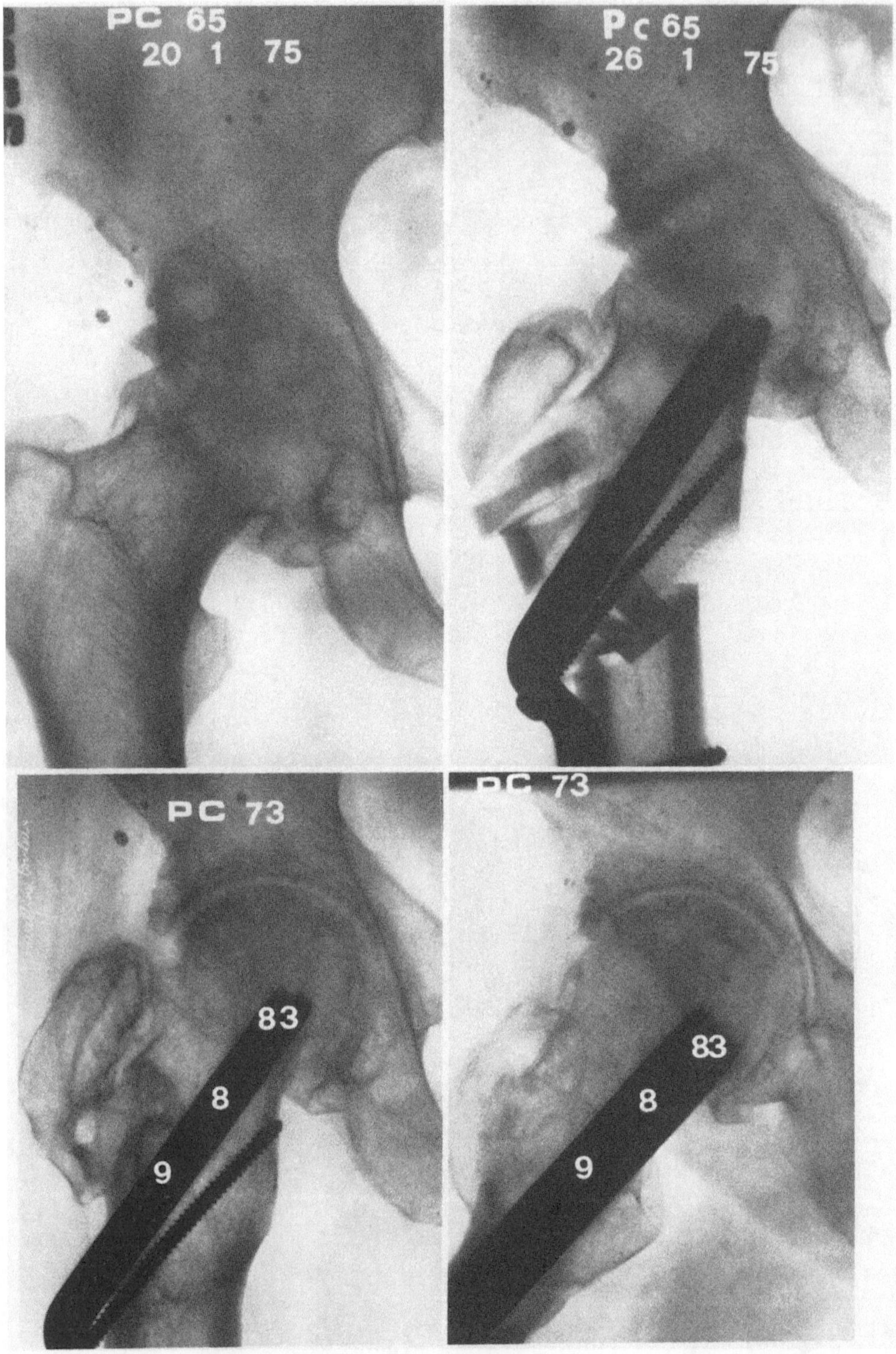

Fig. 71. P.C., aged 65. Effect of valgus osteotomy in coxa equatorialis (WBS is craniomedial; neck-shaft angle is 130°, normal). Clinically, the patient has no limp or pain and the joint has regenerated. Greater trochanter osteotomy is essential to avoid an increase of P_M. The removal of a bone cylinder is necessary to avoid lengthening.

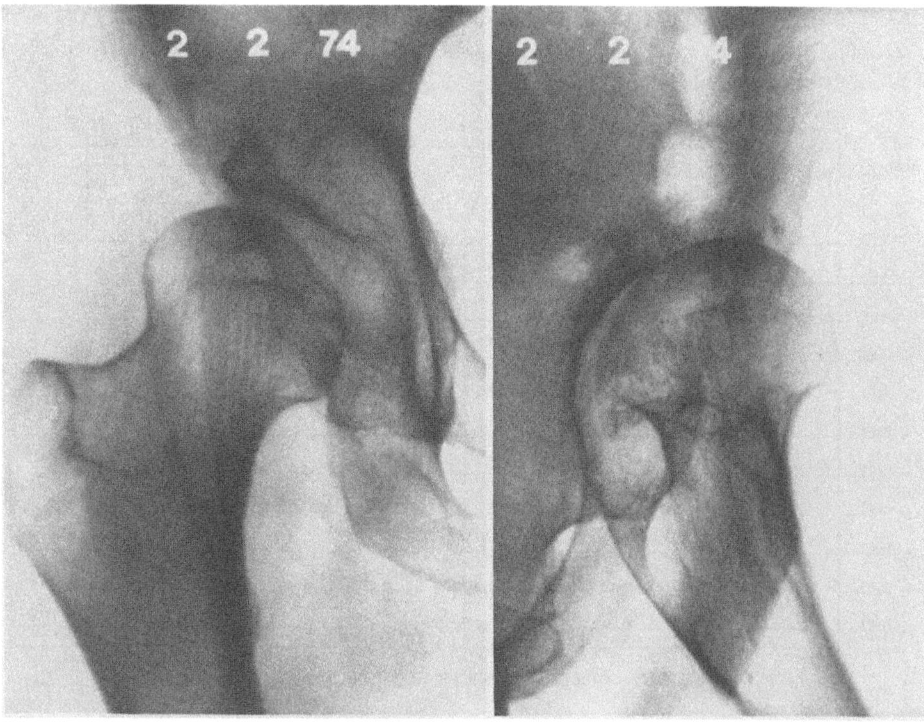

Fig. 72. 2.2.1974. With craniolateral inclination of the WBS the expulsion forces ($Q_R + S$) sublux the head not only craniolaterally, but also anteriorly (see axial view)

a bone graft to fill the osteotomy line. When part or all of the lesser trochanter is inserted at the proximal fragment it will be preserved, because it offers a good medial support for the distal fragments.

The chisel is removed, and along its track in the femoral neck the blade of a 90°-angled plate is inserted. The insertion of the blade into the neck must be gentle in order to avoid incorrect direction. When the elbow of the implant is in contact with the cortex of the metaphysis, its plate is in contact with the lateral surface of the femoral shaft, which, due to the elbow, is also shifted medially. The degree of medial displacement depends on the depth of the elbow (10–20 mm). The femoral shaft must be displaced inward for two reasons: (a) to prevent varus in the knee, and (b) to prevent excessive bending stress and strain in the neck of the femur.

It is advisable to drive a cortical screw into the hole of the elbow, the apex of the screw gripping the calcar femorale. This screw prevents lateral extrusion of the blade during the compression, and with the blade forms a hinge in the femoral neck. This hinge is very convenient when extension is indicated as well as varus. The blade by itself may act as a pivot, and if the cancellous bone is not hard enough, may wobble, preventing achievement of the exact degree of extension. The femoral shaft is positioned to ensure that the patella points directly upwards. A tension device is fixed to the shaft.

When no bone wedge is removed (to reduce the shortening of the femur), a wedge-shaped empty space with an anterolateral base is apparent (Fig. 75). Before tightening the tension device the previously removed part or whole of the lesser trochanter is inserted into this empty space. Four screws, three holding both cortices and the distal one only the lateral cortex, are driven through the plate into the shaft.

The opening in the joint capsule is sutured. The vastus lateralis is stitched to the intermuscular septum and to the free edge of its tendon left inserted on the greater trochanter. The aponeurosis of the iliotibial band and the skin are closed. We use absorbable sutures and six suc-

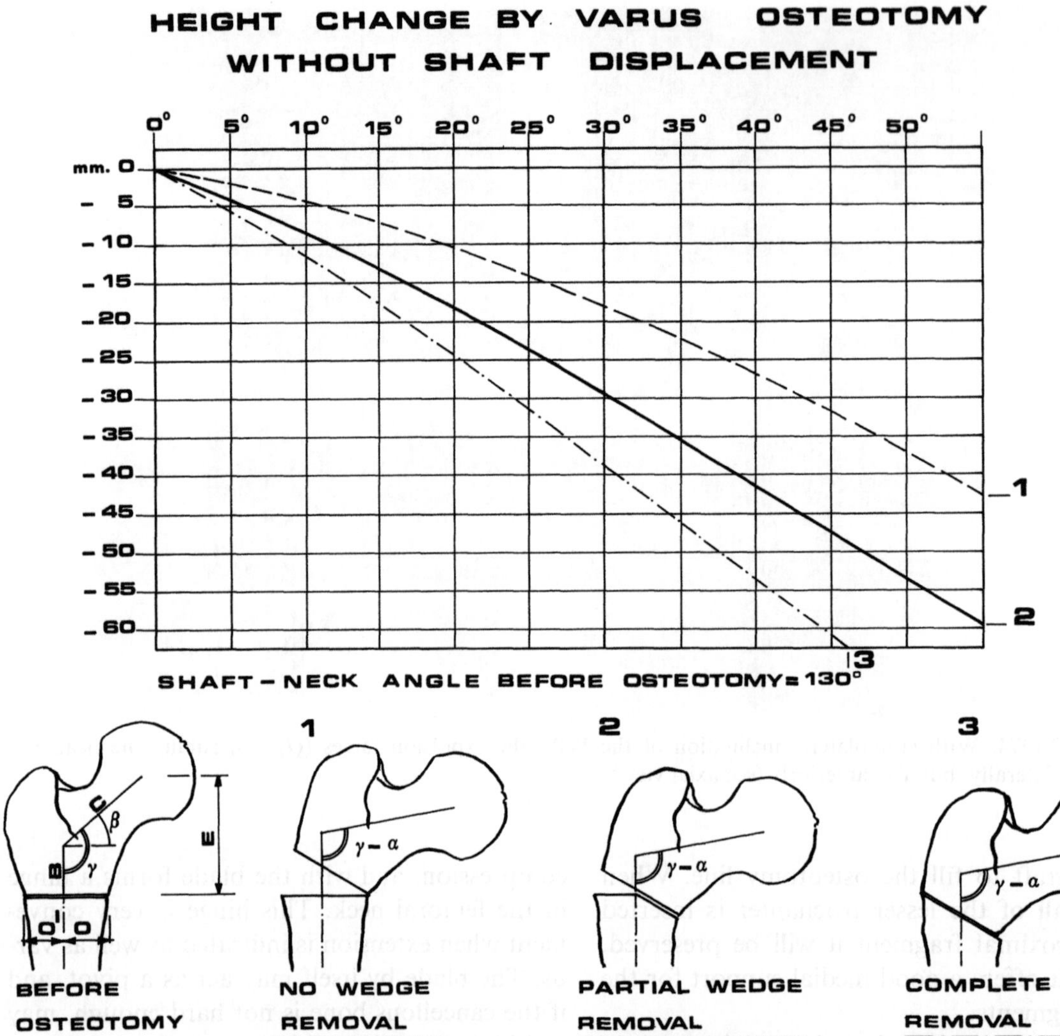

$\Delta h = E\alpha - E$

1 $E\alpha = B\cos\alpha + C\sin(\beta - \alpha) + O'\sin\alpha$

2 $E\alpha = B\cos\alpha + C\sin(\beta - \alpha)$

3 $E\alpha = B\cos\alpha + C\sin(\beta - \alpha) - O\sin\alpha$

Fig. 73. Actual shortening of femur according to the type of varus osteotomy

tion drains, four under the vastus lateralis and two between the vastus lateralis and the tensor fasciae latae, which are left in place for 48 h. The limb, slightly flexed, rests on a rubber splint (Fig. 67).

Postoperative Management

The postoperative treatment is similar to that after valgus-extension osteotomy. Beginning 24 h after operation, the patient moves the hip and the knee freely in bed and does exercises with the upper limbs and the nonoperated limb. Walking with a walker is permitted 4–5 days after operation, with partial weight-bearing (15–20 kg). On the 6th or 7th day the patient walks with two elbow crutches and from the 6th or 7th day is taught active exercises. Passive exercises and physiotherapy are not allowed. Movement must cause no discomfort. On the 15th day the patient leaves hospital. He walks

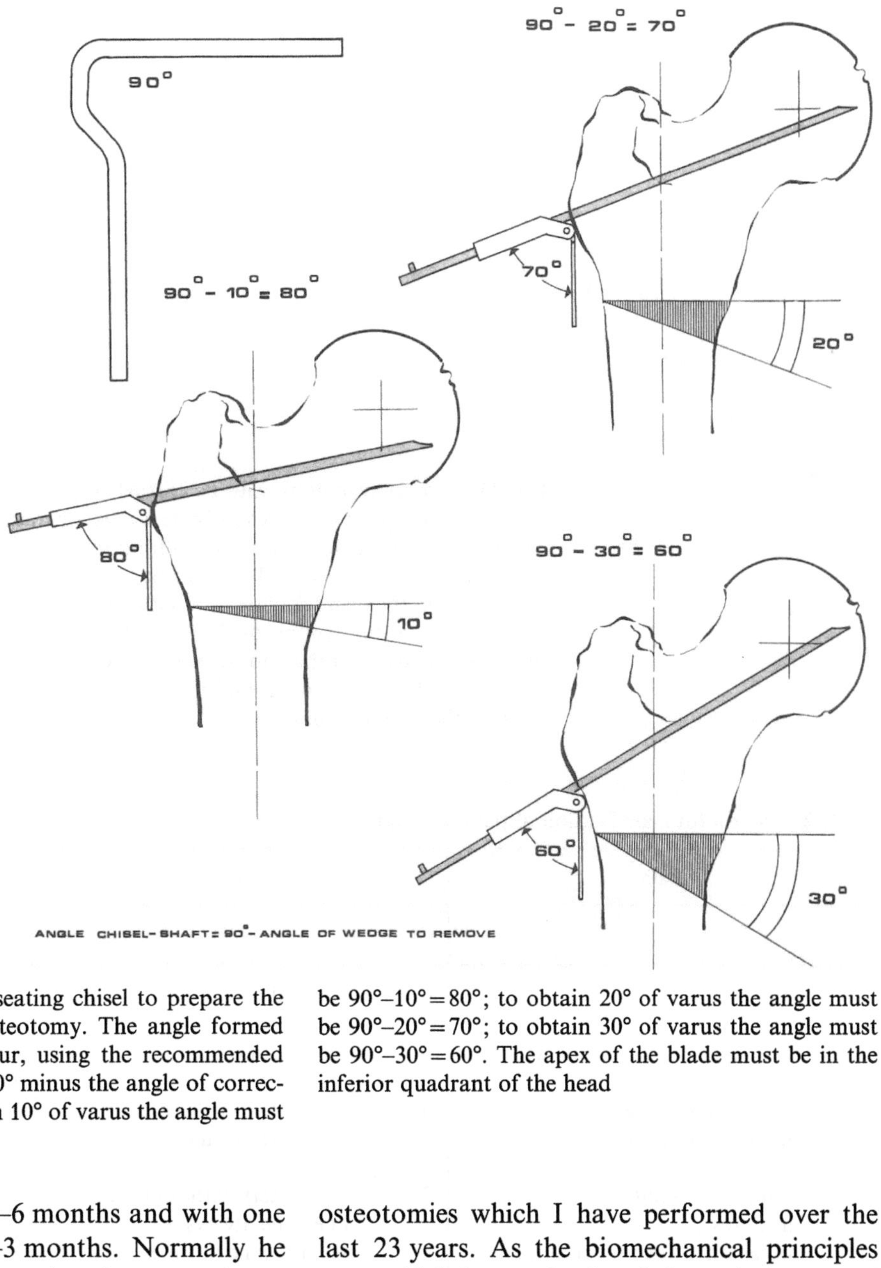

Fig. 74. How to insert the seating chisel to prepare the blade channel for varus osteotomy. The angle formed by chisel and shaft of femur, using the recommended 90°-angled plate, must be 90° minus the angle of correction. For instance, to obtain 10° of varus the angle must be 90°–10° = 80°; to obtain 20° of varus the angle must be 90°–20° = 70°; to obtain 30° of varus the angle must be 90°–30° = 60°. The apex of the blade must be in the inferior quadrant of the head

with two crutches for 5–6 months and with one crutch for a further 2–3 months. Normally he can drive a car $2^1/_2$–3 months after operation.

Results

In 1979 and 1980, four doctors interviewed, examined, and radiographed over 1,000 patients with a minimum period of 3 years since valgus or varus osteotomy of the hip. The longest follow-up in this series was 9 years and the average about 5 years. This group of patients represents approximately one-third of the total number of osteotomies which I have performed over the last 23 years. As the biomechanical principles were still being evolved and the techniques and instrumentation perfected during the early years, these patients operated on between 1971 and 1978 were selected to represent standardized application of principles and techniques.

Results are based upon pre- and postoperative grading according to three categories of hip function based on Merle D'Aubigné [33] (Table 2). The detailed statistics presented in the second edition of my book [6] have for practical application been simplified and reorganized here.

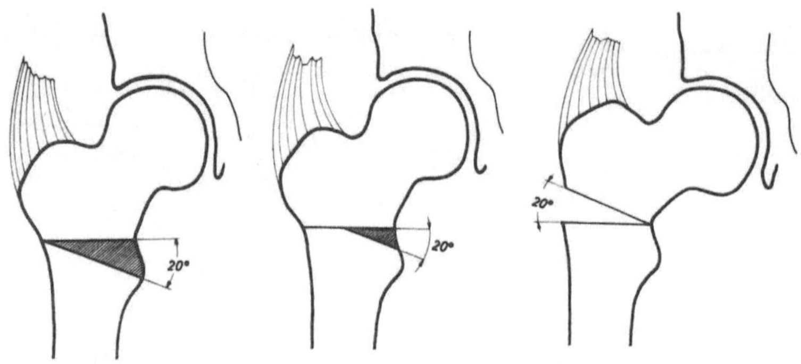

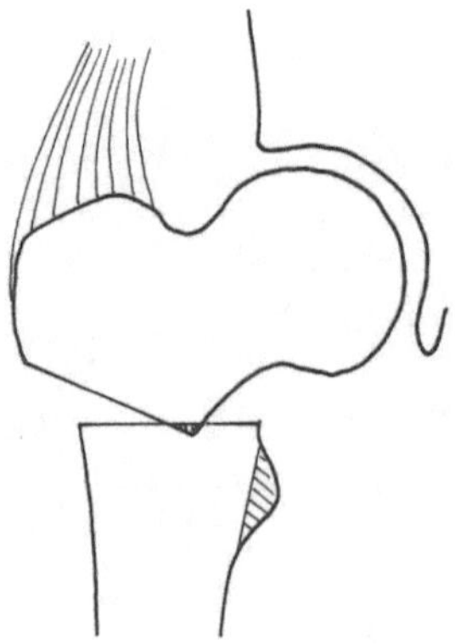

Fig. 75. A varus osteotomy can be carried out by removing a full-thickness bone wedge, removing a half-thickness bone wedge, or transversely dividing the intertrochanteric region of the femur and shifting the superior fragment upward without removing any bone wedge. When a bone wedge must be removed, it is advisable to cut it from the distal fragment, otherwise Adam's arch is weakened. It is always useful to divide the tendon of iliopsoas in order to reduce constant compression on joint. The femoral shaft must be displaced inwards for two reasons: to prevent varus in the knee (in presence of a normal knee) and to prevent excessive bending stress in the neck of femur

Table 2. Criteria for classification of pain, gait, and motion in OA of the hip (Merle D'Aubigne [33])

Pain		Gait		Motion	
Class		Class		Class	
6	None	6	Normal	M	*Mobile* Flexion 60° ABD 15° ADD 15°
5	Occasional ache on full activity	5	Fatigue; no limp		
4	Ache on walking; no discomfort at rest	4	500 meters without cane; one cane at times	HY	*Hypomobile* Flexion 30–60° ABD 15° ADD 15°
3	Pain on walking; ache rest; occasional discomfort at night	3	100 meters without cane; one cane always; second cane at times		
2	Frequent pain at night	2	Two canes always	S	*Stiff* Flexion 30° ABD 15° ADD 15°
1	Chronic pain; severely impaired activity	1	Two crutches always		

Varus Osteotomy

Four indications were followed (see Table 3) and the osteotomies were carried out according to the principles described above.

The complete data are presented in Table 4. An 81% follow-up was achieved despite four deaths. The indications differed in sex predominance and in frequency of cases, but not in actual results.

Table 3. Indications for varus osteotomy

WBS	Type	Head	Osteophytes
1. Horizontal	Concentric	Spherical	Normal
2. Craniolateral	a	Spherical	Early
3. Craniolateral	d_1	Spherical	Early
4. Horizontal	Coxa valga	Spherical	Early

Table 4. Results of varus osteotomy in concentric and craniolateral (CL) types a and d_1 OA

1971–1978: 294 operations performed
4 deaths reported

1980: 238 patients (81%) returned for evaluation
minimum follow-up 3 years

Indication	Number of cases	Average age	Sex predominance
Concentric			
CL a	212	49	86% women
CL d_1	26	53	81% men
		Pain	
Improved	234 (98%)	*Preoperative:*	*Postoperative:*
Same	4 (2%)	236 (99%)	222 (93%)
Worse	0 (0%)	in classes 1–4	in classes 5–6
		Gait	
Improved	216 (91%)	*Preoperative:*	*Postoperative:*
Same	19 (8%)	222 (93%)	188 (79%)
Worse	3 (1%)	in classes 3–4	in classes 5–6
Trendelenburg:		29 (12%)	61 (26%)
		Motion	
Improved	40 (17%)	*Preoperative:*	*Postoperative:*
Same	190 (80%)	26 stiff (11%)	12/26 mobile (46%)
Worse	8 (3%)		No stiff hips created

Typical candidate (49-year-old woman)	*Typical results*
Class 2: pain ($n=106$)	3–4 classes improvement (95; 90%)
Class 3: gait ($n=128$)	2–3 classes improvement (93; 73%)

Table 5. Indications for valgus osteotomy

WBS	Type	Head	Osteophytes
Valgus-extension			
1. Craniolateral	b	Elliptical	Normal-hypertrophic
2. Craniolateral	c	Elliptical	Normal-hypertrophic
3. Craniolateral	d_2	Elliptical	Normal-hypertrophic
Valgus-flexion			
4. Craniomedial	a	Spherical	Normal
5. Craniomedial	b	Spherical	Normal
Pure valgus or trochanteric transfer			
6. Horizontal	Coxa vara	Spherical	Fatigue fracture of neck

Pain relief was very reliable; in fact, dramatic relief was experienced in 90% of cases. Gait improvement was slightly less dramatic, but over 90% of patients showed some change for the better. Trendelenburg gait was created in some cases, but was not pronounced.

The typical patient was a 49-year-old woman with frequent night pain, barely able to walk 100 meters without a cane. After osteotomy she resumed normal activity without a cane and complained of only occasional aching. Motion was generally maintained rather than increased. No stiff hips were created, in spite of a minor (3%) risk of losing some mobility.

Valgus-Extension Osteotomy

Table 5 outlines the indications followed for valgus-extension osteotomy. Craniolateral type b OA with atrophy is no longer an indication for osteotomy, as the results are generally not good, and is reported separately in Table 7.

The valgus-extension osteotomies performed for mechanical, normotrophic OA were successful (Table 6). Over 500 returned for review. Craniolateral type b was the most common indication and women were predominant in all

Table 6. Results of valgus-extension osteotomy in craniolateral types b, c, and d_2 OA

1972–1977:	789	operations performed (normal to hypertrophic)
	27	deaths reported
1980:	578	patients (73%) returned for evaluation (Minimum follow-up 3 years)

Indication	Number of cases	Average age	Sex predominance
Type b	662	34	74% women
Type c	35	32	85% women
Type d_2	92	50	96% men

	Pain		
Improved	562 (97%)	*Preoperative:* 551 (95%) in classes 1–4	*Postoperative:* 527 (91%) in classes 5–6
Same	16 (3%)		
Worse	0 (0%)		
	Gait		
Improved	505 (87%)	*Preoperative:* 511 (88%) in classes 3–4	*Postoperative:* 444 (77%) in classes 5–6
Same	57 (10%)		
Worse	16 (3%)		
	Motion		
Improved	194 (34%)	*Preoperative:* 175 stiff (30%)	*Postoperative:* 46/175 mobile (26%) 16 (3%) became stiff
Same	340 (59%)		
Worse	44 (8%)		

Typical candidate	*Typical results*
Class 2 Pain ($n=287$)	3–4 classes improvement (252; 89%)
Class 3 Gait ($n=332$)	2–3 classes improvement (244;74%)

Table 7. Results of valgus-extension osteotomy in atrophic OA (metabolic disease)

1972–1977:	208	cases of craniolateral type b
1980:	130	patients (62%) returned for evaluation (minimum follow-up 3 years)

Average age	Sex predominance
58 years	85% women

	Pain		
Improved	120 (92%)	*Preoperative:* 127 (98%) in classes 1–4	*Postoperative:* 100 (77%) in classes 5–6
Same	10 (8%)		
Worse	0 (0%)		
	Gait		
Improved	91 (70%)	*Preoperative:* 106 (82%) in classes 3–4	*Postoperative:* 67 (52%) in classes 5–6
Same	29 (22%)		
Worse	10 (8%)		
	Motion		
Improved	44 (34%)	*Preoperative:* 57 (44%) stiff	*Postoperative:* 14/57 mobile (25%) 15 became stiff (12%)
Same	60 (46%)		
Worse	26 (20%)		

Typical candiate (58-year-old woman)	*Typical results*
Class 2 Pain ($n=60$)	3–4 classes improvement (42; 70%)
Class 3 Gait ($n=70$)	2–3 classes improvement
Stiff Hip ($n=57$)	(31; 44%)

groups except the overuse group, type d_2. Note that congenital craniolateral WBS patients, seen in types b and c, presented for treatment earlier than patients with normal anatomy, type d_2. The results, however, were comparable in all groups.

Pain relief was primary and just as dramatic as in the varus cases. Gait improvement was most common without the Trendelenburg side effect. Mobility was generally preserved, although in 8% some was lost. In 3% of cases the hip became stiff, but 26% of previously stiff hips became mobile.

The typical patient was a woman in her early 30s or an man near 50, depending on the type of osteoarthritis. Preoperatively, night pain was frequent and walking was impossible without a cane. Postoperatively, all pain was relieved and normal activity was resumed. The risk of loss of mobility was greater than in varus osteotomy, although 30% of patients had stiff hips before operation.

Table 7 shows that the typical patient (a 58-year-old woman) with osteoporosis, craniolateral collapse of the osteopenic femoral head (type b) and no biological potential for osteophyte formation (atrophic) did not fare so well with valgus-extension osteotomy. Pain improvement was predictable, but complete relief less common. Gait improved but not as much. Motion was unpredictable postoperatively with a significant risk of becoming stiff. The 62% of patients who returned may not include a significant number who sought reoperation elsewhere. Overall, the results speak against osteotomy, which is now contraindicated in these atrophic cases.

The results of combined femoropelvic osteotomies and valgus osteotomy for medial osteoarthritis types a and b are discussed in the second edition of my book [6]. The numbers are too small to be included here.

Discussion and Summary

This paper presents a biomechanical classification of different types of hip morphology as an aid to understanding the natural history of OA and developing consistent preventive or corrective treatment.

The basis of this biomechanical analysis comes from studies reported in the first [2] and second [6] editions of my book *Osteoarthritis of the Hip*. Some points are emphasized here: the effect of craniolateral inclination of the WBS via force S in reducing pain and creating osteophytes; the additive effect of trunk shift in antalgic gait to a precocious appearance of force S; and the result of maximum body response to the painful hip, i.e., Trendelenburg gait, whereby trunk shift decreases overall force magnitude while a dynamic craniolateral inclination maximizes the percentage of force S, thus transmitting painful compressive force P into soft tissues. It is interesting to observe that nature will expend phenomenal energy (massive trunk acceleration in all three planes superimposed upon completely aphasic pelvic gyrations) through Trendelenburg gait in order to accomplish the same stress relief in the hip that is produced by a well-planned osteotomy.

Another concept well worth considering is that a morphologically normal hip can undergo osteoarthritic degeneration due to excessive use, commonly seen in patients with massive obesity or repetitive high dynamic activity. From static analysis in monopodal stance to idealized values in dynamic phases of normal gait, the damaging forces of P and P_R are increased substantially by over 40%. These force increases are proportional to gait acceleration and additive with repetition. Despite the ability of well-conditioned muscles in the professional athlete to absorb high dynamic forces, aided by the shock-absorbing contributions of the knee, ankle, and foot joints, the elasticity of bone, cartilage, ligaments, and the plantar fat pad, and even supported by the best sports footwear, in time the concentrated forces of P will selectively destroy the hip weight-bearing sector. The hip joint can however, easily endure a lifetime of normal usage, as evidenced by the often normal cartilage on spherical heads removed from elderly patients who sustain subcapital fractures due to metabolic osteoporosis.

The results here represent a careful clinical review of approximately 1,000 cases of osteotomy for OA. It is encouraging that the statistics have borne out the importance of biomechanical analysis. The essential role of osteophytes in treatment by valgus osteotomy is underscored by the limited clinical response of atrophic OA cases. As patients return to our clinic with painless, mobile hips osteotomized over 15 years ago, the longevity of this treatment becomes increasingly apparent.

We have outlined specific types of OA where osteotomy has not been successful (e.g., protrusio, atrophic, stiff). Perhaps in these cases prosthesis technology will provide an adequate solution. What is certain is that osteotomy of the hip facilitates biological potential and maximally preserves living tissues when indicated and executed according to the biomechanical principles detailed here.

References

1. Bombelli R (1957) Displasia cotiloidea ed artrosi deformante dell'anca – Revisione statistica su 441 casi di anche artrosiche. Archivio Putti, VIII: 192–198
2. Bombelli R (1976) Osteoarthritis of the hip. Pathogenesis and consequent therapy. Springer, Berlin Heidelberg New York
3. Bombelli R (1979) Klassification der Coxarthrose als

Grundlage operativer Gelenkerhaltung. Biomechanik der cranio-lateralen Hüftarthrosen; Ziel und Technik der Extension-Valgisations-Osteotomie; Ziel und Technik der Extension-Varus-Osteotomie. Ergebnisse. Orthopade 8:245–263
4. Bombelli R (1981) Radiological pattern of the normal hip joint and its biomechanical meaning. In: Draenert K, Rütt A (eds) Morphologie und Funktion der Hüfte, Histo-Morphologischer Bewegungsapparat I. Art and Science, München, pp 113–138
5. Bombelli R (1983) Hinweise zur operativen Gelenkerhaltung bei Hüftdysplasie und Coxarthrose auf der Basis der Morphologie des Oberschenkel-Hüft-Gelenks. In: Rütt A, Küsswetter W (eds) Gelenknahe Osteotomien bei der Dysplasiehüfte des Adoleszenten und jungen Erwachsenen. Thieme, Stuttgart New York, pp 177–213
6. Bombelli R (1983) Osteoarthritis of the hip. Classification and pathogenesis. The role of osteotomy as a consequent therapy. Second revised and entlarged edition. Springer, Berlin Heidelberg New York Tokyo
7. Bombelli R, Santore R (1983) The morpbology and classification of osteoarthritis: an anatomical and biomechanical perspective. J Rheumatol suppl 9:10
8. Bullough P et al. Incongruent surfaces in the human hip joint. Nature 217:1290
9. Chiari K (1955) Ergebnisse mit der Beckenosteotomie als Pfannendachplastik. Orthop 87:14–26
10. Chiari K (1974) Medial displacement osteotomy of the pelvis. Clin Orthop 98:55–71
11. Chiari K, Endler M, Hackel H (1978) Indications et résultats de l'ostéomie du bassin selon Chiari dans l'arthrose avancée. Acta Orthop Belg 44:1–76
12. Endler F (1983) Die biomechanischen Prinzipien bei der Beckenosteotomie nach Chiari unter Demonstration von Langzeitergebnissen. In: Rütt A und Küsswetter W (eds) Gelenknahe Osteotomien bei der Dysplasiehüfte des Adoleszenten und jungen Erwachsenen. Thieme, Stuttgart New York, pp 19–42
13. Goodfellow IV, Mitson A (1977) Joint surface incongruity and its maintenance. J Bone Joint Surg 59/B, 446–451
14. Mittelmeier H, Nizard M (1980) Indication, technique et résultats de l'association ostéotomie fémorale intertrochantérienne-acetabuloplastie à l'aide du coin d'ostéotomie. Annales orthopédiques de l'Est, 27–31
15. Mittelmeier H, Nizard M (1981) Technique de l'ostéotomie fémorale intertrochantérienne à l'aide de plaques coudées autoserrantes. Rev Orthop 81:67
16. Morscher E (1971) Die intertrochantäre Osteotomie bei Coxarthrose. Huber, Bern
17. Müller ME (1957) Die hüftnahen Femurosteotomien. Thieme, Stuttgart
18. Müller ME (1969) Die Varisationsosteotomie bei der Behandlung der Coxarthrose. In: Rütt A (ed) Die Therapie der Coxarthrose. Thieme, Stuttgart
19. Müller ME (1979) Planung einer komplexen, intertrochanteren Osteotomie. Z Orthop 117:145–150
20. Müller ME, Allgöwer M, Schneider R, Willenegger H (1979) Manual of Internal Fixation. AO Technique, 2nd edition. Springer, Berlin Heidelberg New York
21. Pauwels F (1961) Neue Richtlinien für die operative Behandlung der Coxarthrose. Verh Dtsch Orthop Ges, 48 Kongr. Enke, Stuttgart, pp 332–366
22. Pauwels F (1963) Die Bedeutung der Biomechanik für die Orthopädie. IXème Congrès de la Societé Inter de Chir Orthop et de Traum. Wien, 1–7/IX/1963, Tom II
23. Pauwels F (1965) Gesammelte Abhandlungen zur funktionellen Anatomie des Bewegungsapparates. Springer, Berlin Heidelberg New York
24. Pauwels F (1973) Atlas zur Biomechanik der gesunden und kranken Hüfte. Springer, Berlin Heidelberg New York
25. Salter RB (1966) Role of innominate osteotomy in the treatment of congenital dislocation and subluxation of the hip in the older child. J Bone Joint Surg 48/A, 1413–1439
26. Schneider R (1979) Die intertrochantere Osteotomie bei Coxarthrose. Springer, Berlin Heidelberg New York
27. Steel HH (1973) Triple osteotomy of the innominate bone. J Bone Joint Surg 59/A, 1082–1090
28. Swanson SAV (1979) Friction-wear and lubrication. In: Freeman MAR (ed) Adult articular cartilage, 2nd ed. Pitman Medical, Kent, pp 415+460
29. Teinturier P, Levai JP, Collin JP (1981) L'ostéotomie de flexion épiphysaire de hanche dans les coxarthroses évoluées. Analyse évolutive et résultats à 5 ans de recul. International Orthopaedics (SICOT), 5, 217–223
30. Tönnis D (1983) Indikation und Ergebnisse der Dreifachosteotomie nach Tönnis. In: Rütt A, Küsswetter W Gelenknahe Osteotomien bei der Dysplasiehüfte des Adoleszenten und jungen Erwachsenen. Thieme, Stuttgart New York, pp 103–111
31. Wagner H (1965) Korrektur der Hüftgelenkdysplasie durch die sphärische Pfannendachplastik. Intern Symposium Beckenosteotomie-Pfannendachplastik. Thieme, Stuttgart
32. Wagner H (1976) Osteotomies for congenital hip dislocation. In: The Hip, Proc of the Fourth Open Scientific Meeting of the Hip Society. Mosby, St. Louis, p 45
33. Merle d'Aubigne R (1952) Reposition with arthroplasty for congenital dislocation of the hip in adults. J Bone Joint Surg 34/B, 22–29

Intertrochanteric Osteotomy in Osteoarthritis of the Hip Joint

R. SCHNEIDER

Introduction

We feel that in the present age of prosthetic replacements, it is important to draw attention to the possibilities of intertrochanteric osteotomy as a joint-preserving operation for patients with osteoarthritis of the hip. In many cases, an osteotomy can be successfully repeated years later. If this is not possible, one can always carry out a total hip replacement.

This article is based on the experience gained from 786 intertrochanteric osteotomies performed since 1959. On the basis of a follow-up examination of a group of 108 osteotomies, on the average 13 years after operation performed 1959–1962, we concluded that in spite of the early broader and less precise indication for surgery, we had achieved about 50% satisfactory results. Our experience with total hip replacement shows the complication rate after a comparable period to be also about 50%; however, the failures after total hip replacement pose far greater therapeutic problems, which in many cases have only unsatisfactory solutions. We realize that due to the continuous advances in the techniques of THR, considerable improvement in the late results can be anticipated in the future. Until such time as there is evidence of a definite improvement, we must carefully evaluate all patients to see if they are suitable candidates for intertrochanteric osteotomy before a total hip replacement is carried out. There are certain prerequisites for a successful intertrochanteric osteotomy. The desired joint regeneration after intertrochanteric osteotomy can take place only in viable and reactive bone. During the early postoperative period pain-free movement of the joint must be possible to ensure nourishment of the cartilage. In addition, the surgery must not only be correctly planned, but also correctly executed. Early pain-free movement and maintenance of the correction have become possible only since the introduction of stable internal fixation based on the principle of interfragmentary compression. Intertrochanteric osteotomy requires a longer convalescence than total hip replacement, and therefore it makes far greater demands on the patient, who must begin movement early and yet avoid weight-bearing. Careful psychological assessment and preparation of the patient is important. Apprehensive, tense, poorly compliant patients and misanthropes immediately jeopardize the results, and must therefore be excluded.

There are indications, especially for the classic valgization osteotomy, where success of intertrochanteric osteotomy can be predicted with a great degree of certainty.

It is equally important to recognize the patients with a less certain prognosis, such as those in whom it is difficult to evaluate the viability and the reactivity of the femoral head. In patients with radiologically almost identical situations we have had good and bad results. In the future, with the use of angiography and scintigraphy, it may become possible to be more accurate in predicting the prognosis.

In 1963 we showed on the basis of 100 consecutive patients with osteoarthritis of the hip undergoing conservative therapy for an average of 17.3 months that the average spontaneous course of osteoarthritis is one of progressive deterioration. Despite the fact that these were relatively mild cases, not yet ready for surgery, their pain increased, their walking distance decreased from 3.8 to 2.1 km, their functional leg length remained the same, their range of flexion decreased from 60° to 47°, their range of rotation decreased from 15° to 9°, and their extension decreased from 165° to 161°.

Thus in evaluating the results of surgery in difficult cases, we must always keep in mind the natural history of the disease.

Indications

One can only determine the indications for an intertrochanteric osteotomy successfully if one knows the mechanical and biological possibilities of this operation.

Although Pauwels' basic concepts (Pauwels 1965) are common knowledge, from a practical clinical point of view the following considerations are equally important.

Pathogenesis

Under physiological stress conditions, a balance exists between breakdown and formation of bone and cartilage. Only mechanical overstress can interfere with this balance and lead to a disorganization of the cartilage until it wears out completely. This cartilage is supported normally by vascularized bone which is not only able to react but also does so, first with sclerosis, and later with cyst formation, deformation, and osteophyte formation. This type of mechanical overload can be the sole cause of secondary osteoarthritis. In an isolated case of secondary osteoarthritis, the role of the different factors may be difficult to assess, particularly in the presence of relative tissue insufficiency.

In the past the progression of osteoarthritis was accepted as inevitable and irreversible. Now it is known that the elimination or improvement of mechanical overload restores the disturbed equilibrium and makes it possible for regenerative forces to restore a severely damaged joint by transformation and regeneration (Figs. 1, 2).

The nature of the mechanical overload includes two components which must be recognized:

1. The pathological increase in total pressure from
   - Weight increase, heavy work.
   - Too steep a femoral neck angle with shortened lever arm of the abductors.
   - Adduction contracture with lengthening of the medial load caused by a shift of the center of gravity away from the femoral head during walking and standing. Compensatory lurching designed to decrease load is made more difficult or impossible.
   - Flexion contracture with the additional pressure of the hip extensors.
   - Muscle spasm and contracture in response to pain.
2. The pathological distribution of a total pressure normal in itself by
   - Too small a weight-bearing area. Example: acetabular dysplasia. Lateral, frontal, and central acetabular insufficiencies must be distinguished.
   - Incongruity of the joint due to head deformation. Examples: Slips of the epiphysis, dysostoses, partial head necroses, traumatic head defects.
   - Incorrect orientation of the head in the acetabulum. Example: coxa antetorta with a tendency to anterior subluxation, coxa vara, long neck of femur with tendency to coxa retrotorta. This situation leads to increased horizontal force vectors at the head orientation away from the acetabular roof. In this way, particularly in the case of small heads or medial acetabular insufficiency, a medial osteoarthritis of the hip joint with overloading of the acetabular floor and a tendency to protrusion can develop as a result of too wide an incisura acetabuli.

In practice a combination of both components of mechanical overload is almost always present. Consequently the therapy one plans must be based on an analysis of the degree of the joint overload present so that suitable mechanical corrections can be carried out. The procedures available to achieve these mechanical corrections are intertrochanteric osteotomy and tenotomy.

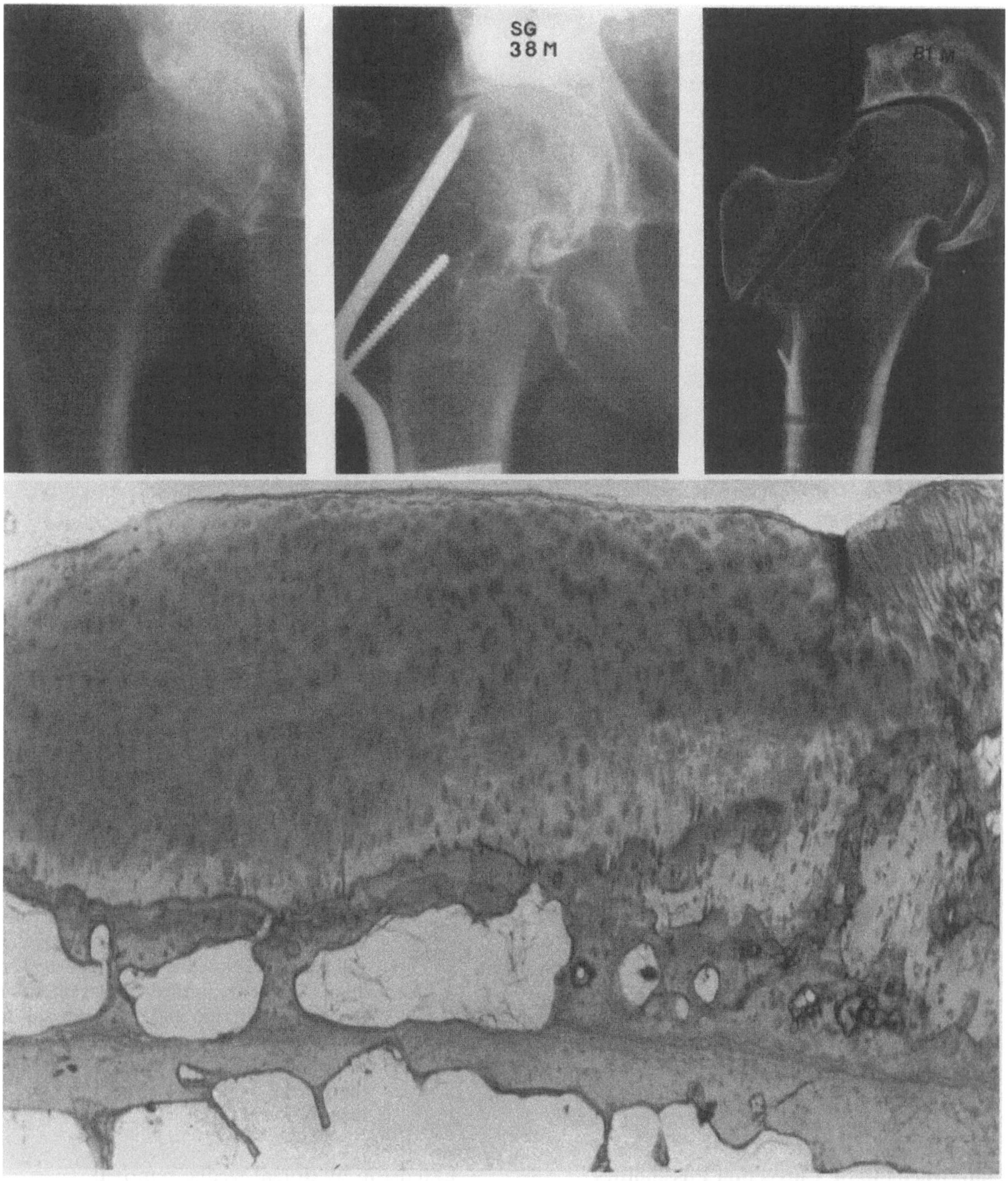

Fig. 1. A 66-year-old salesman. Moderate joint regeneration 38 months and 81 months after valgization oblique displacement osteotomy. Patient died of cardiac failure 81 months after surgery. Histological investigation of the femoral head performed by Prof. P. Riniker, Locarno, demonstrated islands of newly formed fibrocartilage in the main weight-bearing zone. Under the newly formed cartilage, residues of spongy, old cartilage are visible. S. Krompecher of Debrecen, who examined these pictures in 1967, stressed that this is a neoformation of cartilage, and not merely regeneration

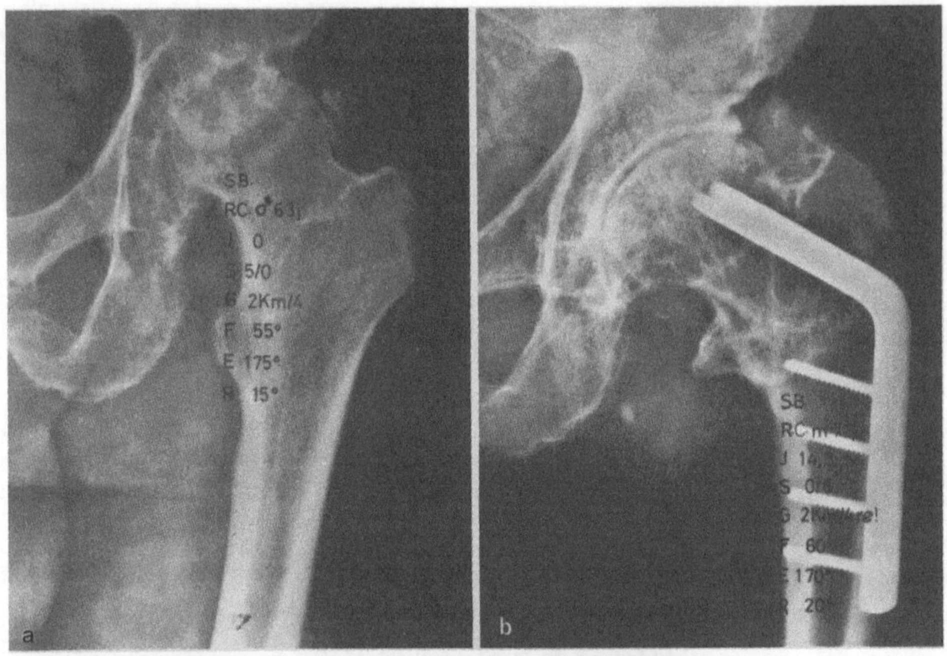

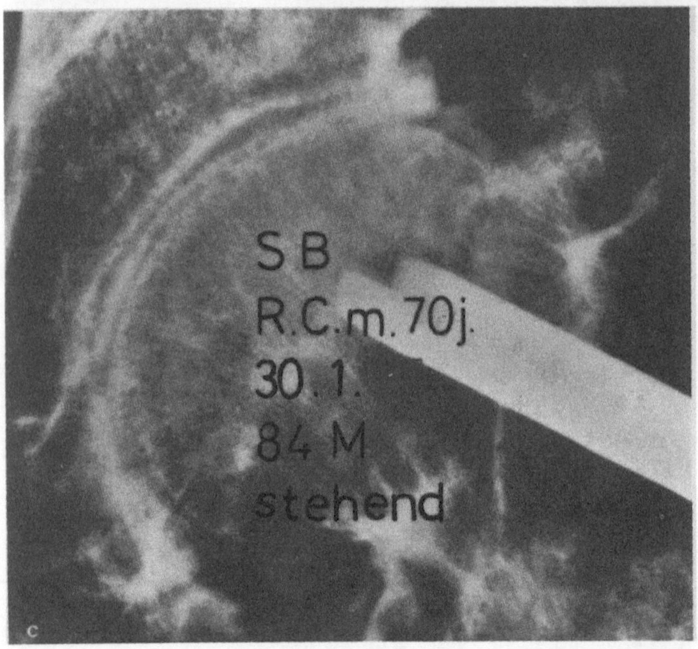

Fig. 2.1 a–c. A 63-year-old farmer. **a** Severe osteoarthritis of the hip joint with corresponding pain. **b** Fourteen years after varization-extension osteotomy the patient is still pain-free. Note the good joint regeneration. The newly formed cartilage both on the acetabular side and the head side is shown in the arthrogram. **c** After 7 years, while the patient was weight-bearing. For the legend for abbreviations used on X-rays see Results (p. 155)

Intertrochanteric Correction Possibilities

Intertrochanteric osteotomy permits 12 different corrections:

- Valgization by lateral wedge removal
- Varization by medial wedge removal
- Inward rotation relative to the axis of the femur
- Outward rotation relative to the axis of the femur
- Extension by dorsal wedge removal
- Flexion by ventral wedge removal
- Leg shortening by resection of a segment, by varization, or by oblique osteotomy and medial displacement
- Leg lengthening by valgization or oblique osteotomy and lateralization
- Medial displacement of the femoral shaft
- Lateral displacement of the femoral shaft
- Forward displacement of the femoral shaft
- Backward displacement of the femoral shaft

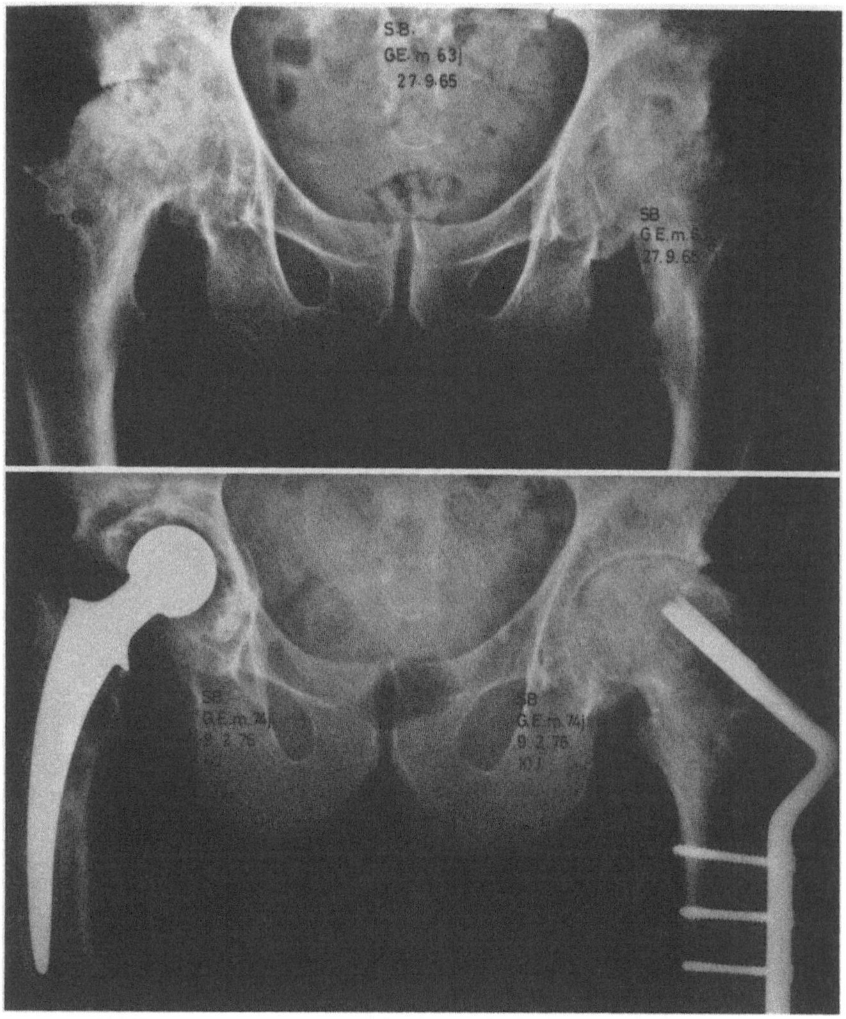

Fig. 2.2. A 63-year-old farmer. Severe bilateral osteoarthritis of the hip joint. Left intertrochanteric osteotomy in 1963, right total hip replacement in 1970. On the left, $10^1/_2$ years after osteotomy, the hip is free of pain and functions efficiently. Good radiological joint regeneration despite relative overstressing of the joint. On the right, 6 years after total hip replacement the prosthesis became loose and painful, and had to be revised. For abbreviations, see Results

Of these 12 possibilities, only the last two are of no practical significance. Usually a combination of several is necessary (Figs. 3, 4).

Analysis of the Mechanical Effect of the Commonly Used Intertrochanteric Osteotomies

Valgization

Valgus osteotomy enables medial parts of the head to bear weight and is, therefore, always indicated if a large osteophyte (capital drop) is present medially and an overload is present in the region of the acetabular corner.

Two mechanisms operate in valgization:

1. Increase in the weight-bearing area.
2. Medialization of the supporting point away from the acetabular corner lengthens the lateral lever arm and shortens the medial (Fig. 5).

Valgization inevitably reduces the lateral lever arm by opening the CCD angle and makes the vector of the abductors more vertical. Medialization of the supporting point by shifting

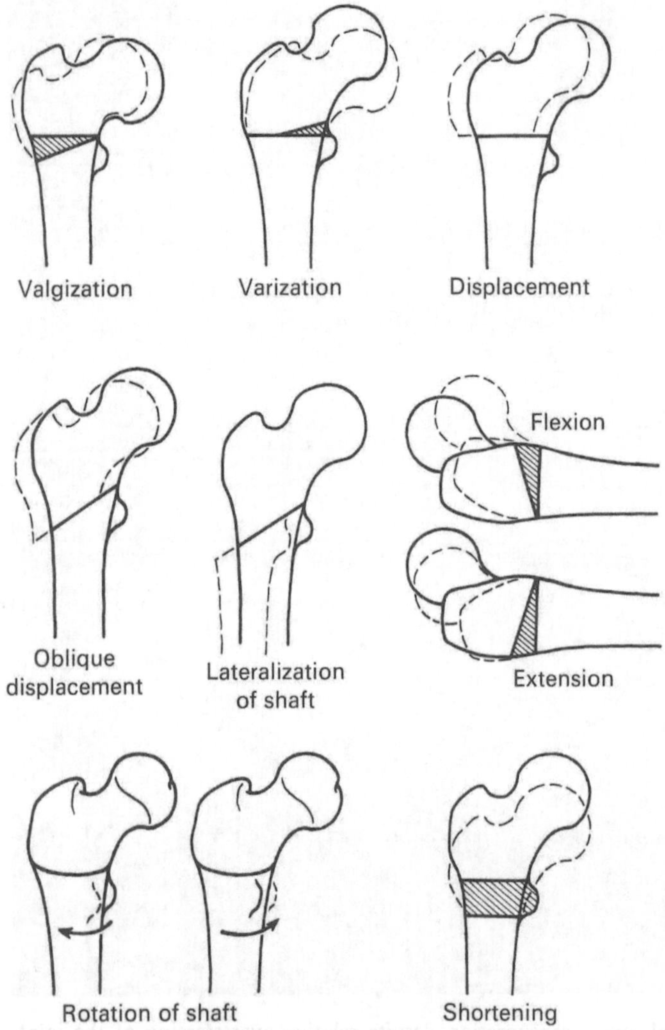

Fig. 3. The commonly used corrective maneuvers in an intertrochanteric osteotomy. Frequently valgization, varization, and displacement are combined with extension osteotomy and rotational correction of the shaft. Medial displacement of the shaft always comes under varus osteotomy and lateralization of the shaft under valgus osteotomy. The direction and the extent of the displacement of the shaft are determined by the initial loading at the knee joint and by the size of the correction angle

it to the medial osteophyte partly compensates for the inevitable disadvantages of valgization. In addition, by lateralizing the greater trochanter one can further lengthen the lever arm. This restores normal relationships (Fig. 6).

Valgization produces lateral displacement of the weight-bearing line of the leg and leads to a certain valgus overload of the knee joint.

Our experience shows that if we start with a normal leg axis, up to 20° valgization will not cause valgus overload of the knee with secondary osteoarthritis. A varus knee will be influenced favorably. In the case of a previous genu valgum or of valgizations above 20°, valgus gonarthritis could arise, and therefore lateralization of the femoral shaft becomes necessary.

Valgization also causes lengthening of the leg and thus increases muscular tension. Therefore, if valgization is significant it is necessary to prevent leg lengthening by resection of a segment of bone. Frequently, tenotomies of the iliopsoas muscle and the adductors are also required.

By shortening, by tenotomy, by lateralization of the trochanter and by lateralization of the femoral shaft one can overcome all the disadvantages of valgization and at the same time allow the considerably improved pressure distribution in the joint to exert its beneficial effect to the full.

Valgization osteotomy can also be indicated without medial head osteophytes, if a fixed adduction contracture is present. The adduction

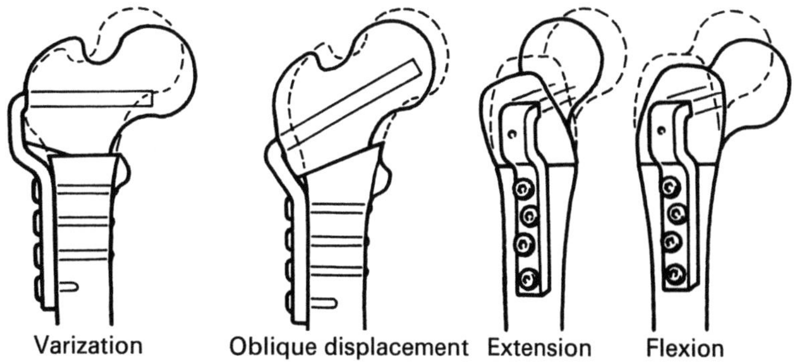

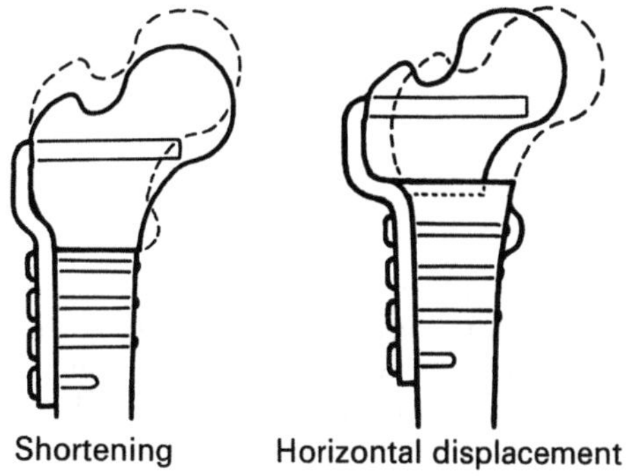

Fig. 4. Shortening mechanisms intertrochanteric osteotomies. Shortening occurs in varization, in oblique medial displacement osteotomy, in extension and flexion osteotomy, in removal of a horizontal segment of bone for shortening, and even, but to a lesser extent, in the mere medial displacement of the shaft and fixation with compression devices. Shortening generally means reduction in muscle strength and consequently in total pressure

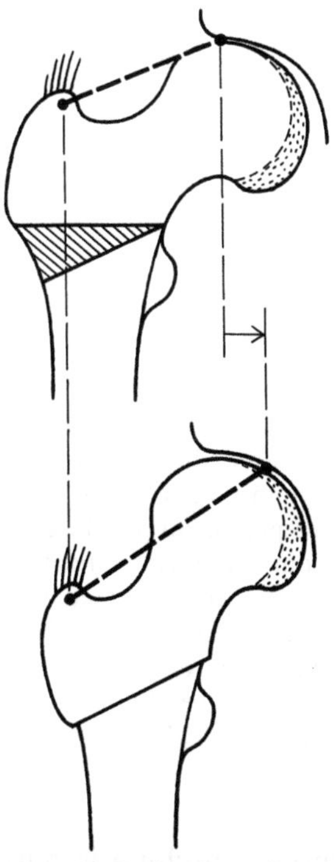

Fig. 5. Elimination of overload of acetabular corner by valgization. The positioning of the medial head osteophyte can compensate for the shortening of the lateral lever arm caused by valgization or even lengthen the lateral lever arm. Considerable decrease in joint pressure due to better pressure distribution in the joint and decrease in total pressure due to the relief of Duchenne limping by valgization (limp associated with an adductor contracture)

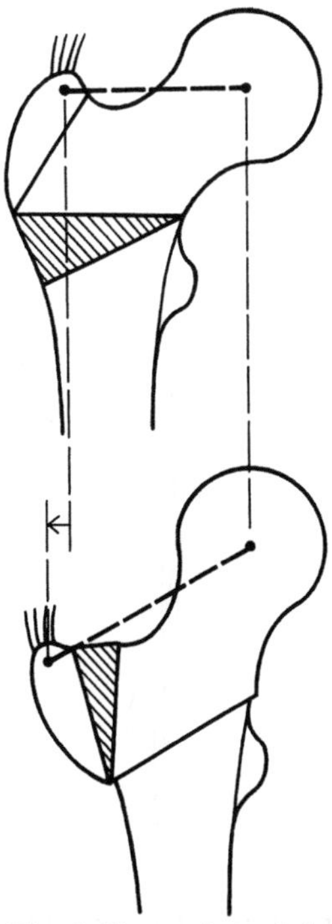

Fig. 6. Shortening of the lateral lever arm by valgus osteotomy can be compensated by lateralization of the trochanter (R. Bombelli, P. Maquet)

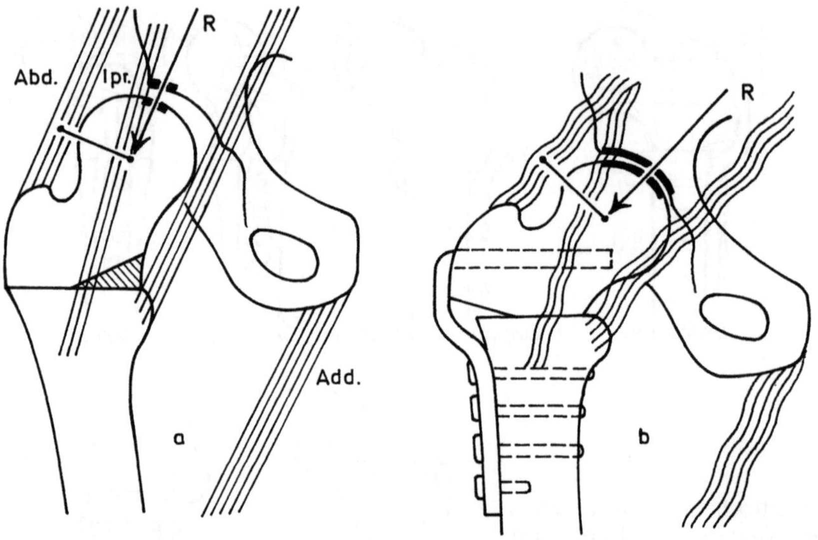

Fig. 7a, b. Effect of varus osteotomy according to M.E. Müller. Better centering of the head in the acetabulum results in reduction of the specific loading of the joint cartilage, as well as in reduction of total pressure through more advantageous lever arm conditions, a more horizontal direction of the force vector of the abductors, reduction in the muscle pressure through shortening, and a change in the head-neck stress with corresponding structural transformation

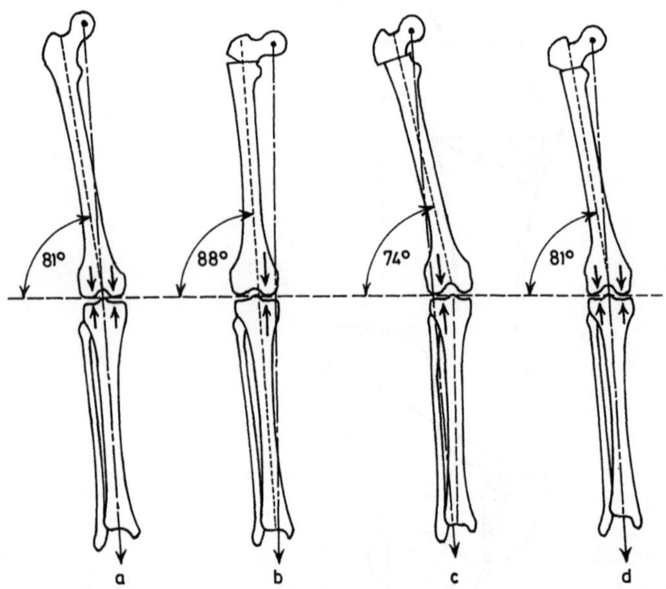

Fig. 8a–d. Effect of varus osteotomy and medial displacement on overloading of the knee joint. Pure varization produces varus overload. Pure medial displacement produces a valgus overload. A combination of varization and medial displacement normalizes load conditions at the knee joint (M.E. Müller). Conversely, valgization produces valgus overload of the knee joint, which can be eliminated by lateralization of the femoral shaft

contracture lengthens the medial lever arm and thus causes a great increase in the total pressure (Fig. 9).

It also prevents Trendelenburg lurching, which makes it impossible for the patient to shift the center of gravity vertically above the involved femoral head, and in this way almost completely abolishes the abductor pressure. The single fact that Trendelenburg lurching is rendered impossible makes valgus osteotomy a valuable, total-pressure-reducing measure. This applies, however, only if no abduction deformity with functional lengthening of the leg occurs as a result of the valgization. A leg that is too long hinders or prevents the pressure-reducing lurching. Therefore, it is important in valgus osteoetomy to make sure that any excessive lengthening of the limp is prevented by suitable shortening of the shaft.

Varization

Varization was originally recommended by Pauwels, who based his reasons in recommending the procedure on the lever law for reduction of total pressure and on the improved centering in the acetabulum for better pressure distribution. Today we feel that varization is rarely indicated in advanced osteoarthritis of the hip in the adult. The validity of the Pauwels varization theory depends of the gait pattern. It applies to the limp-free normal gait, but less in the presence of the antalgic Duchenne limping. As soon as varization leads to an adduction position of the leg, a pressure-increasing lengthening of the medial lever arm takes place, which results in a compromise of the varization effect.

Thus varus osteotomy is indicated only if the range of abduction exceeds the preoperatively planned varization angle. One of the best indications for varus osteotomy is a dysplastic acetabulum and an almost normal femoral head, i.e., without appreciable osteophytes. The improved centering of the head in the acetabulum leads to a favorable pressure distribution. In addition, the vectors of the abductors become more oblique away from the edge of the socket and become oriented more towards the floor of the acetabulum, which further facilitates better pressure distribution. Varization leads automatically to a certain leg shortening. Shortening that is not due to an adduction contracture facilitates Trendelenburg lurching, which further increases joint decompression (Fig. 7).

A clear indication for varus osteotomy is functional leg lengthening due to a fixed abduction contracture.

Through shortening of the leg, varization osteotomy relaxes important muscle groups (gluteus maximus, iliopsoas, abductors, adductors, tensor fasciae latae, etc.) (Fig. 8).

The total pressure is thus immediately and probably permanently reduced. The price one pays is a certain impairment of joint stability. In younger women especially, the limp due to shortening, coupled with a decrease in stability

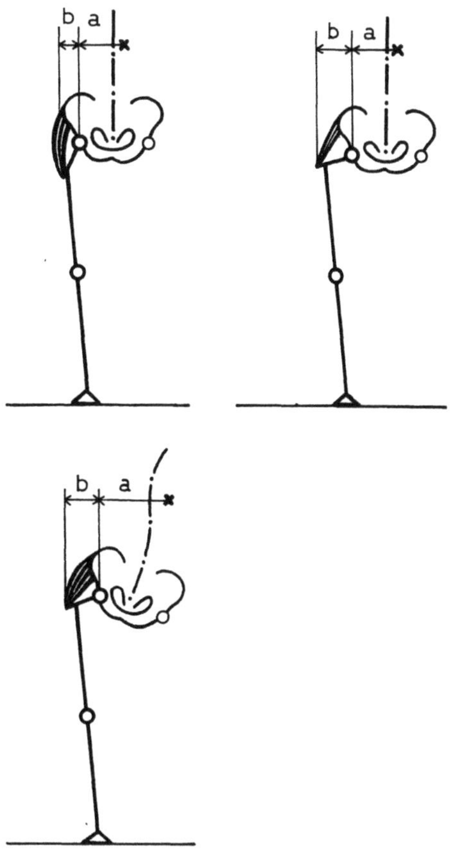

Fig. 9. Reduction in the total pressure by varization in accordance with Pauwels' law of levers. Varization relieves load only when satisfactory abduction is possible. If varization leads to an incorrect adduction position, the center of gravity is shifted from the vertical above the femoral head, away from the involved side which lengthens the medial lever arm, and produces joint overload (Osborne and Fahrni 1950)

in standing, and the lurching may prove to be very annoying. Therefore in extensive varus osteotomies one should consider simultaneous distal displacement of the greater trochanter.

Extension Osteotomy

The classical Pauwels theory of reduction in joint pressure and better pressure distribution relates entirely to the force and congruity conditions in the frontal plane.

We are most anxious to include in our plan of treatment also the conditions and correction possibilities in the sagittal plane. The correction possibilities in head lesions or partial head necroses are greater in the sagittal plane than in

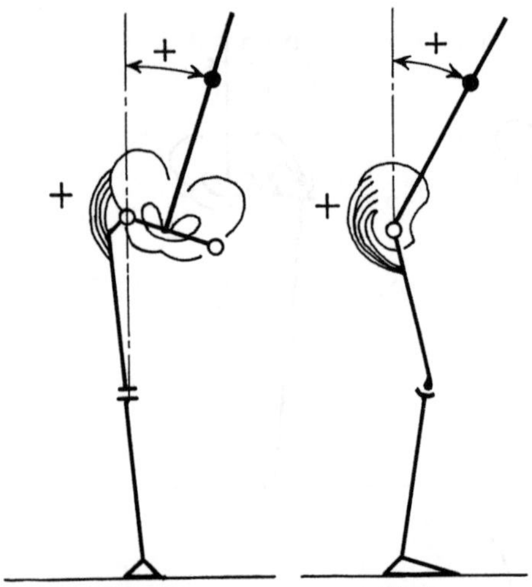

Fig. 10. Increase in the total pressure in both adduction contracture and flexion contracture of the hip joint. In both cases the center of gravity of the body is shifted from the vertical above the femoral head. Decrease in the total pressure can be achieved by a valgus extension osteotomy

the frontal plane, since it is possible to achieve about 60° of extension and about 35° of flexion. In osteoarthritis of the adult hip, usually there is loss of extension, and flexion osteotomy plays almost no role at all. Extension osteotomy, on the other hand, is most effective.

Extension osteotomy has five functions:

1. It eliminates or reduces the loss of extension and thus makes an upright body posture possible. It reduces the total joint pressure by returning the body's center of gravity to the proximity of the vertical above the femoral head. This eliminates the additional pressure of the powerful hip extensors (mainly gluteus maximus). It relieves the hip joint in the same way as valgization does in the case of an incorrect adduction position (Fig. 10).
2. Depending on the degree of mobility in the hip joint, particularly if the loss in extension is relatively small, extension osteotomy allows rotation of the head in the joint in the sense of flexion. For this reason, some people, for example in France, refer to an extension osteotomy as flexion osteotomy. In practice, part of the correction causes improved extension of the leg and part flexion of the femoral head. Since it is customary to designate our osteotomies in accordance with the change in position of the distal fragment relative to the proximal one, we would like to retain our designation. In varization, for example, rotation of the head takes place in the sense of valgization, and yet it has not occured to anybody to designate varization as valgization. Through the flexion of the head the anterior parts of the head are rotated into the main weight-bearing zone of the acetabular roof. If these parts of the head are still spherically intact and have good cartilage, the joint congruity is improved, which results in a further decrease in the specific surface stress, i.e., a better pressure distribution and decrease in load (Fig. 11).
3. The removal of the dorsal wedge results in a moderate muscle relaxation due to shortening of the leg but this does not lead to any insufficiency of the hip.
4. Extension osteotomy displaces the femoral head dorsally relative to the femoral axis. In eccentric, ventrally situated overload damage of the joint with a tendency to lateral and ventral subluxation of the head, as one encounters in acetabular dysplasia, extension osteotomy is an excellent means of centering the head. It is comparable to the varization effect in the frontal plane (Figs. 12, 25).
5. Since the extension osteotomy is frequently performed with a right-angled plate, we must note the corresponding varization effect. It is easy to understand how extension of flexion of 90° reduces every CCD angle to 90° if a right-angled plate is employed with the blade in the plane of the femoral neck axis. The varization effect can be calculated according to the following formula:

$$\frac{\text{CCD angle} - \text{plate angle} \times \text{angle of extension}}{90} = \text{varization angle}$$

This varization effect must be known so that it can be taken into account in planning the operation. (From the formula it is clear that with a 120° or 130° hip plate the varization effect is almost completely cancelled out.)

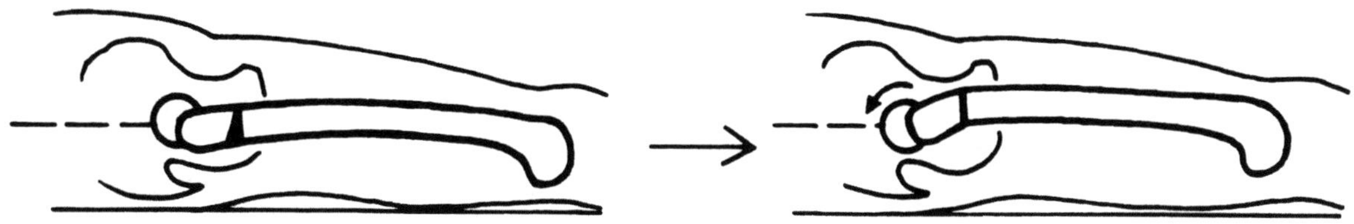

a) Free mobility

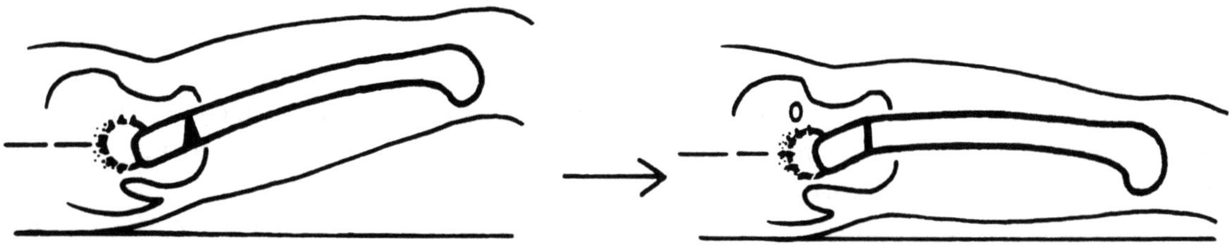

b) Stiffness and flexion contracture

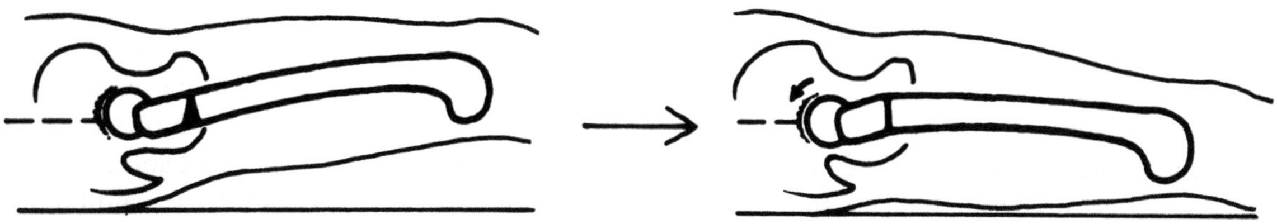

c) Osteoarthritis of the hip joint

Fig. 11 a–c. Effect of extension osteotomy. **a** In a freely mobile hip, the head is rotated into flexion. **b** In the case of a stiff hip joint only the leg is extended. **c** In a stiff hip joint with loss of extension (normal case in osteoarthritis of the hip joint) the head is partly flexed and the leg is partly extended

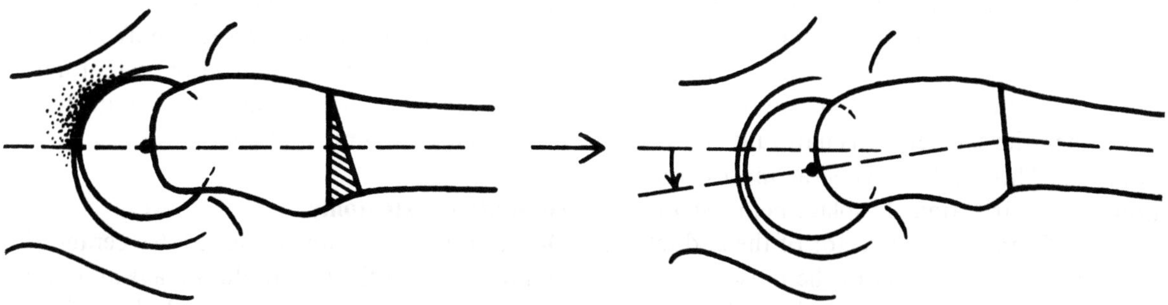

Fig. 12. The effect of extension osteotomy on the centering of the head in the hip joint. Extension osteotomy orients the head dorsally relative to the axis of the femur and can eliminate a frontal overloading of the joint

Flexion Osteotomy

A ventral wedge is removed and the craniodorsal sections of the femoral head are rotated into the main weight-bearing zone. Excision of the ventral joint capsule with the iliofemoral ligament and tenotomy of the psoas tendon aids extension. A prerequisite for flexion osteotomy is preserved normal extension. Fortunately, there is frequently no flexion contracture in cranioventral lesions of the head (partial necroses, traumatic defects, incongruences from subchondral dysostoses). Flexion osteotomy displaces the femoral shaft with the lesser trochanter dorsally, causing an increase in tension of the iliopsoas muscle. It is therefore advisable to perform a tenotomy of the iliopsoas.

Displacement Osteotomy

The first intertrochanteric osteotomy was called a displacement osteotomy by McMurray. He believed that the decompression of the joint was achieved by supporting the pelvis on the shaft fragment at the ischial tuberosity. Although his explanation of joint decompression is wrong, we continue to refer to displacement osteotomy as a McMurray osteotomy, which is wrong. McMurray introduced his osteotome through a small incision and kept the hip immobilized in a spica cast until healing was complete. Incorrect positions of the head were corrected spontaneously during plaster application, so that very frequently, abduction, extension, and inward rotation were achieved, as well as medial displacement. It seems important to draw attention to these mechanisms if the McMurray operation is to be evaluated correctly.

Medial displacement of the femoral shaft effectively reduces the length of the muscles acting in the medial direction, such as the adductors and the quadratus femoris muscle. Evaluation after horizontal displacement osteotomies has shown that slight varization almost always occurs and that the compression osteosynthesis leads to a certain shortening.

This slight leg shortening of the horizontal displacement osteotomy is further increased when one adds extension, which is frequently the case. If the displacement osteotomy is oblique, then the shortening is naturally more pronounced. This leads to general muscle reluxation, as in varization. Displacement osteotomy has no influence on the vector of the abductors, but there is further relief of the muscular forces acting in the medial direction through the influence of the displacement on the function of the iliopsoas muscle. This strong muscle attached to the lesser trochanter is normally an inward rotator (von Lanz 1949). Its inward rotator function, which is more pronounced in coxa vara and if the femoral shaft is long, is compensated for by the pull of the small external rotators and the gluteus maximus, which produce a force that is directed obliquely and medially. Medialization of the lesser trochanter, i.e., of the attachment of the iliopsoas muscle, neutralizes its inward rotatory function or even reverses its action to make it an outward rotator. This explains the observation that after displacement osteotomy alone, without any change in rotation, there is often an "inexplicable" tendency toward outward rotation. In our opinion the iliopsoas muscle is responsible for this. The neutralization of the iliopsoas muscle as an inward rotator and consequently of the small outward rotators as antagonists reduces the force directed centrally, and therefore has a decompressing effect in cases of medial osteoarthritis of the hip with progressive tendency to protrusio acetabuli (Fig. 8).

In a way similar to valgization, displacement osteotomy shifts the weight-bearing axis laterally. It aggravates a valgus knee, improves a varus knee, but is of no consequence for a normally stressed knee joint. It is logical to make it part of every varization osteotomy, because in this way the varus effect produced by varization is neutralized (Fig. 8). The displacement osteotomy line runs horizontally in combination with varization, obliquely in combination with valgization if a shortening effect is desired in order to compensate for lengthening caused by the valgization. The indication for a medial displacement in combination with valgization is medial osteoarthritis of the knee.

Lateralization of the femoral shaft is necessary in more extensive valgization osteotomies, e.g., of 30°, or when valgization is indicated in the presence of genu valgum.

Derotation Osteotomy

Derotation osteotomy designed to center the femoral head in the acetabulum plays an important role in young people with pathological coxa antetorta (excessive anteversion). In osteoarthritis of the hip joint in the adult, rotational corrections are carried out to correct malposition of the leg and in this way protect the lumbar spine, the sacroiliac joint, the knee joint, and the ankle joint. Internal rotation deformity must be prevented at all costs.

Tenotomy

Osteotomy of the greater trochanter for reduction of abductor pressure and tenotomies of the adductors, the iliotibial tract, and the iliopsoas muscle, or even neurectomy of the obturator nerve, i.e., operations of the Voss type, are rarely used today as sole corrective measures. They are frequently essential, however, in combination with intertrochanteric osteotomy. According to Bombelli (1976), tenotomy of the iliopsoas muscle should be included regularly in valgization osteotomy. The recovery of the function of this muscle during the first year following tenotomy is always impressive.

Judet et al. (1965) have also routinely performed iliopsoas tenotomy. They believe that they have found no significant difference between the results of the horizontal and the oblique (McMurray) displacement osteotomies.

Analysis of Biological Effect

An intertrochanteric osteotomy activates a reparative process. This consists of hyperemia and an increase in the rate of bone remodeling. Osteotomy spares the joint by effectively unloading it. Nissen has shown that this leads to clinical success for at least a short period of time.

An intertrochanteric osteotomy brings about a change in position, which changes the loading on the bone. A restructuring according to Wolf's law must therefore inevitably take place. The pathologically changed areas together with the old normal structure are resorbed and remodelled. If the osteotomy has resulted in favorable stress conditions, then a durable new formation of the femoral head results. Osteophytes are included in this new formation. Cysts and sclerosing tissue can disappear completely. Pain-free movement immediately after surgery is essential if this desirable transformation is to occur. This emphasizes the great importance of a stable osteosynthesis.

We must also mention the papers of Arnoldi et al. (1972) and Phillips (1966), who felt that osteoarthritic pain in the hip was caused by venous hypertension in the femoral head. The opening up of the metaphysis and its cancellous bone, as in displacement osteotomy or in simple trochanteric osteotomy, would have a pain-reducing effect through a simple decompressive effect on the venous hypertension. We are not in a position to express an opinion on this. Our impression is that large displacements are generally favorable. Whether this venous pressure theory does offer an explanation for this is not clear. The fact that Hawk (1970) has found this intramedullary pressure to be dependent on the arterial inflow and that Hayashi (1973) has determined an increase in the arterial inflow by up to a factor of 10 by postoperative scintiscan appears to indicate that this is not the case. In our experience the biological effect of osteotomy can be enhanced by surgical curettage of large cysts in the head or acetabular roof and by filling them with cancellous bone as described by Camera (Fig. 20, p. 157).

Operation Plan

The plan of operation is based on the radiological and clinical findings. In the presence of a fixed deformity correction of the deformity has absolute priority. In the absence of a deformity, the decision between varization or valgization depends to a great extent on the residual range of movement. If abduction or adduction is obviously restricted by pain, then the final decision on the extent of the correction must be made under general anesthesia before the actual surgery is begun.

Varization is indicated if abduction is at least 20° and if in this position there is a good fit of the head in the joint. Frequently, abduction is appreciably improved by flexion of the hip, which would be a very clear indication for simultaneous extension osteotomy of the order of magnitude of the flexion carried out in assessing maximum abduction. The X-ray picture with the hip in abduction yields information about congruity. Varization is generally contraindicated if in abduction a narrowing of the joint space occurs at the level of the acetabular corner.

Valgization is indicated in cases with limited abduction, a large rounded head, or a head with a medial osteophyte. The extent of valgization is determined by the degree of adduction under anesthesia. If an excessively large medial osteophyte blocks adduction, it may have to be resected before a valgus osteotomy is possible. Abduction deformity must be avoided. Lateralization of the femoral shaft, shortening of the leg, and trochanteric osteotomy facilitate adduction, which is improved postoperatively by adduction exercises. Bombelli (1976) has shown that radiological improvement of congruity in the adduction picture is not necessary; the subsequent head remodelling leads to spontaneous improvement of congruity. If adduction is better in flexion, simultaneous extension osteotomy is indicated.

Extension osteotomy is always indicated if there is a flexion deformity or if abduction or adduction is considerably better in flexion. It is also indicated if functional contour X-rays indicate a better sphericity of the cranioventral portion of the head, because this increases congruity and helps in joint decompression.

Displacement osteotomy is indicated in cases where neither varization nor valgization offers any advantages. It often has to be combined with an extension. We have found the oblique displacement osteotomy particularly effective, because it leads to the relaxation of all distally attached muscles. It is our experience that horizontal displacement osteotomy is clearly indicated in medial osteoarthritis of the hip joint. It can be readily combined with valgization and, if required, with extension.

Flexion osteotomy can be considered only if no loss of extension exists. It is indicated for destructive head processes (traumatic or vascular in origin) in which contour X-rays show the craniodorsal parts of the head to be intact.

Technique

X-Ray Investigation

The X-ray projections which we require in order to evaluate a patient for an intertrochanteric osteotomy are referred to as the function projections. The patient is positioned supine with both hips extended. For the X-ray in abduction the hips are maximally abducted and internally rotated and either held in this position by an assistant or fixed with sandbags. The pelvis must remain as orthograde as possible. The beam is centered vertically on the upper symphysis rim. For the functional picture in adduction, the legs are extended, inwardly rotated as far as possible, and crossed. The leg on the affected side remains on the table.

The above abduction and adduction projections serve to assess the behavior of the joint space and the positioning of the head in the acetabulum. We look for good positioning with optimal joint congruity. The width of the joint space plays a subordinate role in the considerations of indication for intertrochanteric osteotomy. Marked widening of the joint space in the abduction picture must not be interpreted as a positioning with a thicker, more intact cartilage layer. On the contrary, this indicates an effusion and that the joint fluid is being forced cranially between the head and acetabulum by the tightly stretched caudal capsule.

If medial *arthritis* is present, then in obtaining preoperative X-rays of the affected hip the beam must be centered on the head. As a rule, only the operated side is checked postoperatively. In medial arthritis, because of projection distortion, symphysis-centered views must not be compared with head-centered ones.

In acetabular dyplasia the additional faux-profile view as described by Lequesne is useful, since it permits evaluation of the ventral portion of the acetabular roof.

If on clinical examination the patient has a clear-cut hip problem, no obvious lesions can be seen on the X-ray picture, then we must check very closely the sphericity of the femoral head. Very small differences, usually associated with certain structural irregularities in the cranial head segment, indicate head necrosis. In these cases contour photographs have been found to be very useful. As a rule two images are sufficient:

1. To obtain these contour views the patient lies flat on his back. The leg on the side to be investigated is raised to 45° with the knee kept in extension. An exact AP-directed central beam is centered on the femoral head. In this way the cranioventral area of the head

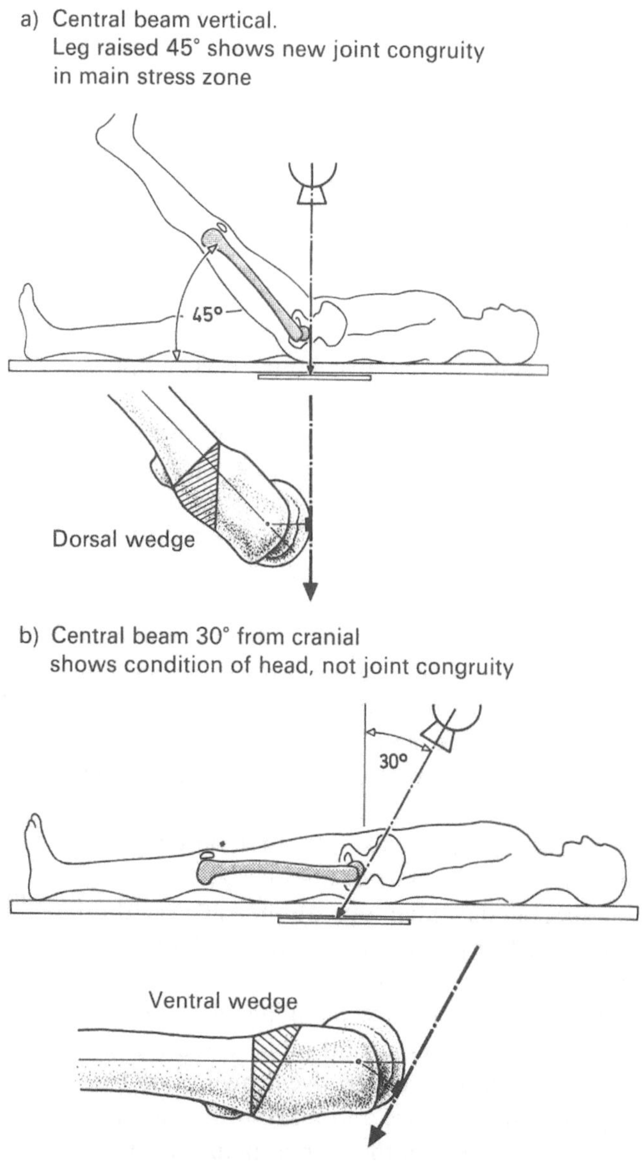

Fig. 13 a, b. Technique for obtaining the contour projections of the hip. **a** Representation of the cranioventral head contour and the corresponding joint congruity in extension osteotomy with removal of dorsal wedge. **b** Representation of the craniodorsal head congruity: The removal of a ventral wedge causes the dorsally situated head segment to be positioned in the main weight-bearing zone

is struck tangentially and is rendered visible. This also allows us to evaluate the congruity of the main weight-bearing zone as it will be after removal of a dorsal wedge of 45°.

2. The patient lies flat on his back, the knees are extended and the legs are in neutral rotation. The central beam is centered on the femoral head, but is directed about 30° obliquely from cranial to caudal. It strikes the abdominal skin approximately at the level of the classic appendectomy scar. This projects the craniodorsal head segment. Since the X-ray beam strikes the film obliquely and the distance from the object to the film is increased, the head appears to be oval and enlarged. In spite of this the state of the head segment represented can be assessed. The state of joint congruity as it will become after removal of a corresponding ventral wedge for a flexion osteotomy cannot be deduced from this projection, but it is safe to assume that it will be favorable if no deformity of the head contour is present (Fig. 13).

Lauenstein projections are frequently difficult to obtain because of the restricted movement. We recommend them only in exceptional cases. In patients with arthritis secondary to dysplasia with good joint mobility, they yield interesting information on the location of the wearing of the head and on the degree of decentralization of the head.

For reasons of economy we have not made full-length X-rays of the legs in the standing position in order to determine the line of weight-bearing.

Preparation for Surgery

General rules for elective bone surgery apply. The patient must be well; patients who are convalescing from a general illness are unsuitable for surgery. The skin of the area to be operated on must be free of any inflammatory or traumatic changes, and it should be covered on admission to hospital with a bacteriostatic or bactericidal substance with prolonged action, in order to prevent contamination by hospital bacteria. Shaving with a sterile razor is carried out only shortly before surgery and only adjacent to the operative area. The operation is performed under general or spinal anesthesia. We have found *dextran 70* to be the best for thromboembolic prophylaxis. The first bottle is administered at the start of anesthesia, the second on the 1st day after operation, and the third on the 3rd day after operation. Antibiotic prophylaxis is contraindicated.

Careful preoperative planning of the operation is the most important preparation one can make. We make preoperative drawings by tracing the X-ray picture and mark in the intended correction angles in the frontal plane. They can be cut out so that the extent of shortening and lengthening can be determined. We determine, with the aid of a special template, the plate which we are going to use as well as the required length of the blade. Clinical evaluation of the weight-bearing axis is adequate. We determine this by observing the alignment of the leg in the standing position. This allows us to determine which displacements are permissible.

Surgery

The operation is performed on a regular operating table. The patient is positioned supine. The involved hip and leg are draped free. We prefer waterproof draping so that irrigation can be used during surgery without fear of contamination. The draping must be such that the anterior superior iliac spines, the patellae, and the medial malleoli are palpable. The cleansed skin in the operation field is covered with a thin, plastic sheet.

The skin incision is lateral and extends 20–30 cm distal from the tip of the greater trochanter. In extensive valgization osteotomies it must be made considerably longer than in varization osteotomies, especially if the tension device is to be used. The skin and subcutaneous tissue are incised in one plane. Hemostasis is secured with electrocoagulation. All vessels must be coagulated, since meticulous hemostasis is the best prophylaxis for postoperative hematoma. This is of particular importance since dextran increases the tendency to postoperative hematoma formation. At the end of surgery subcutaneous hemostasis is checked once more, so that not a single bleeder remains unchecked. The fascia lata is opened for the length of the skin incision. Care should be taken not to damage the vastus lateralis muscle. The linea innominata, the distal limit of the trochanteric mass, is palpated, and a Hohmann retractor with a narrow tip is inserted dorsal to the trochanter. The vastus lateralis is then detached from its insertion into the linea innominata of the greater trochanter. This dorsoventral cut reaches the linea aspera distally through the fascia. Once the fascia overlying the vastus lateralis is cut the muscle is pulled ventrally with a sharp rake and with a broad periosteal elevator, the vastus lateralis muscle is then reflected from the bone and the septum. The perforating vessels should be isolated, crossed, clamped and ligated. The heavy bleeders in the vastus lateralis muscle at its insertion in the intertrochanteric region must be coagulated as the cut is made. The intertrochanteric area is exposed with a periosteal elevator. Posteriorly the gluteus maximus is released from the linea aspera over a distance of 4 cm. Once this is done it is possible to palpate with a finger the lesser trochanter. A Hohmann retractor with a wide tip is then introduced dorsally in order to protect the

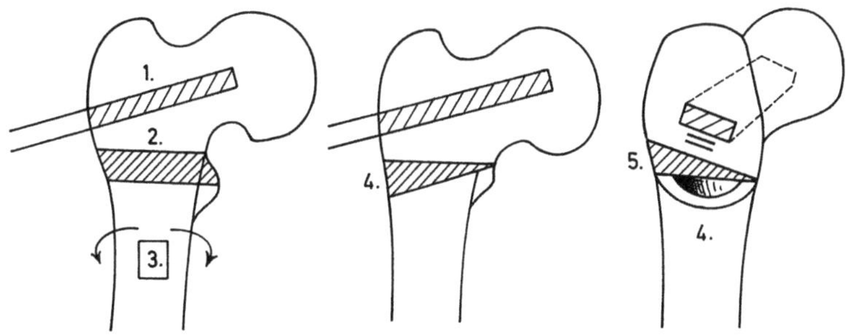

Fig. 14. Technical steps of a valgization osteotomy to be fixed with either a 120° or 130° plate. *1* Determine the position of the blade within the femoral head, driving in the seating chisel. *2* Horizontal osteotomy above the lesser trochanter. In the case of more extensive valgization (above 20°) or in a patient with an especially long femoral neck, a bone segment is removed from the intertrochanteric area to shorten the leg. According to Bombelli the lesser trochanter can be sacrificed. *3* Rotational correction before removal of the valgization wedge. *4* Remove the valgization wedge from the distal fragment. *5* Removal of the dorsal extension wedge from the proximal fragment with the cut parallel to the seating chisel. It is imperative that the rotational correction be made before removal of the wedge from the distal fragment

sciatic nerve. A second Hohmann retractor is introduced medially round the femur. The calcar is exposed with a curved periosteal elevator. The dissection is then continued to expose the anterior part of the joint capsule. Once this is done, a Hohmann lever with a narrow tip is inserted over the anterior lip of the acetabulum. This will maintain the anterior exposure of the hip. The capsule is incised in line with the neck. This avoids damage to any vessels which supply the femoral head. The joint is examined and any loose bodies are removed. The capsule is left open. The area of the bone where the osteotomy is to be made is exposed, and with the help of the preoperative sketch the wedges to be removed are marked in the bone. The site of blade entry is chosen so that there will be at least a 15-mm bony bridge between the blade and the osteotomy. A Kirschner wire is now placed along the inferior aspect of the neck to mark the anteversion. A second Kirschner wire is now inserted into the greater trochanter to mark in the frontal plane the position of the seating chisel. Its angle with a shaft axis has been predetermined in the preoperative drawings. It must also be inserted parallel to the first Kirschner wire which marks its anteversion or direction in the horizontal plane. In order to achieve the desired correction in the sagittal plane, the flap of the seating chisel guide is held at the appropriate angle to the femoral shaft. The seating chisel is then hammered into a depth of about 4 cm, with constant checking its direction against the guide wire. At this point small corrections in the sagittal plane are still possible with the aid of the slit hammer. If all is well, the seating chisel is driven in to the calculated depth of the blade. If it is driven in correctly, it will not meet any appreciable resistance. It should then be backed out with the slit hammer for about 1–2 cm to make sure it is not stuck. It is much easier to knock out the seating chisel before the osteotomy is made, because the mass of the femur is still intact. Next make the intertrochanteric osteotomy with the oscillation saw, following the precut markings in the bone. It is important to use a new, undamaged blade and to let it run without pressure. This first osteotomy cut is usually made at 90° to the axis of the shaft.

In a valgus osteotomy, first correct the rotation and then cut a wedge with a lateral base from the distal fragment. If shortening is required, the wedge becomes a trapezium. In the case that extension is necessary the corresponding wedge with a dorsal base is removed from the proximal fragment. Once the valgization wedge has been removed, the rotation of the leg can no longer be corrected (Fig. 14).

In a varization osteotomy, we remove the wedge from the proximal fragment. If the saw blade is held exactly parallel to the seating chisel and a 90° plate is used, then the wedge cut will automatically be correct. This also applies in

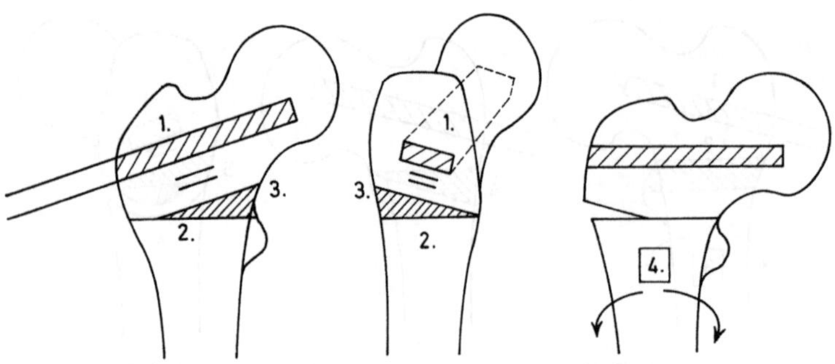

Fig. 15.1. Technical procedure in the planning of varization osteotomy using a 90° angled plate. *1* Prepare the seat for the blade within the femoral neck. Its position is determined by the extent of the planned varization and, if necessary, extension. The blade position ultimately determines the corrections in the frontal and sagittal planes. *2* Horizontal osteotomy above the lesser trochanter. *3* The required wedge is removed from the proximal fragment parallel to the seating chisel. In order to prevent greater shortening than necessary, the medial wedge is cut only from half the width of the osteotomy. *4* Because of the horizontal position of the osteotomy cut in the distal fragment, the rotation correction can be performed even after removal of the wedge from the proximal fragment

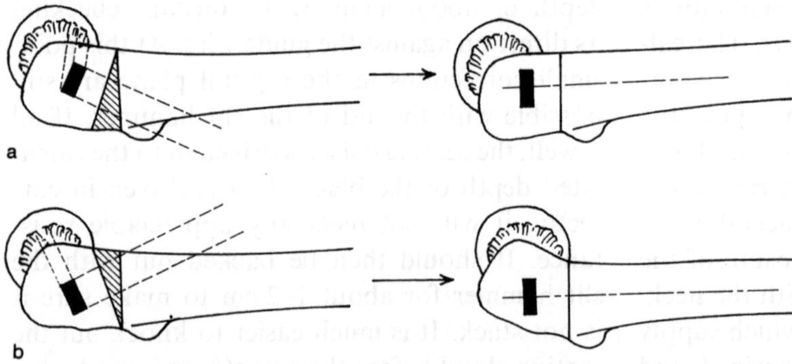

Fig. 15.2 a, b. The position of the blade for both the extension and flexion osteotomy. **a** In extension osteotomy the seating chisel is introduced as far ventrally as possible. **b** In flexion osteotomy the blade has to be introduced as far dorsally as possible. Observance of these facts ensures that the best possible congruity of the osteotomy surfaces is attained

the case of simultaneous extension. In order to minimize the shortening, we recommend to cut the wedge only from the center of the osteotomy area and to insert it in the lateral defect before compression with the tension device. Because the osteotomy in the distal fragment is vertical to the shaft axis, rotational correction of the leg can also be made after removal of the wedge without the danger of any incongruity in the contact area (Fig. 15).

One should not, however, attempt any rotational corrections once the tension device is fixed to the bone. After removal of the wedge, the seating chisel is knocked out. The previously selected plate, held in the plate holder, is first pushed by hand a few centimeters into the precut channel, and then completely hammered in.

Reduction of the osteotomy occurs automatically as the plate is held against the lateral cortex of the femoral shaft. One or two Verbrugge forceps are used to hold the reduction. Next check leg length and rotation. Interfragmentary compression can be performed in different ways. The maximum loading path of 2 mm of the DC holes of a DC plate is normally not sufficient; therefore, even if a DCP is used, the tension device is required. With a round-hole 90° plate the tension device is a must. Axial interfragmentary compression can also be achieved with the 120° and 130° plates, but the proximal fragment must first be fixed to the plate with a screw. The more elegant way of achieving interfragmental compression with the 120° and 130° plates is to use the obliquity of the osteotomy. If the most distal screw is screwed in before the plate touches the proximal part of the femoral shaft (a distance of about 0.5–1.0 cm), the insertion of the proximal screws will then produce interfragmental compression.

Finally, the position of the leg is checked once again. The vastus lateralis muscle is reattached. The joint capsule is left open. The tendon of the iliopsoas muscle can be cut. A 4-mm suction drain is placed under the vastus lateralis muscle in such a way that its tip lies behind the osteotomy. The fascia is then closed. A second suction drain is placed subcutaneously, and the skin is sutured. At the end the degree of abduction is checked, and if it is insufficient, a tenotomy of the adductor longus tendon is carried out, and if necessary also of the adductor magnus tendon. These are performed through a stab incision. A skin suture is usually not necessary.

Finally, while the patient is still on the operation table both legs are raised vertically and massaged vigorously from toes to groin. Compression bandages are applied from toes to the groin on the operated side, and up to the knee joint on the other side. For greater details of the surgical technique we refer the reader to the AO (ASIF) Manual of Internal Fixation (Müller et al. 1979).

Postoperative Treatment

We have found that postoperative treatment plays a much greater role in determining the success of intertrochanteric osteotomy in osteoarthritis of the hip joint than it does in total hip replacement. In the early postoperative days it is important to give the patient confidence in his stable internal fixation. Because of fear that something could slip after the "bone cutting", patients tend to contract their muscles in order to splint the hip. This in itself is painfree, and the patients are content, but the physician must not allow the patient to lie tense and stiff. Rotation of the foot and stretching exercises of the quadriceps muscle are not sufficient. From the first postoperative day onward, assisted flexion exercises must be performed. This is possible without pain only in patients who relax; usually the first attempt at flexion causes pain. In our opinion it is most important that the surgeon explains to the patient that this pain originates solely from the muscles in spasm. The patient will gain confidence and relax once he realizes that the pain disappears after repeated assisted flexion movements. Usually within a few days at least half of the preoperative range of flexion is regained. It is most important that the patient learns to relax. The assisted movement exercises should be of the nature of relaxation exercises. For psychological reasons, it is important that early on in the postoperative period these exercises be not simply delegated to a physiotherapist. We know from our own experience that a correctly performed osteotomy can fail if the surgeon does not give personal attention to the patient's postoperative rehabilitation.

Early movement brings great advantages, but early ambulation does not. Unfortunately, high hospital costs require patients to be discharged at the start of the 3rd week, so that they must get up at the end of the 1st week. Partial weight-bearing with correct heel to toe contact must be learned. We aim at a loading of 15–25 kg. The patient should check this frequently with the aid of a bathroom scale. This partial weight-bearing with two elbow crutches should be carried out for at least 3 months. Subsequently the patient should use a cane on the opposite side for a further 3 months. Time to return to work varies. Patients who do heavy physical work may not be fit to return to work for 9–12 months.

Results

Large series, by their very nature, make accurate reporting of results difficult. In our series of 786 intertrochanteric osteotomies for osteoarthritis of the hip joint, because all were executed and followed up by the same surgeon, the number and type of secondary revision operations are known. This total includes a group of 109 operations in 100 patients performed between 1959 and 1962. This group was carefully examined after 2–5 years and after 12–15 years (Tables 1–3). After 2–5 years 95 patients could be followed up, after 12–15 years only 35. We tabulated our results under pain, ability to walk,

Table 1. Quality of results (12- to 15-year follow-up)

Result	Patients Operations			
I. Follow-up examination	Good or satisfactory	33	37	(65%)
	Unsatisfactory	2		
II. Death without reoperation (results from questionnaire)	Good or satisfactory	27	34	
	Unsatisfactory	4		
III. Poor results with reoperation (after an average of 8 years)		34	38	(35%)
Total hip replacement			34	
Arthrodesis			4	

Table 2. Osteotomy type related to results (12- to 15-year follow-up)

	Valgus	Varus	Displacement	Addition extension
I. Follow-up examinations (25 F, 10 M)	13	20	4	23/37
II. Death without reoperation (27 F, 4 M)	13	10	11	23/34
	26	30	15	
III. Reoperation	20	17	1	20/38

leg length discrepancy, range of flexion, loss of extension (fixed flexion deformity) and rotation (Table 1). Of special interest are the 35 long-term survivors (Table 3). Note their average age and ability to walk.

In 60 cases, an *extension osteotomy* (average 30°) was performed simultaneously with varization, valgization, or just with displacement. It is of interest to note that simultaneous extension was performed in 51% of the cases with poor results in whom reoperation was necessary, whereas in the good or satisfactory cases the corresponding figure was 69%.

The Influence of Extension Osteotomy on Flexion and Extension. Despite the removal of a dorsal wedge on average of 30°, after 2–5 years extension had improved by only 5°. In 48 cases without a dorsal wedge, it deteriorated by 2°. Flexion was affected only to a small degree. With extension osteotomy it was reduced on average by 4°, without extension osteotomy it improved on average by 5°.

The Influence of Bilateral Disease. Basically, all parameters are influenced in the same way in bilateral disorders as in unilateral disorders, but they were on average 15°–20° worse.

Incidence of Revision Surgery. Of the 677 operations performed since 1 June 1962, 154 (22.7%) were unsatisfactory and required a second operation. There were 129 total hip replacements, 12 arthrodeses, and 13 secondary intertrochantric osteotomies. Total hip replacement had to be performed on the average 5.3 years after surgery, arthrodesis in 1.4 years, and secondary intertrochanteric osteotomies after 3.8 years.

Table 3. Parameters used in evaluation of intertrochanteric osteotomy

	Time of operation (100 patients; average age 59.5 years)	After 2–5 years (95 patients)	After 12–15 years (35 patients; average age 69.6 years)
Pain (Merle d'Aubigné scale)	2.5	5.4	5.3
Ability to walk	1.7 km	4.9 km	4.0 km
Difference in leg length	−1.8 cm	−1.3 cm	−1.0 cm
Range of flexion	48°	48°[a]	47°
Loss of extension	15°	13°	13°
Range of rotation	3°	20°	20°
Rotation attitude	18° outward	–	16° outward

[a] This mean value for the range of flexion is misleading. The analysis of the individual cases shows 52 improvements, five unchanged, and 38 deteriorations. Among the improvements there are two of 50° and 55°, among the deteriorations three of 60°, 70°, and 80°. In the latter both the indication and the technique applied were in correct.

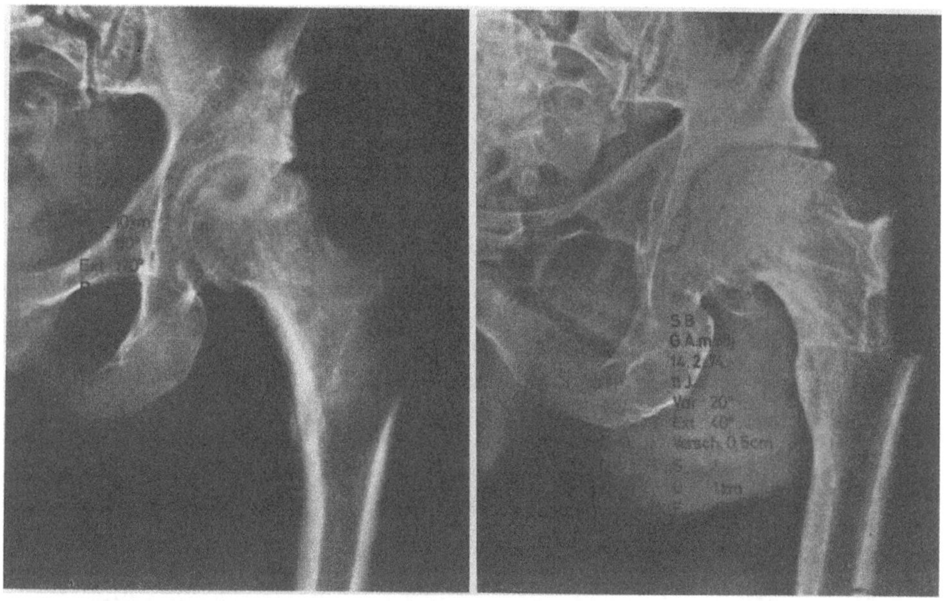

Fig. 16. Severe osteoarthritis of the hip with loss of the joint space in a 56-year-old factory worker. Note the absence of a distal head osteophyte in the main weight-bearing zone. Nine years after varus-extension-displacement osteotomy. Good radiological joint regeneration has been maintained

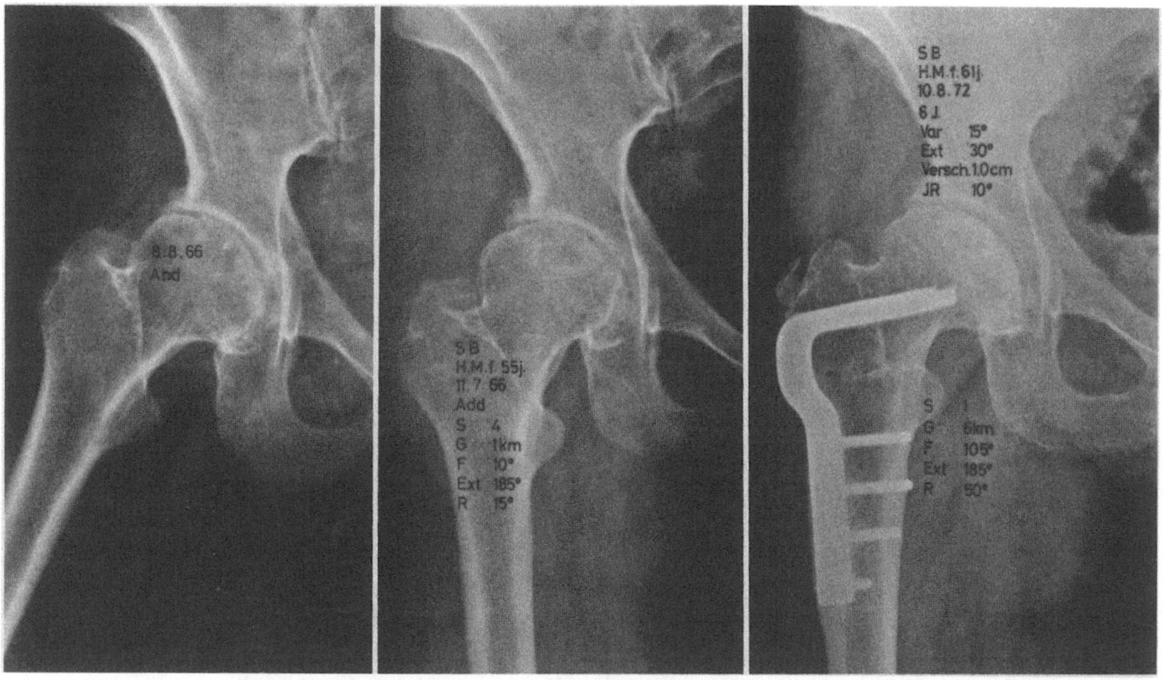

Fig. 17. A 55-year-old housewife. Abduction with congruent joint space maintained in the abduction picture. Indication for varization. Six years after varization of 15° in combination with extension of 30°, medial displacement of 1 cm, and inward rotation of 10°. The patient is almost completely free of complaints. Flexion gain of 95°(!), rotation gain of 35°

Legend to Symbols Used on X-Rays

S=pain; *0*=no pain (*6* on Merle d'Aubigné scale), *5*=severe permanent pain (*0* on Merle d'Aubigné scale). *G*=ability to walk unaided or with one cane; *F*=range of flexion; *E*=extension, 180°=complete extension, 160°=loss

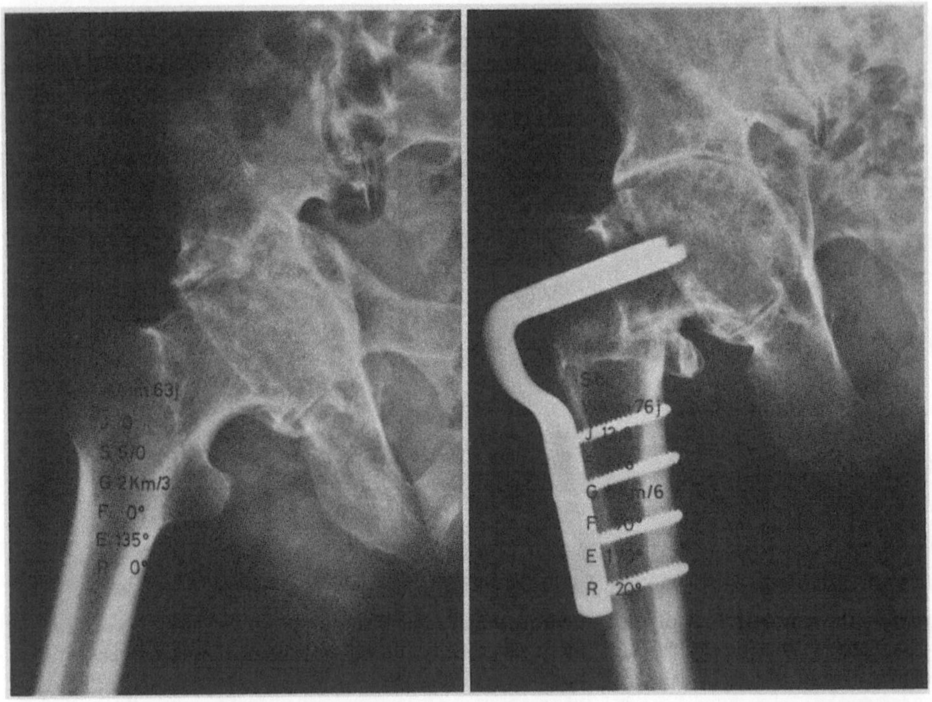

Fig. 18. Primary osteoarthritis of the hip in a 63-year-old man with abduction and flexion contracture. Completely stiff joint with severe pain. Intertrochanteric varus-extension osteotomy performed to correct the deformity of the leg. After 13 years, there is a range of flexion of 70°. Range of rotation is 20°. The leg lies in the correct position with a loss of extension of only 10°. The patient is free of pain and can walk 5 km

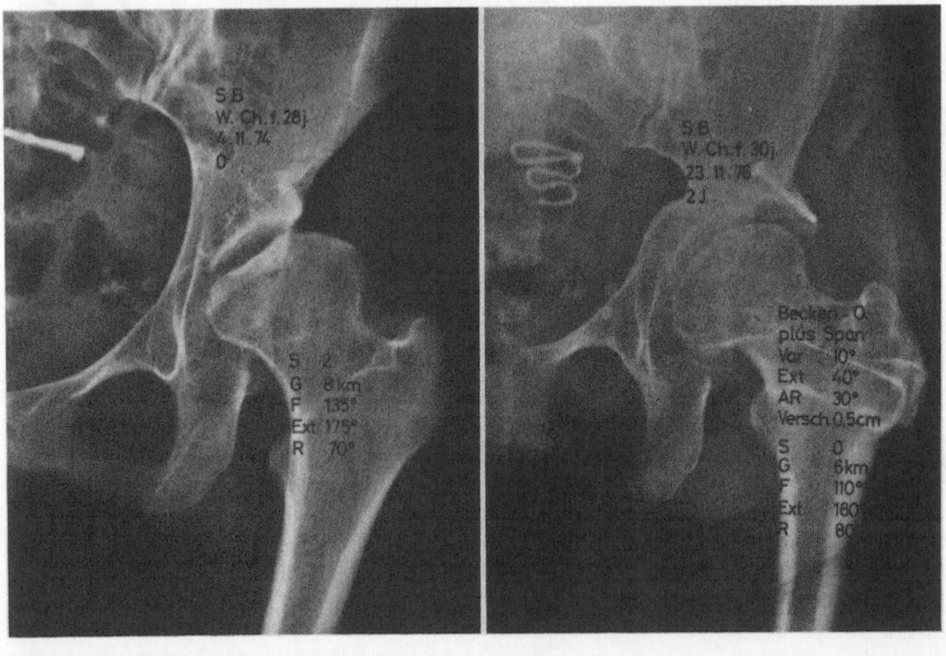

Fig. 19. Severe painful dysplasia of the hip in a 28-year-old woman. Severe lateral and frontal acetabular insufficiency. Acetabular roof-plasty by pelvic osteotomy with additional bone graft. Varus-extension osteotomy at same time. Two years after surgery, the condition of the joint has improved considerably and the patient is symptom-free

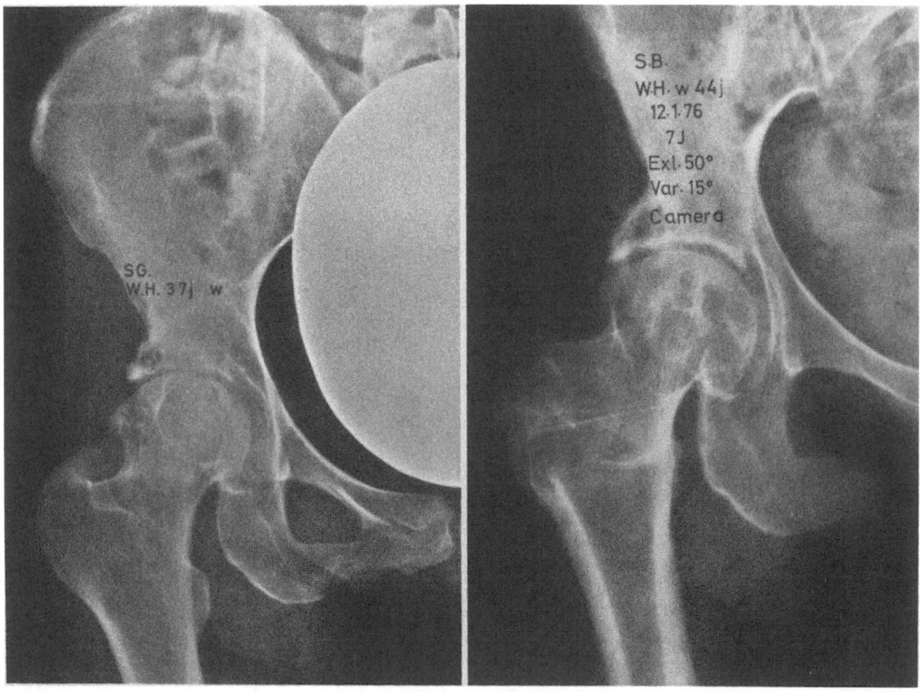

Fig. 20. A 37-year-old farmer's wife. Early head depression with painful severe subchondral dysostosis. Narrowing of joint space to 1.5 mm. Seven years after varization of 15° and extension of 50°, with simultaneous cancellous grafting of the large head cyst. The head appears beautifully spherical and sharply outlined. The joint space has widened to 3–4 mm. Patient is symptom-free

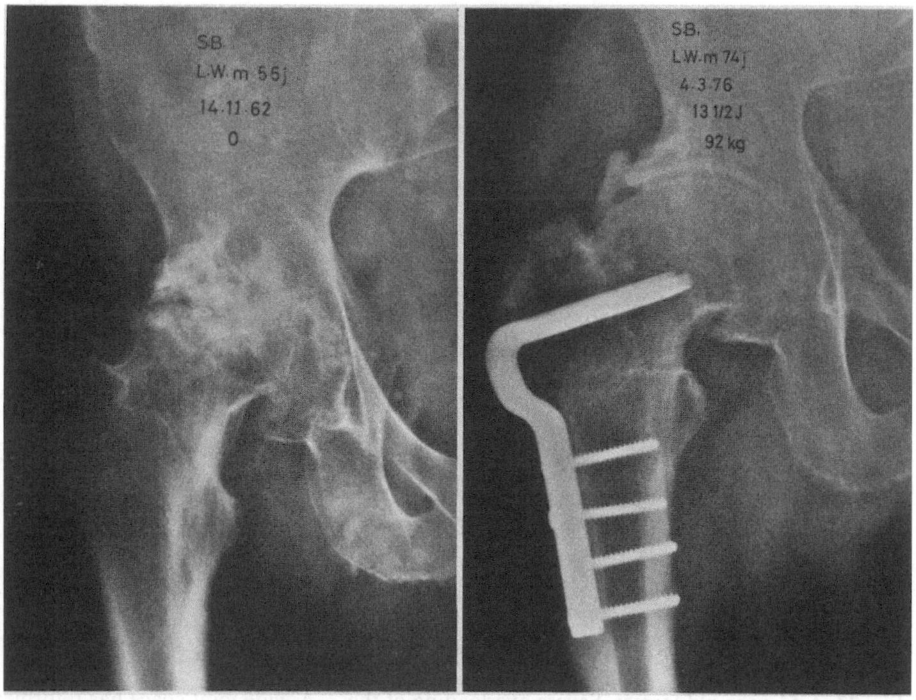

Fig. 21. An obese, 55-year-old businessman. Severe joint damage. At $13^1/_2$ years after varization of 20°, inward rotation of 10°, and adductor tenotomy there is good joint regeneration. A joint space with a 3 mm width has been maintained. Striking disappearance of the pathological contractures and complete absence of symptoms

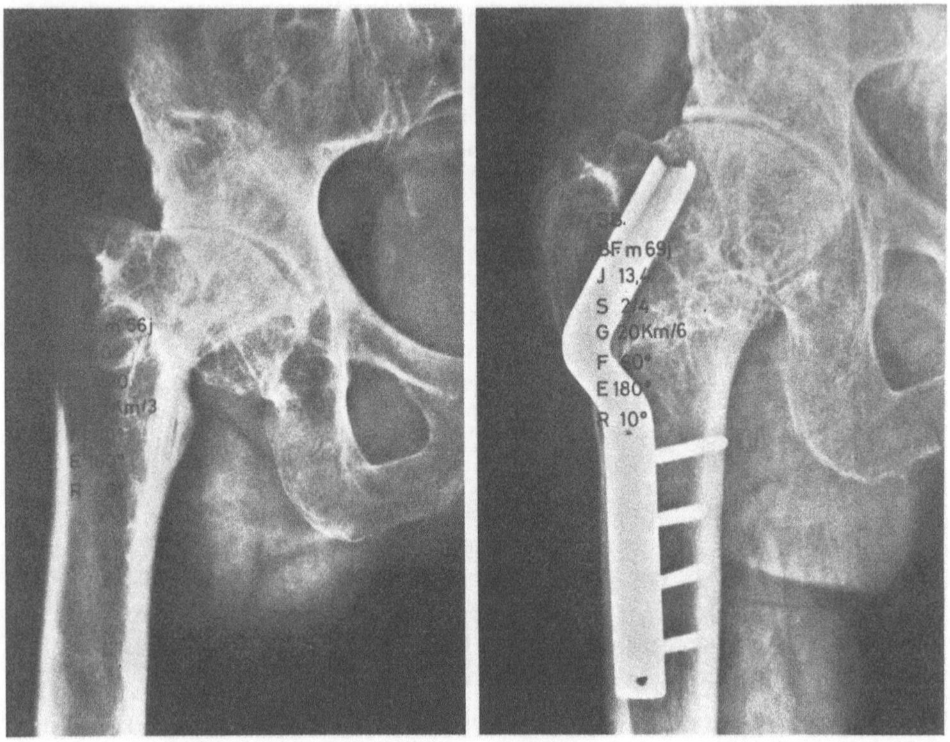

Fig. 22. A 56-year-old farm worker. Coxa vara after a slipped capital epiphysis. Ideal indication for valgization. After 13 years the joint space measures 3–4 mm and is congruent. The pathological structural changes secondary to arthritis have disappeared

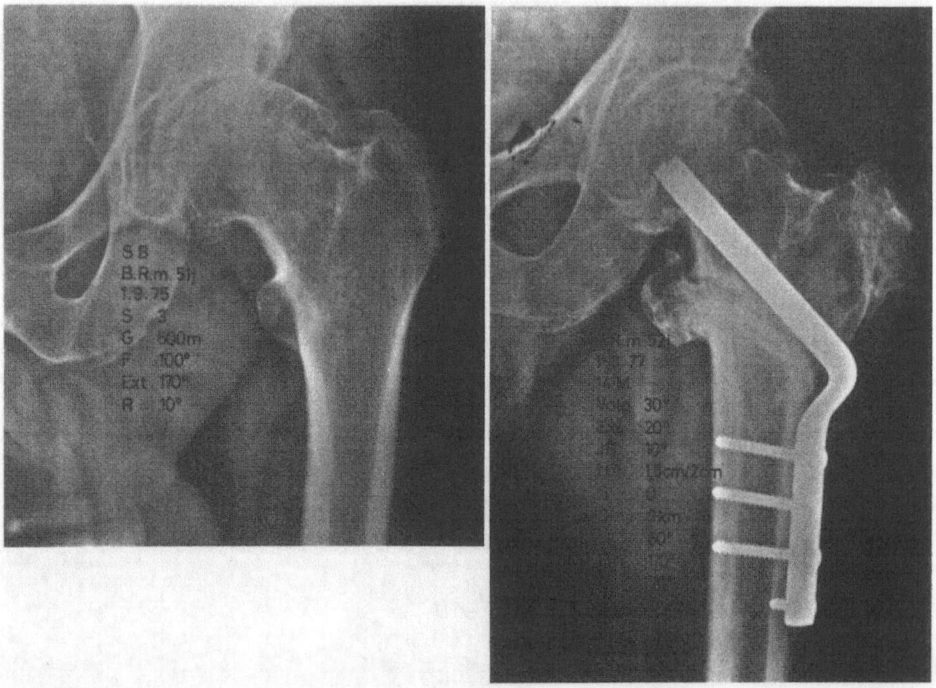

Fig. 23. A 51-year-old farmer. Severe overloading of the acetabular corner. Fourteen months after performance of a valgus-extension osteotomy with lateralization of the trochanter, and osteotomy of the lesser trochanter. A wide joint space has reformed, and the arthritic structural damage has regressed markedly. The pain has disappeared and walking ability has improved considerably

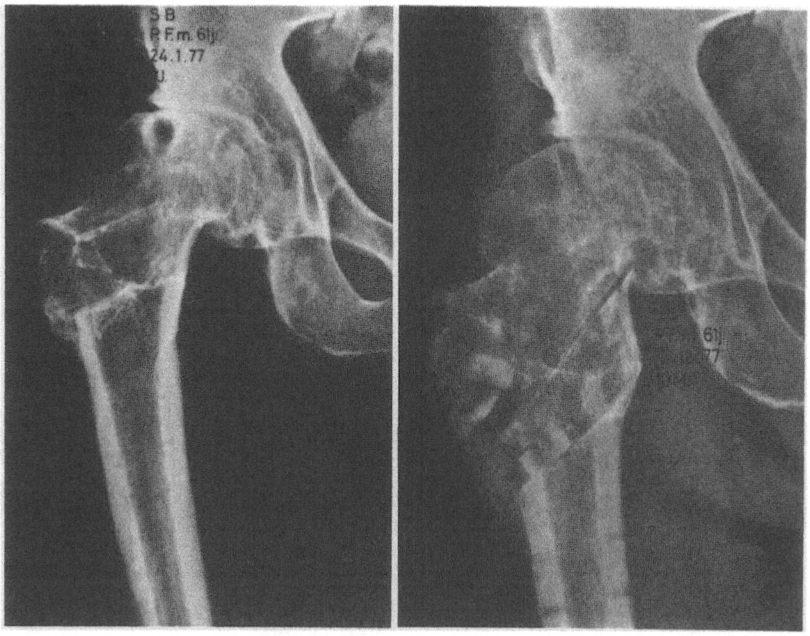

Fig. 24. A 61-year-old administrative clerk. Unsatisfactory result 7 years after varization. Note the formation of a medial head osteophyte. This is a good indication for a second osteotomy. The Bombelli type valgus osteotomy with lateralization of the shaft was performed. Valgization of 30°, extension of 20°, and shortening of 1 cm with sacrifice of the lesser trochanter. Increasingly good mobility and freedom from pain. Plate removed after 10 months. Good regeneration of joint space

of extension of 20°; R = range of rotation; M = months; J,j = years.

In some figures the extent of the surgical correction is also given (Versch. = displacement, R. = rotation, Var. = varus, Valg. = valgus, Displ. = displacement and Displ. Ext. = extension osteotomy). In the contour films (Figs. 26, 27, 28.2), F/flexion designates the extent of hip flexion at the time the X-ray was taken.

S.G./S.B. = patient at the author's clinic in Grosshöchstetten/Biel. Reference is made to Figs. 16–29 in the Discussion.

Complications

Infection

If we define an infection as a prolongation of the treatment period or impairment of the final result, then we have experienced only four infections (0.5%). Two of the infections involved the same patient, who apparently had a decrease in resistance. One side could be salvaged by a cobra plate arthrodesis. On the other side, 5 years after the arthrodesis, we attempted a total hip replacement which unfortunately failed and the patient ended with a girdlestone. In a second patient the hip underwent spontaneous fusion with a satisfactory result. In a third patient we had to carry out on the 9th postoperative day a debridement with suction drainage. The final result was perfect.

Postoperative Hematoma

Postoperative hematomas, like infections, are not as serious a complication in intertrochanteric osteotomy as in total hip replacement. Only in six cases did a hematoma have to be surgically drained. It should be stressed, however, that a painful distended wound secondary to a hematoma must be drained surgically. Hematoma formation is unquestionably related to early movement, but it is a small price to pay for the benefit of early mobilization.

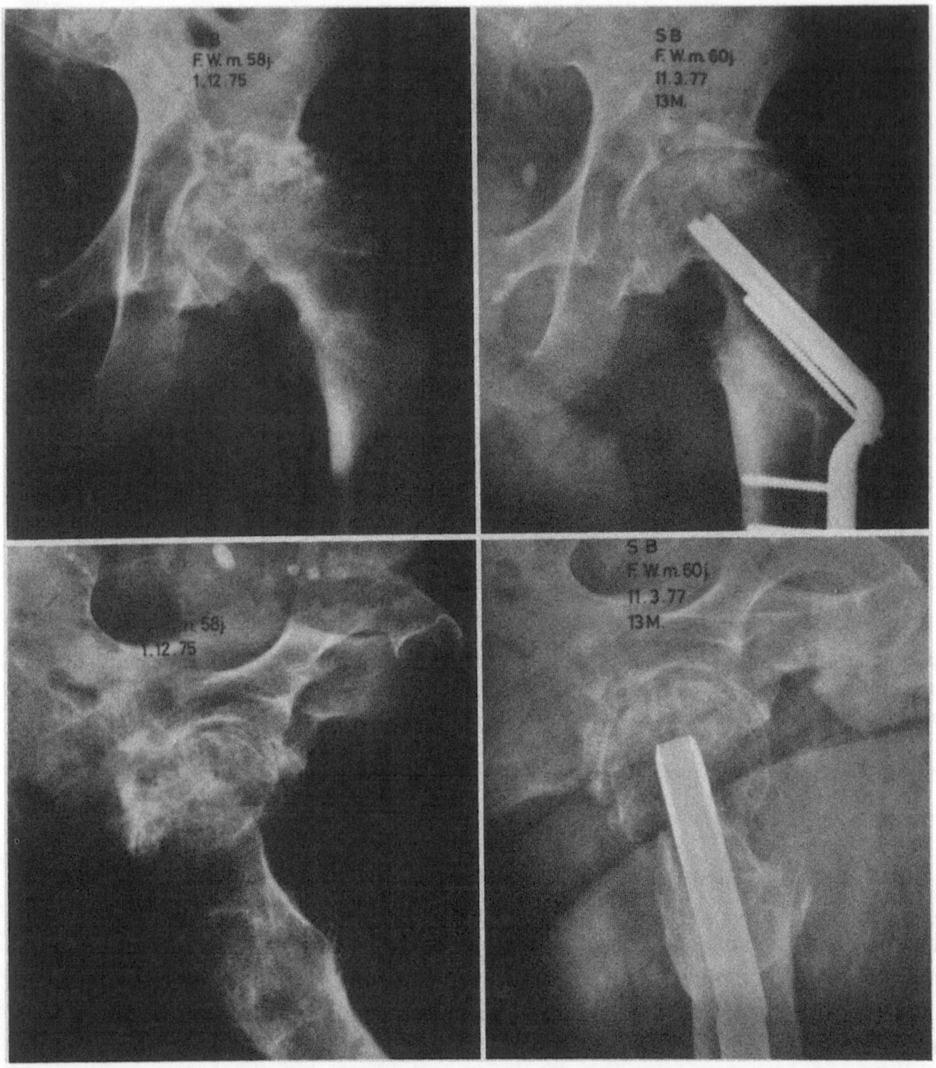

Fig. 25. A 58-year-old business man. Severe osteoarthritis of the hip with severe cranial and ventral wear of the head. Caudal head osteophyte present. This is a good indication for a valgus-extension osteotomy. After 13 months the patient is symptom-free and the joint is undergoing regeneration. The head osteophyte has been integrated. Extension osteotomy has resulted in an impressive centering of the head. The ventral joint overload has been eliminated

Phlebothrombosis and Pulmonary Embolism

Before 1971 we lost three patients to pulmonary embolism, but since then, at the time of writing, we have not had any further cases. Deep phlebothrombosis occurs clinically in about one-quarter of all cases. Postoperative swelling of the leg must be interpreted as phlebothrombosis, even in the absence of color changes or other signs. In our experience most of these symptoms disappear within a year.

We ascribe the reduction in the incidence of fatal pulmonary embolism to the systematic use of dextran prophylaxis. Regular elevation of the legs at the end of surgery, massage from toes to groin, compression bandages, active leg muscle exercises, and breathing exercises are valuable supportive measures if carried out as early

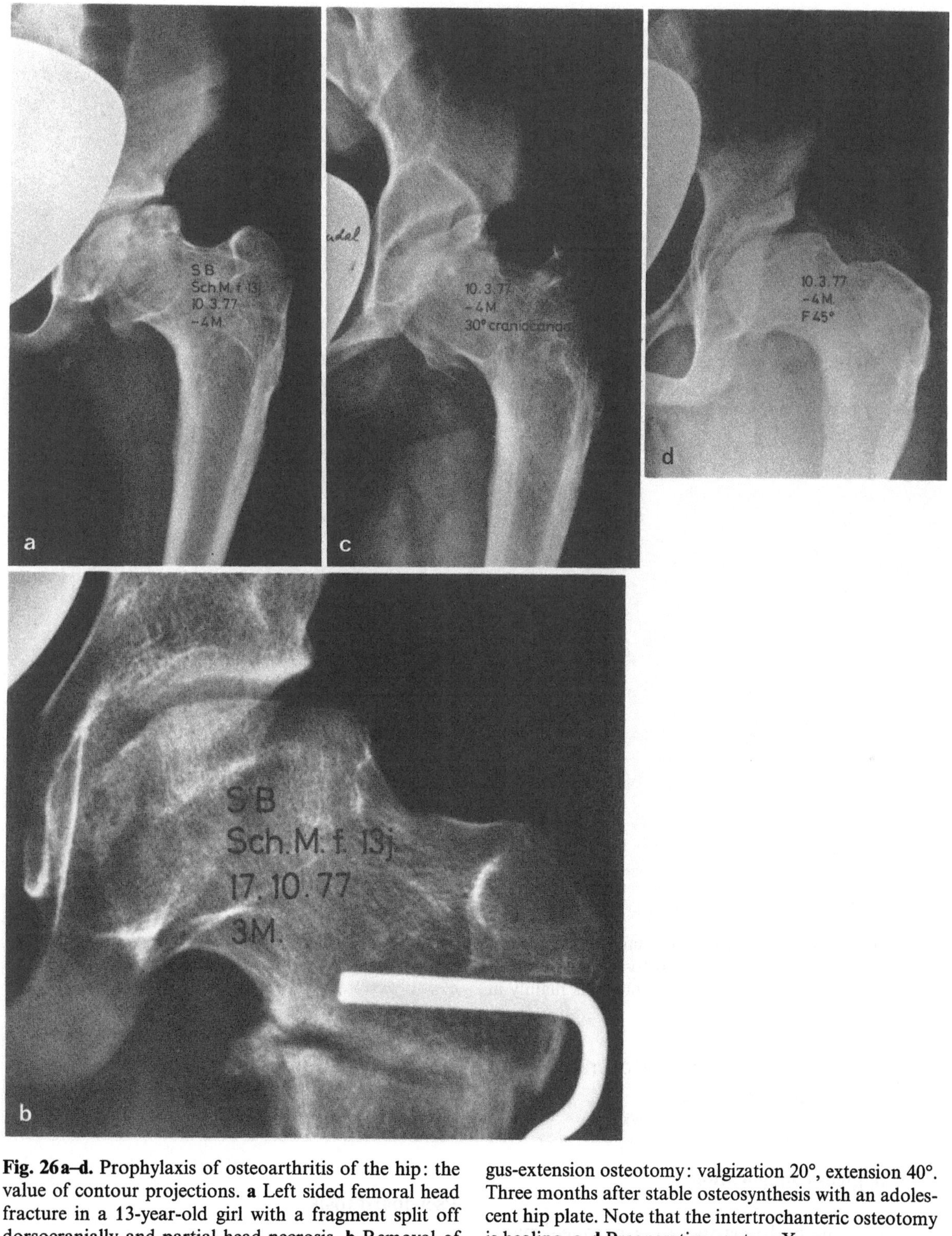

Fig. 26a–d. Prophylaxis of osteoarthritis of the hip: the value of contour projections. **a** Left sided femoral head fracture in a 13-year-old girl with a fragment split off dorsocranially and partial head necrosis. **b** Removal of joint incongruity and symptoms by intertrochanteric valgus-extension osteotomy: valgization 20°, extension 40°. Three months after stable osteosynthesis with an adolescent hip plate. Note that the intertrochanteric osteotomy is healing. **c, d** Preoperative contour X-rays

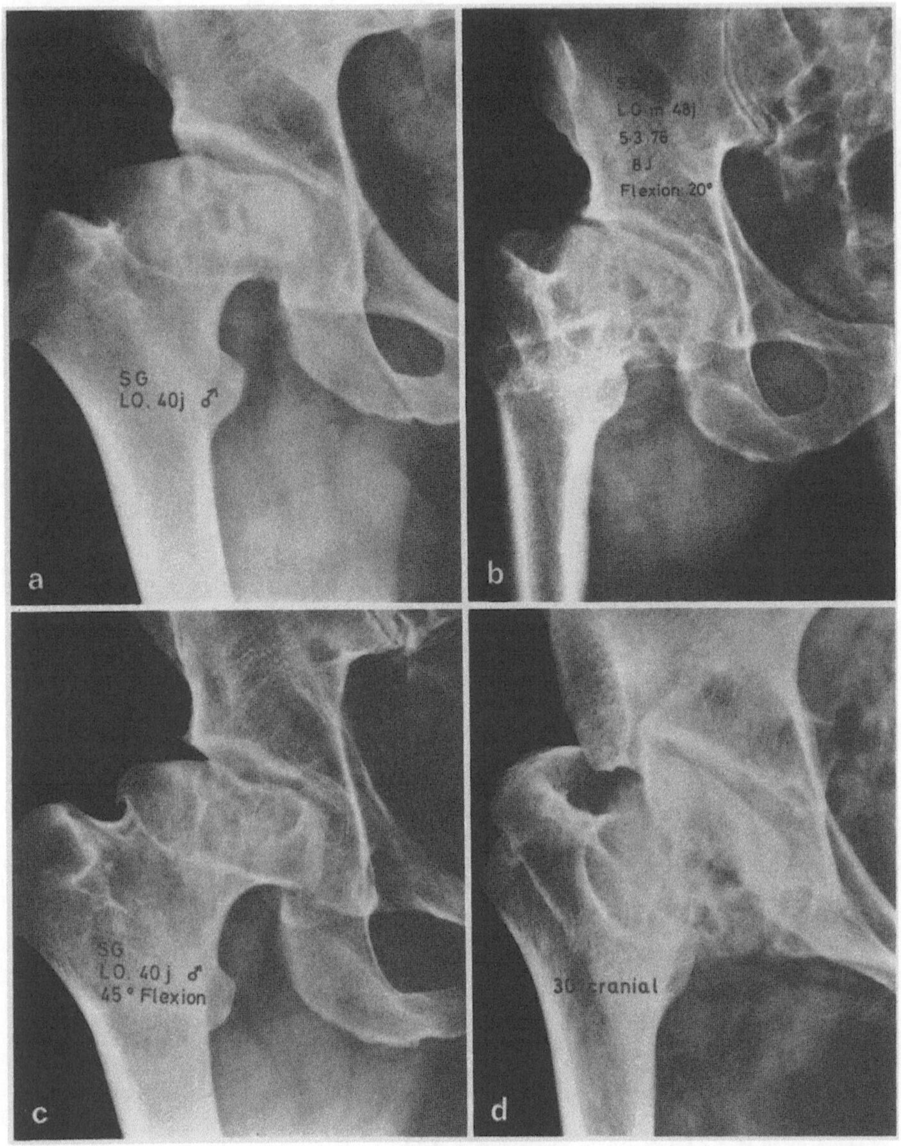

Fig. 27a–d. A 40-year-old businessman. **a** Severe head deformity with subchrondral dysostosis. According to the contour X-rays (**c, d**), the deformity was mainly in the cranioventral region. **b** Eight years after flexion osteotomy the joint is fairly congruent

as possible. During the first postoperative night the bladder must be emptied.

Neurological Complications

Twelve cases had postoperative peroneal paresis, which became permanent in two patients. Examination of the sciatic nerve, particularly its lateral portion, did not reveal any signs of nerve damage. As explanation we postulate either peripheral pressure damage or intraneural hemorrhages. We observed no lesions of the femoral nerve.

Pseudoarthrosis

Two early cases developed a pseudoarthrosis and had to be reoperated. Both healed. In two cases, the blade was pulled out in the immediate postoperative stage. Despite the necessary oper-

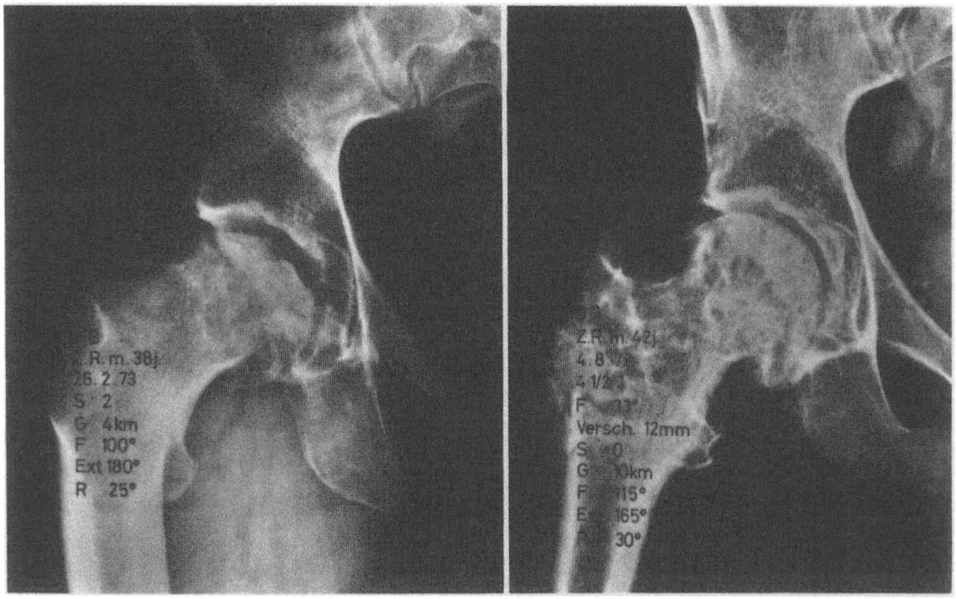

Fig. 28.1. A 38-year-old building foreman. Severe idiopathic head necrosis mainly of the cranioventral portion. According to the contour projections (not shown), the dorsal portion of the head contour is relatively intact. At $4^1/_2$ years after intertrochanteric flexion osteotomy of 30° the patient is free of symptoms. There is a loss of extension of 15°. Sphericity of the head in the main weight-bearing zone is restored, and the width of the joint space is normal

ation one of these two patients ended up with a particularly good late result!

We must emphasize that as long as one avoids technical errors the AO technique makes it possible to prevent pseudoarthoses completely.

Discussion

Analysis of our results shows that if the indications are good the results of the different intertrochanteric osteotomies are the same as far as pain, ability to walk, range of flexion, extension, and range of rotation are concerned. In the late result no significant difference can be found between valgization, varization, and displacement osteotomy. The addition of extension appears to be beneficial. After 12–15 years one can expect 50% satisfactory permanent results. The results published in 1974 by Plass and in 1977 by Watillon et al. are slightly better. The reasons for this are that our follow-up period is longer, our patients on the average older and the surgery was performed between the years 1959–1862 when our understanding of the indications was less clear.

The correlation between freedom from pain and improvement in range of rotation is impressive. In the good cases it is remarkable that the degree of rotation, the loss of extension, and the functional leg length remain unchanged with the course of time. Just like the walking ability, these values were improved by intertrochanteric osteotomy.

We did not find any improvement in the average range of flexion as a result of intertrochanteric osteotomy. This parallels the experience of other authors.

The range of flexion achieved did not increase with the course of time. The average values given for the range of flexion were misleading because some spectacular restrictions are balanced by just as many increases. In the majority of instances the poor results were due to incorrect indications. These consist of cases with progressive, destructive changes due to inflammation which have a well-preserved range of flexion and end up with stiffness even after intertrochanteric osteotomy. We are also anxious to

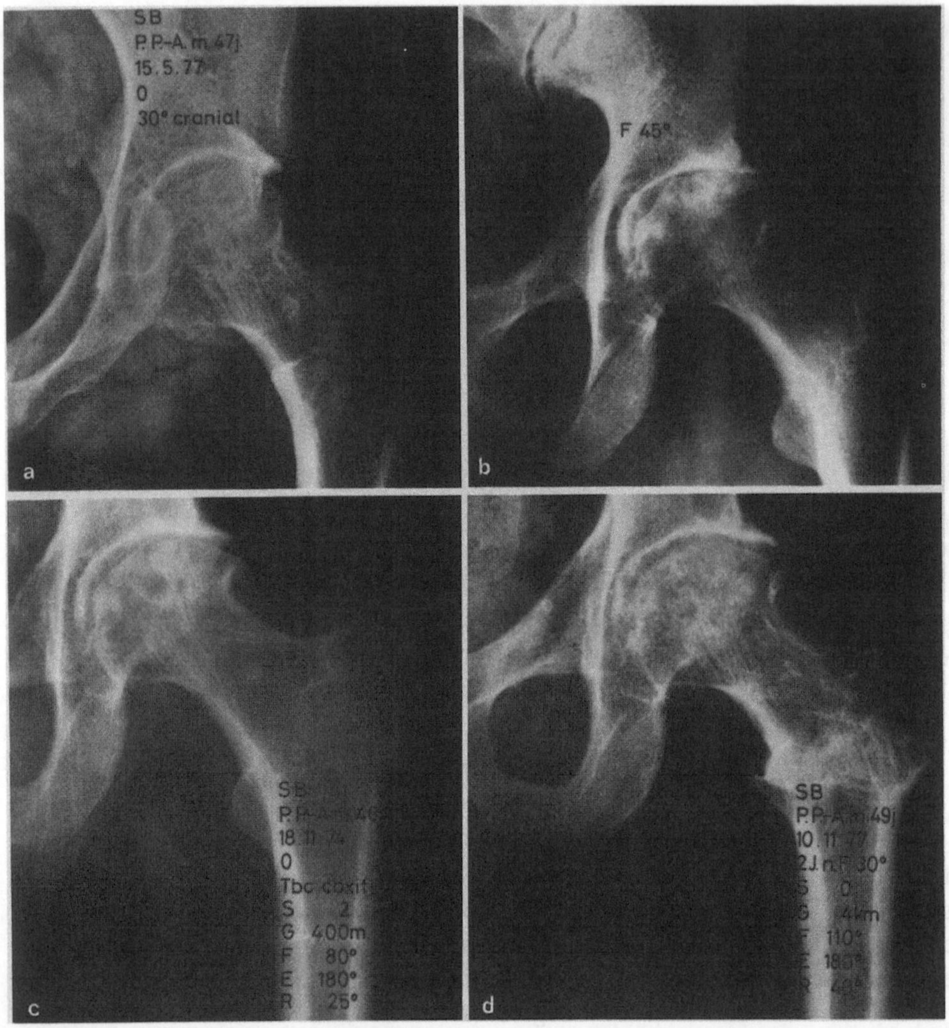

Fig. 28.2 a–d. A 47-year-old watchmaker with a history of tuberculous coxitis on left side at the age of 20. At 46 pain with severe limitation of walking (**c**). On the basis of contour X-rays (**a, b**), a flexion osteotomy of 30° was performed. Two years later the patient was symptom-free, with a gain in flexion of 30°. Extension was full. Note also the good radiological joint regeneration (**d**)

point out all the cases in which the range of flexion increased significantly. We feel that the range of flexion alone cannot be used as a parameter to decide for or against an osteotomy. Two of our patients with deformity and a completely stiff hip underwent intertrochanteric osteotomy simply to realign their limb. They achieved gains in flexion of 60° and 70° respectively after 12 and 14 years. At the same time they were free from pain and showed good joint regeneration radiologically (Figs. 17, 18). We agree completely with Schneider und Weill (1975) that a good permanent clinical result is always accompanied by radiological evidence of joint regeneration. We agree also with H. Wagner (personal communication 1976), who maintains that if one succeeds in restoring function, the structures will recover spontaneously. We have referred to the histology of one of our cases, which according to S. Krompecher (personal communication 1967) showed evidence of neoformation of cartilage.

The question of whether valgization or varization should be used has been further clarified. Valgization (Pauwels II) is indicated in the case of large deformed heads, in advanced osteoar-

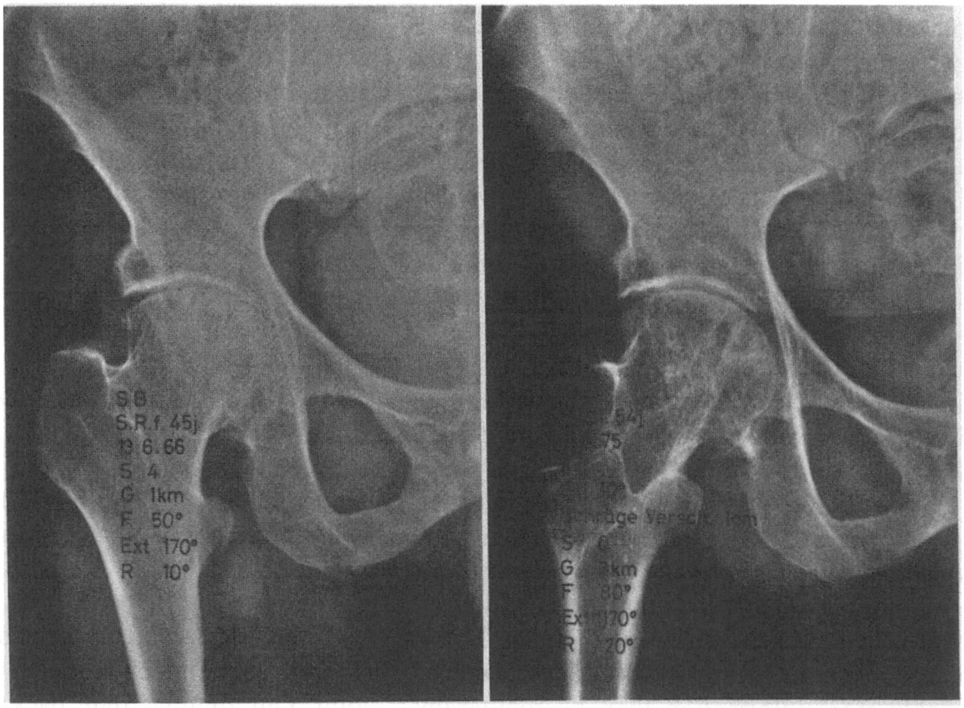

Fig. 29. A 45-year-old domestic. Primary osteoarthritis of the hip of the medical type. Severe pain. Nine years after an oblique displacement-extension osteotomy the medial narrowing of the joint space has disappeared and there is a gain in flexion of 30°. The patient is pain-free

thritis of the hip with medial head osteophytes, in patients with adduction contractures, and in medial types of osteoarthritis (Figs. 22–25). Many authors agree with the correctness of these indications (e.g., M. Watillon, F. Hoet, P. Maquet, M. Schneider, D. Weill, R. Bombelli). In 1959, M.E. Müller advised me to perform valgization in the cases with large heads. Opinion varies on the extent of valgization. We use as a guide the range of adduction possible under general anesthesia and, if necessary, at the time of surgery after surgical removal of the distal acetabular rim osteophytes which block adduction. Bombelli does not hesitate as a rule to perform 30° valgization. It appears that his Italian patients, who suffer predominantly from osteoarthritis secondary to dysplasia, tolerate more extensive valgization. At any rate, Bombelli advises in such extensive valgizations to lateralize the diaphysis, lateralize the trochanter, cut the psoas, and prevent an increase in leg length by removal of a segment of bone. We agree with Bombelli that a radiological joint incongruity in the sense of widening the lateral joint space in the adduction is not a contraindication to valgization. Abduction contracture following valgus osteotomy must be prevented.

Varus osteotomy is indicated if the leg can be abducted at least 20°. Frequently, to achieve maximum abduction it is necessary to flex the hip. This abduction position must be checked radiologically. It must not result in joint incongruity in the sense of a more marked narrowing of the space at the level of the acetabular corner. H. Willenegger, whose cases have been published by Plass (1974), has had good results with varus osteotomy. Adduction contracture secondary to varus osteotomy must be avoided. The mechanism of joint overload secondary to adduction contracture was extremely well described in 1950 by Osborne and Fahrni (Fig. 9).

After reviewing our experience of 17 years we are convinced that it is not enough to think only in terms of the frontal plane. There is no doubt in our minds that McMurray achieved corrections of malposition during plaster immobilization after osteotomy and thus accidentally performed extensions in many cases. The elimination of a flexion contracture reduces the total pressure by removing the compression force of the gluteus maximus. The degree of femoral head flexion depends on the range of movement of the hip. Thus it is possible to rotate more intact frontal parts of the head into the main weight-bearing zone (Figs. 16, 19, 20). Retroversion of the femoral head, which is associated with extension osteotomy, probably plays a role in the centering of the head in the acetabulum in the cases with eccentric frontal joint overloading (Fig. 25).

The rotational corrections possible in the sagittal plane are of greatest value in patients with damage to the head by the breakdown of large cysts, in dysostoses, in traumatic head defects, and in partial head necroses (Figs. 26, 27, 28). Our two contour X-ray projections yield considerably more information than do tomograms. They clearly support flexion osteotomy in the case of cranioventral head defects and extension osteotomy in the case of craniodorsal head defects. The value of intertrochanteric flexion osteotomy was confirmed in 1975 by Willert and Safert. Before considering total hip replacement or arthrodesis in relatively young patients with head necrosis, one must exhaust all these therapeutic possibilities. The technique of contour radiography is described by Hafner and Meuli (1975). The X-ray with the hip in flexion permits direct assessment of the joint congruity that can be achieved with an extension. If congruity is improved by simultaneous abduction or adduction, in addition to the extension osteotomy corresponding degrees of varization or valgization must be planned.

These combined corrections in two planes can be performed reliably only with the aid of the AO technique (Olsson 1974). The AO hip plates have a fixed angle between blade and shaft. The position of the blade in the femoral neck, which ultimately determines the corrections, must be calculated carefully with the aid of the preoperative drawings. During insertion of the seating chisel one must constantly check the direction of the neck axis and the inclinations of the chisel in the frontal and sagittal plane. The angle measurements are indicated by Kirschner wires which are drilled into the bone to serve as guides. If the blade is correctly inserted into the neck, once the wedges are resected the reduction of the plate to the lateral side of the femoral shaft will automatically bring about the desired correction and reduction of the osteotomy. It is important to compress the osteotomy with a tension device, which imparts great stability and makes early pain-free mobilization possible. The importance of this has also been stressed by other authors, such as Judet et al. in 1965. In our experience, correct AO technique practically eliminates the risk of pseudroarthrosis. Under stable conditions, not even an infection will represent any great danger to healing after osteotomy.

Figures 1 and 2 prove that the radiological widening of the joint space is due to neoformation of functional cartilage on both sides of the joint. Our findings date back 10–15 years and were established at a time when many other authors considered the radiologically apparent widening of the joint space after intertrochanteric osteotomy to be only a projection phenomenon.

Summary

An intertrochanteric osteotomy can be a success only if the indications are correct. A well-motivated and confident patient and properly supervised postoperative care are also important. In summary, we feel that a varus osteotomy is indicated if joint congruity is good and if there is a good range of abduction. If there is loss of extension or if abduction is better in flexion, then extension osteotomy must also be performed. Apart from this, regardless of the range of movement, varus-extension osteotomy is indicated in all cases of fixed abduction and flexion. In contrast to congruity, which is essential in a varus osteotomy, the width of the joint space is not important.

Valgus osteotomy is indicated in advanced osteoarthritis with loss of abduction, in the presence of a medial head osteophyte, where the head is largely deformed, after slipped capital epiphyis or Perthes, in medial osteoarthritides with a tendency to protrusion, and generally in cases with a fixed adduction deformity. If there is often also a loss of extension, the valgus osteotomy should be combined with an extension osteotomy. Joint congruity plays a smaller role in valgus osteotomy than in varus osteotomy, and the width of the joint space is not an important consideration when one is weighing the indications.

Medial displacement of the shaft belongs by its very nature to varus osteotomy, and lateralization to valgus osteotomy. In this way, provided that the knee joint is normal, we avoid pathogenic displacement of the weight-bearing axis. When varization is performed with a valgus knee, medial displacement is hardly necessary and similarly, lateralization of the shaft is not needed when valgization osteotomy is performed in a patient with a varus knee.

The corrections in the frontal plane (Pauwels) must be supplemented by any possible corrections in the sagittal plane. Extension osteotomy is useful in correcting flexion deformity and to achieve a reduction in total pressure. Extension and flexion osteotomy, provided that joint mobility is satisfactory, serve to improve congruity and thus pressure distribution. The contour radiographs (Schneider) indicate that relatively intact spherical cranioventral or craniodorsal heads are positioned in the main weight-bearing zone. These osteotomies have been found to be especially useful in cases with traumatic head defects or partial head necroses. Correct preoperative planning of an intertrochanteric osteotomy includes selection of the type of plate to be used. Reliable corrections are only possible with the use of the AO technique. The position of the blade within the femoral neck as well as its appropriate point of entry are determined prior to the osteotomy. This, in combination with a fixed predetermined angled device, guarantees the planned corrections. Stable internal fixation with compression not only prevents secondary displacement, but also allows early mobilization, which we consider important. The correct surgical technique prevents pseudoarthroses.

Unfortunately, in assessing the prognosis of an intertrochanteric osteotomy there are still factors which are difficult to determine. We are talking here of the evaluation of reactivity, i.e., of the transformation potential of the femoral head and the assessment of inflammatory factors. Nevertheless, experience has shown that long-lasting (over 10 years) good results can be expected in half the cases. Therefore all patients with hip disease who are going to undergo surgery must be carefully evaluated to see if they are suitable candidates for an intertrochanteric osteotomy.

References

Arnoldi CC et al. (1972) Venous engorgement and intraosseous hypertension in osteoarthritis of the hip. J Bone Joint Surg 54B/3

Bombelli R (1976) Osteoarthritis of the hip. Springer, Berlin Heidelberg New York

Hafner E, Meuli HC (1975) Röntgenuntersuchung in der Orthopädie. Huber, Bern Stuttgart Wien

Hawk HE, Skim S (1970) The nature of the intramedullary pressure of bone. Surg Forum 21:475–477

Hayashi M (1973) Studies on the circulation of the femoral head using catheter semiconductor radiation detector. J Jap Orthop Ass 47/7:581–617

Judet R, Judet J, et al. (1965) L'osteotomie de MacMurray dans le traitement des coxarthroses. Rev Chir Orthop 51/8:681–697

von Lanz T (1950) Anatomie und Entwicklung des menschlichen Hüftgelenkes. Verh Dtsch Orthop Ges Enke, Stuttgart, p 26

Maquet P (1974) Coxarthrose protrusive. Etude biomécanique et traitement. Acta Orthop Belg *40*/fasc 2

Maquet P (1977) La latéralisation du grand trochanter, Congrès Société Belge de Chirurgie Orthopédique, Charleroi

Müller ME (1971) Die hüftnahen Femurosteotomien. Thieme, Stuttgart

Müller ME (1975) Intertrochanteric osteotomies in adults: planning and operating technique. In: Cruess, Mitchell (eds) Surgical management of degenerative arthritis of the lower limb. Lea & Febiger, Philadelphia

Müller ME, Allgöwer M, Schneider R, Willenegger H (1979) Manual of internal fixation. Springer, Berlin Heidelberg New York

Olsson S (1974) Intertrochanteric osteotomy of the femur with AO technique for osteoarthritis of the hip joint. Acta Orthop Scand 45:914–925

Osborne GV, Fahrni WH (1950) Oblique displacement osteotomy for osteoarthritis of the hip joint. J Bone Joint Surg [Br.] 32:148–160
Pauwels F (1965) Gesammelte Abhandlungen zur funktionellen Anatomie des Bewegungsapparates. Springer, Berlin Heidelberg New York
Phillips RS (1966) Phlebography in osteoarthritis of the hip. J Bone Joint Surg 48B:280–288
Plass U (1974) Spätergebnisse nach intertrochanteren Osteotomien. Z Orthop 112:699–703
Schneider R (1966) Mehrjahresresultate eines Kollektivs von 100 intertrochanteren Osteotomien bei Coxarthrose. Helv Chir Acta 33/fasc $\frac{1}{2}$:185–205
Schneider R (1977) Die intertrochantere Extensions- und Flexionsosteotomie bei traumatischen Hüftkopfdefekten. Unfallheilkunde 80:177–181
Schneider M, Weill D (1975) La place de l'ostéotomie intertrochantérienne valgisante (Pauwels II) dans le traitement chirurgical de la coxarthrose. Principes biomécaniques. Resultats. Rev Rhum 42/1:53–57
Watillon M, Hoet F, Maquet P (1977) Analyse de résultats d'ostéotomies de Pauwels dans la coxarthrose évoluée (804 cas, 3–30 ans). Congrès Société Belge de Chirurgie Orthopédique, Charleroi
Willert HG, Safert D (1975) Die Behandlung segmentaler, ischämischer Hüftkopfnekrosen mit der intertrochanteren Flexionsosteotomie. Z Orthop 113:974–994

Results of Intertrochanteric Osteotomy in the Treatment of Osteoarthritis of the Hip *

E. Morscher and R. Feinstein

Introduction

Osteoarthritis is the result of a disturbance of the biomechanical equilibrium between the resistance of the joint (cartilage) and the amount of stress in the joint. The primary aims of an intertrochanteric osteotomy are to improve joint congruity and to diminish load. Intertrochanteric osteotomy follows Pauwels' [11, 12] law of the load of the joint ("laws of the lever arm"). According to Bombelli [3], intertrochanteric osteotomy also functions to remove harmful biomechanical forces and to create favorable ones. The type of osteotomy performed (valgus, varus, medial displacement, etc.) depends on the results of a precise clinical and radiographical examination of the affected hip. Additional procedures such as tenotomy, osteotomy of the pelvis, and lateral and/or distal displacement of the greater trochanter may be indicated, depending on the biomechanical problems encountered. Exact planning and performance of the osteotomy are essential for success. In addition, stable internal fixation of the osteotomy according to the principles of the AO (ASIF) permits early mobilization with its advantages. Intertrochanteric osteotomy has both immediate and late effects. The immediate effects consist of:

1. Diminishing the pressure in the bone marrow. Both Phillips [13, 14] and Arnoldi [1, 2] demonstrated elevated intraosseous pressure in osteoarthritic joints.. Decompression of the bone marrow is probably the most effective mechanism of bringing about relief from the typical arthritic pain, such as that suffered at night and when starting to walk.
2. By opening the capsule one can decrease the intraarticular pressure and evacuate the effusion which is usually present in painful arthritic joints.
3. Releasing muscle spasms.

The late effects of an osteotomy are:

1. Definite diminution of the joint pressure, which gives the joint a chance to regenerate.
2. According to Wolff's law, the change in loading leads to a change of the internal trabecular architecture of the femoral head and the acetabulum.

Towards the end of the 1960s many orthopedic surgeons – particularly in Europe – believed that with time, total hip arthroplasty would become the only solution for every type of arthritis affecting the hip joint. The statistical data from the ten largest Swiss orthopedic departments show that in the subsequent years the number of total hip arthroplasties rose and the number of intertrochanteric osteotomies fell (Fig. 1). There was at first a real "arthroplasty boom", but since 1973 the number of total hip replacements has remained constant. More recently, there appears to have been a resurgence of the intertrochanteric osteotomy because of the many failures of total hips and their concomitant necessary revisions. This development was predictable from the decline of hip fusions and other operative interventions. More than 10 years ago, the major disadvantages of intertrochanteric osteotomy as compared to hip arthroplasty were the uncertainty of the result and the difficult postoperative rehabilitation with relatively little improvement in joint motion. Even pain relief could not be guaranteed. The fact that planning and technique of an osteotomy demands much more knowledge of biomechanics of the hip joint than the relatively simple and purely technical procedure of insertion of a total hip replacement probably induced

* Paper received in 1980

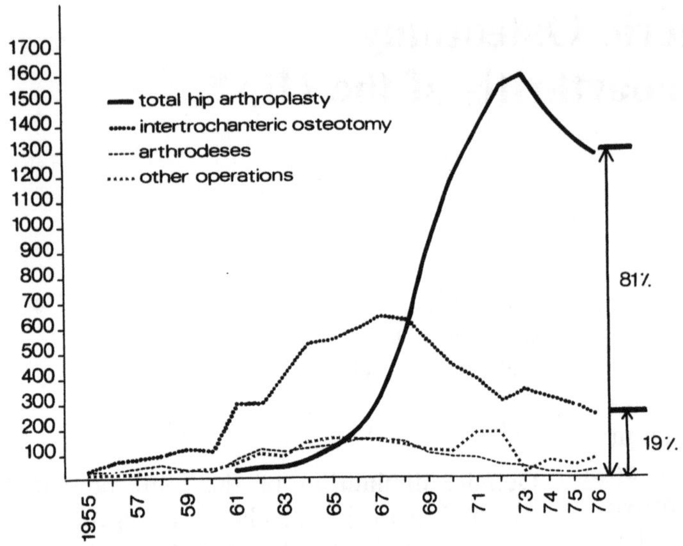

Fig. 1. Statistics on operative interventions in osteoarthritis of the hip in the ten largest orthopedic departments in Switzerland, 1955 to 1976

a large number of surgeons to abandon the intertrochanteric osteotomy. There is, however, no doubt that the intertrochanteric osteotomy still has a definite place in the treatment of osteoarthritis of the hip, particularly as the arthroplasty has not completely fulfilled all the expectations.

The tremendous advantage of the intertrochanteric osteotomy lies in the quantitatively and qualitatively small risk of complications and in the fact that in case of failure no bridges have been burnt and other procedures are possible, e.g., an arthrodesis, an arthroplasty or eventually a Girdlestone procedure.

In 1970, when the total hip arthroplasty seemed to be completing its conquest of Europe, the Swiss Orthopaedic Association chose the subject "Failures of Intertrochanteric Osteotomies" as the main theme of its annual meeting which was held in Basel. The ten largest orthopedic departments collaborated in compiling the results of 2251 intertrochanteric osteotomies performed between 1954 and 1967 and making them available for study. All clinics entered their data on standard questionnaire sheets which were then fed into a computer for analysis [7].

Toward the end of the 1960s, many orthopedic surgeons were of the opinion that with time, total hip arthroplasty would become the ultimate solution for every type of arthritis of the hip. However, we were convinced that intertrochanteric osteotomy would continue to find a definite place in the therapeutic regimen, particularly in young patients. The chief aim of the study of the 2251 operations was to analyze the bad results and the errors committed during treatment in the hope in this way to delineate the precise indications for intertrochanteric osteotomy. We also wished to learn more about the dangers and complications.

In order to determine the reliability of the results of the Swiss Multicenter Study (SMS), particularly with regard to indications and technique, we have followed up 263 patients of our own who were operated on between 1968 and 1976 (ODB), and compared the two sets of results.

Selection of Cases

The studies were limited to patients with radiologically proven osteoarthritis of the hip joint who were aged 20 years or more. The minimum follow-up was 1 year.

Age, Sex, and Stage

In the SMS, 37% of the patients (844/2,251) were between 50 and 59 years old, and 28%

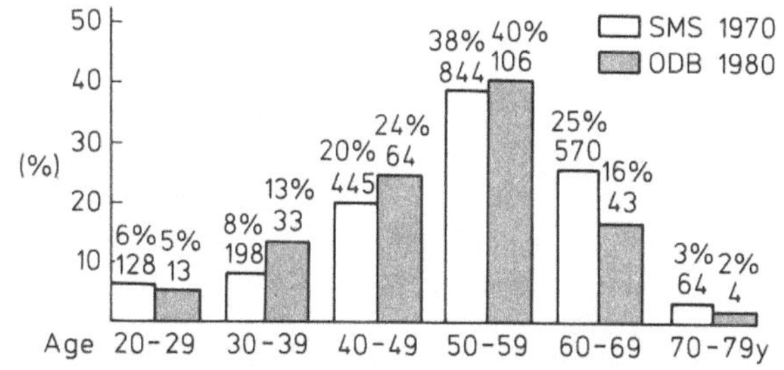

Fig. 2. Age distribution of the intertrochanteric osteotomies in the Swiss Multicenter Study (SMS) and of the Department of Orthopedic Surgery of the university of Basel, Switzerland (ODB)

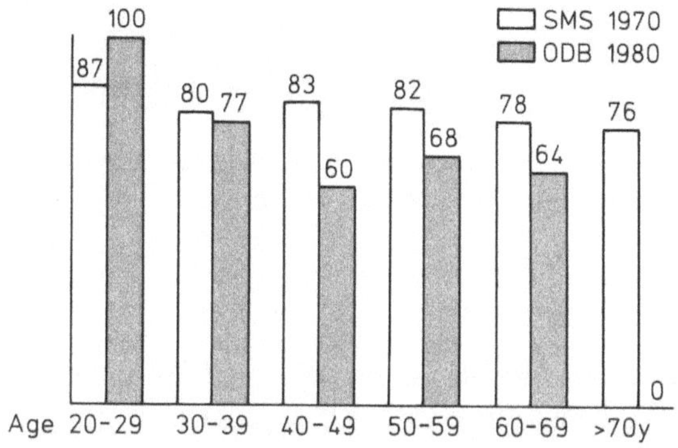

Fig. 3. Percentage of good results in the SMS 1970 (2,251 cases) and the follow-up of the ODB (263 cases) in relation to age

were older than 60; this latter proportion fell to 18% in the years 1968–1976 (Fig. 2).

A total of 1149 operations were carried out in men, (64.4%) and 802 in women (35.6%).

Since it became more and more apparent that the earlier the osteotomy, the better the result, an attempt was made to correlate the severity of the osteoarthritis with the result of surgery. We designated as late those hip joints with a total range of movement no greater than 90°, those with marked narrowing of the cartilage space, and those with evidence of avascular necrosis and collapse.

In the SMS there were 818 early and 1,134 late cases; 299 cases could not be clearly designated as one or the other. Thus more patients with advanced osteoarthritis were operated on, and as expected, they comprised an older population. The patients with early osteoarthritis were mostly between 20 and 30 years old, whereas those with advanced osteoarthritis were mostly in the age-group of 50 and older. The incidence of severe osteoarthritis rose with age, so that in patients of 60 years and more, severe osteoarthritis was twice as common as early osteoarthritis. Even at that time it was evident that total hip replacement would have its place for patients with advanced osteoarthritis, so that patients of 60 and older frequently received an endoprosthesis rather than an intertrochanteric osteotomy.

In our recent follow-up study we observed about the same percentage of good results in the age-group 20–40 years as in the SMS. Thereafter the quota of good results decreased markedly (Fig. 3).

Psychological Factors

We attempted to carry out a rough psychological assessment of the patients in order to weed out those patients who seemed to have absolutely no physical findings to substantiate a failure of the procedure. In 76 cases, psychological factors had to be accepted as the cause of failure. Psychological factors played a very prominent role in the return to work of a postoperative patient. Our study demonstrated that patients with good results showed work tolerance improved by 1.8%, whereas those patients who showed reduced tolerance were found to have 6.5% incidence of adverse psychogenic factors.

Etiology

The greatest problem in determining the indication for an intertrochanteric osteotomy today lies in the relative uncertainty of the prognosis of this operation. We must therefore consider the favorable and unfavorable factors for an intertrochanteric osteotomy. In this connection the cause of the osteoarthritis has a definite bearing on the end result. In many cases, on the basis of either history or X-ray, it was possible to establish with certainty the cause. In the SMS, 906 (43%) of all operatively treated cases

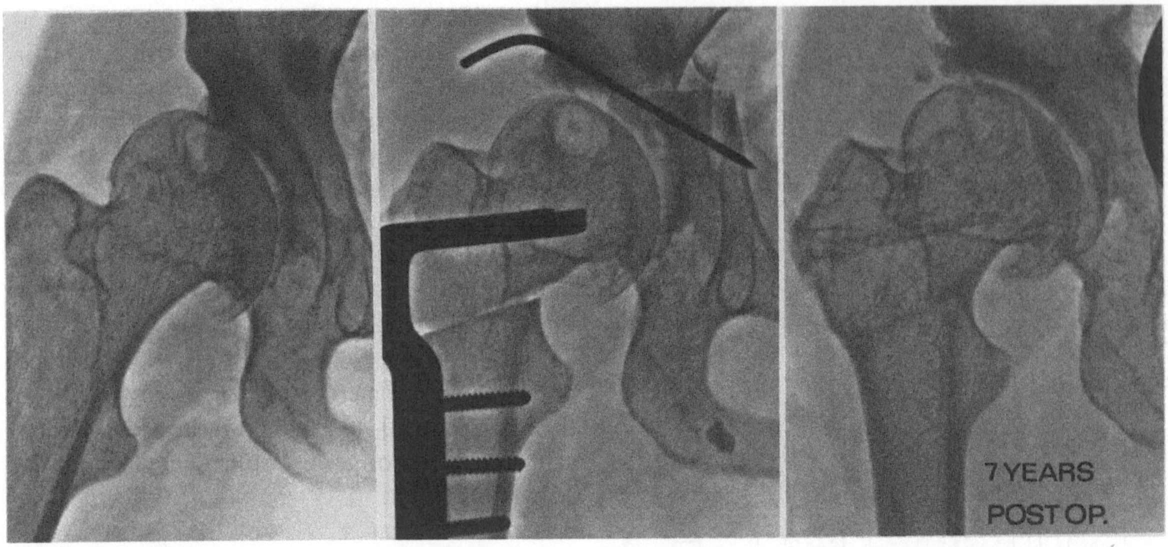

Fig. 4. X-rays of 36-year-old female patient with osteoarthritis of the hip due to hip dysplasia. Good result 7 years after intertrochanteric varus osteotomy combined with Chiari osteotomy of the pelvis

either had primary osteoarthritis or the etiology could not be defined precisely. Of the secondary types of osteoarthritis, those due to slipped capital epiphysis (20%) and those secondary to congenital dislocation of the hip (18%) were by far the most common. These numbers, however, do not represent the general incidence of etiologies of osteoarthritis of the hip joint, as the material was preselected and not all types of osteoarthritis were suitable for intertrochanteric osteotomy. Because of this very fact it is striking that the statistics from orthopedic clinics consistently show a high incidence of slipped capital epiphysis as an etiological factor of osteoarthritis. The high incidence of slipped capital epiphysis in patients undergoing intertrochanteric osteotomy may be the result of the fact that osteoarthritis secondary to slipped capital epiphysis is particularly suitable for intertrochanteric osteotomy if treatment is required. Thus, we should not wonder why other series report a much lower incidence of slipped capital epiphysis as a cause of osteoarthritis.

Pauwels [11, 12] based his indications for an intertrochanteric osteotomy on biomechanical principles, and recommended varus osteotomy in coxa valga with subluxation. In cases of subluxating hip where the femoral head has a pronounced capital drop osteophyte, Bombelli [3] advocates extreme valgus osteotomy.

Some authors are sceptical of the value of intertrochanteric osteotomy in protrusio acetabuli. If at all, a valgus osteotomy is indicated [5]. For osteoarthritis secondary to enchondral dysostosis, Perthes' disease, or slipped capital epiphysis, most orthopedic surgeons suggest simply medial displacement or valgus osteotomy.

Since osteotomies performed for osteoarthritis caused by Paget's disease or rheumatoid arthritis usually ended up in failure, these conditions represent a contraindication for an intertrochanteric osteotomy.

Of patients in the SMS with osteoarthritis secondary to hip dysplasia 68% were treated by varus osteotomy and in 88% had a good to excellent result. In the past 10 years a combination of intertrochanteric varus or valgus osteotomy with a Chiari pelvic osteotomy has become more and more popular, particularly in the treatment of osteoarthritis of the hip secondary to dysplasia with a shallow acetabulum (Fig. 4). In our experience this combination – performed as a one-stage procedure – was especially successful. In cases where the functional X-rays do not show any improvement in the congruency either in abduction or in adduction, even a pure Chiari osteotomy can still lead to an excellent result.

In every case, however, exact planning according to functional X-rays (AP views in abduction and adduction and other projections) is mandatory.

Type of Osteotomy and Fixation

The etiology of osteoarthritis plays a definite role in the choice of operative procedure. In the SMS, varus osteotomy was performed in 41% of cases and valgus osteotomy in 36%. A pure medial displacement osteotomy [6] was carried out in 18% of cases. Patients with osteoarthritis secondary to a slipped capital epiphysis were treated with valgus osteotomy in 42% of cases, and those with hip dysplasia and a luxating hip with a varus osteotomy in 68% of cases. Hips with osteoarthritis secondary to Perthes' disease had a valgus osteotomy performed seven times as often as a varus osteotomy, whereas in patients with enchondral dysostosis, protrusio acetabuli, idiopathic necrosis, rheumatoid arthritis, and even coxa vara there was an equal incidence of valgus and varus osteotomies.

Up to the end of the 1950s the straight plate of Bosworth, Kessel or Blount was used as the implant of choice for internal fixation. Thereafter, all Swiss clinics began to use the AO angled plate [8–10] for the internal fixation of intertrochanteric osteotomies. Of the valgus osteotomies fixed with a straight plate, 5.7% ended up with a secondary varus deformity.

Complications

In the SMS there were 227 complications (10.08%). Six patients died (0.28%); two succumbed to a pulmonary embolus, one to a severe infection, two to myocardial insufficiency, and in one the cause of death was not clear. In our own series of 236 patients there were no deaths. The relatively low incidence of fatalities is the result of rapid mobilization, which became possible once rigid internal fixation came into use.

Thrombophlebitis and thromboembolism occurred in 47 cases (2.08%). None occurred in patients under 40, whereas in those between 60 and 80 years of age the incidence was 3.6%. We have no doubt that postoperative anticoagulant therapy, which was carried out most of the time, greatly contributed to the low incidence of this dreaded complication.

Local infections were divided into two groups, deep and superficial:

1. Deep infections were severe infections which required reoperation.
2. Light or superficial infections were infections with only soft tissue manifestations which cleared up prior to discharge from hospital and which did not require repeat surgery.

Altogether there were 16 deep (0.71%) and 42 superficial (1.89%) infections.

Superficial infections had no bearing on the end result, whereas most deep infections did: Only 50% of the patients with deep infections ended up with a good result, compared with the average of 84% good results in the whole series. We should mention here that as a rule no prophylactic antibiotics were used. There were 37 pseudarthroses (1.55%). They were more common after valgus osteotomy (1.7%) than after a varus osteotomy (1.5%) or pure medial displacement osteotomy (0.9%). They were more common in the early years of the SMS series, with an incidence of 2.7% between 1955 and 1961, but only 1.1% between 1962 and 1967.

In our recent study (1970-1976) there were no pseudarthroses. This illustrates improvement in the surgical technique as surgeons gained experience with the rigid methods of internal fixation. Most of the pseudarthroses were the result of poor operative technique, such as the use of the oscillating saw without cooling, poor reduction of the fragments, improper use of internal fixation, or premature weight-bearing. Most (80.5%) of the pseudarthroses required reoperation and had a considerably poorer end result. Only 25% of intertrochanteric osteotomies with a pseudarthrosis were considered good.

Operative errors occurred 33 times (1.46%). Most of them consisted of fractures of the proximal fragment due to too small a distance between the osteotomy and the hole for the blade of the plate.

Clinical Results

In the overall assessment of an operation for osteoarthritis, no great discrepancies arose between the assessments of the result by the patient and by the doctor. For the patient, the yardstick of success was the relief of pain, whereas the doctor looked more for objective indices such as changes in range of movement and in the radiological appearance. It is absolutely clear that from the patient's point of view no relief of pain or an increase in pain is equated to absolute failure of the procedure. This was the case in 16% of our patients, but the other 84% were pain-free or afflicted with pain that was only minimal or at least considerably less than prior to surgery (Fig. 5).

As one would expect, the patients were much less accurate in their assessment of function of the operated hip. A more accurate assessment is the objective measurement of the range of movement and walking capacity. It is a fact that an intertrochanteric osteotomy does not as a rule lead to a substantial increase in the range of movement. In any case, an operation which leads to a reduction in the total range of movement greater than half of the preoperative range

	Pain		Walking capacity	Mobility
None	662	(84%)		
Better	1,182		1,380 (61%)	394 (17%)
Unchanged	283	(16%)	565 (25%)	983 (72%)
Worse	124		306 (14%)	271 (11%)

Fig. 5. Results of the 2,251 intertrochanteric osteotomies in the SMS for pain, walking capacity and mobility

must be considered a failure. The walking ability with osteoarthritis is related primarily to the amount of pain. This became evident by the fact that 61% of our cases walked much better following the intertrochanteric osteotomy, whereas only 17% noted a better range of movement.

Socioeconomic Factors

Among the patients of the SMS, 37.9% did heavy manual labor, 43.8% did work of moderate severity, and only 18.3% were engaged in light physical work.

It was interesting to note that 83% of patients with hip luxation were engaged in light or moderately heavy work. In contrast, only 49% of patients with slipped capital epiphysis were engaged in moderate to light work. This means that patients with hip luxations or rheumatoid arthritis avoid heavy work.

Heavy work worsens the prognosis after intertrochanteric osteotomy. Five or more years after surgery, the heavy workers had a bad result in 45.5% of cases, those doing moderately heavy work in 38.6%, and white-collar workers in only 15.9%.

Among our patients, 70.8% returned to their pre-operative occupation, but 10% had to change jobs in order to be able to continue working. However, there is no doubt that psychogenic factors also play a very prominent role in the return to work.

We were also able to demonstrate that work tolerance decreases markedly with the rise in age. Only 6% of those in their 20s were not able to work. The figure rose to 15% of those in their 50s and to 21% of those over 60 years of age.

Radiological Findings

In order to learn more about relevance of the radiological features in determining the indication for intertrochanteric osteotomy the X-rays

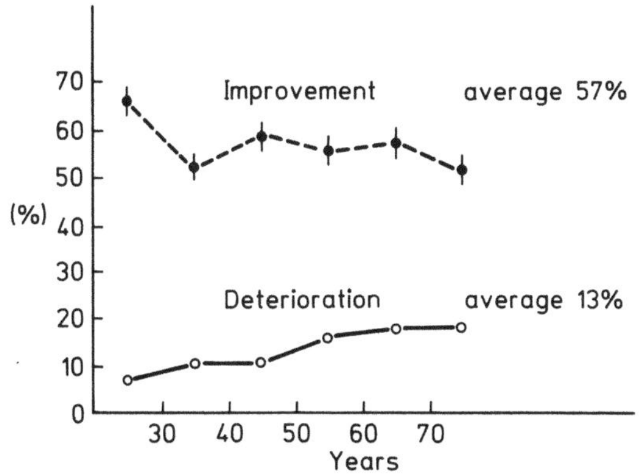

Fig. 6. Radiological appearance of the osteoarthritis of the hip joint after intertrochanteric osteotomy (SMS) in relation to age

of the SMS were subjected to a special analysis (performed by H. Vasey, Assistant Professor, Orthopedic Department of the University of Geneva). The postoperative radiological course of osteoarthritis was assigned to one of three simple groups: improved, unimproved, or worsened. The course of the osteoarthritis was gauged according to the fate of cartilage space, the state of osteophytes, the subchondral sclerosis, cysts, joint congruency, and finally on the basis of the survival or destruction of the femoral head.

The radiological appearance related to age at the time of the operation revealed that the rate of improvement after 40 is fairly constant, whereas after 50 there is an increase in the rate of deterioration (Fig. 6).

The presence of bilateral disease had a clear negative influence on the end result. This was not the case, however, when both hips were subjected to surgery. In patients with bilateral disease where only one side was operated upon, we found clear-cut radiological deterioration more frequently than in cases where both sides were operated on. We must point out, however, that the second operation was as a rule undertaken only when the first one had been successful; therefore there may have been a natural preselection of these cases.

With time, there is a progressive deterioration of the radiological results. Our study is based on the comparison of the initial with the final results, which enables us to exclude transient improvements from our statistics. The rate of deterioration increased from 10% in the first 2 years to 14% in the 3rd and 4th postoperative years. Thereafter the rate remains pretty well constant, but shows further deterioration around the 7th and 8th postoperative year with the rate rising to 18%. After 9 years, about one-third of the patients showed definite radiological signs of deterioration. The percentage of radiological improvement remained stationary for a longer period of time. We have noted a deterioration of the improvement at the end of the first 5 years, so that at the end of 9 years there was a fall from 57% to 42% of patients who were improved.

The radiological findings of deterioration correlate with the overall results of the intertrochanteric osteotomies. We can allow ourselves the following generalization: Those joints in which the osteoarthritis develops as a result of a mechanical disturbance of the joint usually do well following intertrochanteric osteotomy. Patients in whom the osteoarthritis develops secondary to inflammatory states, secondary to derangements of cartilage metabolisms, etc., do not as a rule respond favorably to an osteotomy.

As already mentioned, we found a good and clear correlation between the radiological appearance and the clinical result if we consider pain and range of motion of the joint as clinical parameters of success. This was especially true when a special group of 148 cases declared as failures were compared to 98 cases considered as successes. We found narrowing of the cartilage space, sclerosis, and development of cysts, but the development of osteophytes has no bearing on the end results. However, cases of osteoarthritis which do not show sclerosis and cystic changes invariably have a poor prognosis. Atrophic osteoarthritis is therefore unsuitable for osteotomy [3]. The same is also true for those patients who postoperatively persist in showing a lack of congruence between the hip and acetabulum. Loss of cartilage space, development of sclerosis of subchondral bone, and cyst formation are characteristic signs of overload in weight-bearing areas of the joint. Therefore an operation which is designed to decrease load by either affecting the load itself or distributing it over a greater surface area cannot give a good result if there is no evidence that the joint overload was diminished, at least at the start. Furthermore, failure is much more likely to occur when at the end of intertrochanteric osteotomy there is poor coverage of the femoral head. This is the reason why in recent years, Chiari osteotomy has been performed more and more.

In summary, we can state that there is an excellent correlation between the radiological appearance and the clinical result after intertrochanteric osteotomy. Occasional patients with a good radiological appearance could be declared failures because of their poor clinical results, but the converse, namely clinical success in the presence of radiological failure, was very rare.

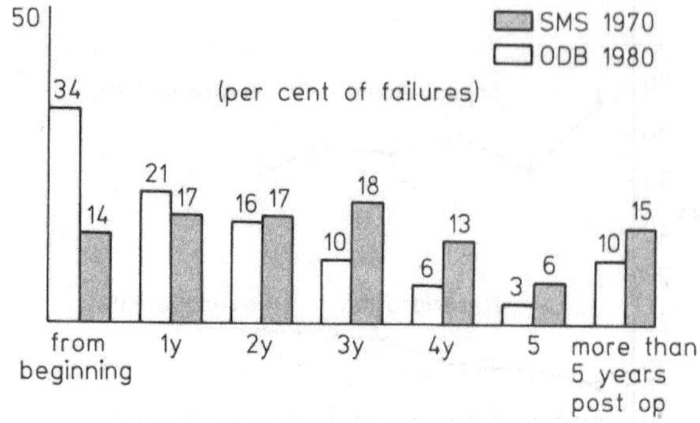

Fig. 7. Percentage of failures of intertrochanteric osteotomies in relation to time after operation

Discussion

It was rather disappointing for us to learn from our recent study (1968–1976) that the subjective assessment of the success of the surgery by patients over 40 years of age was worse than in the SMS. Only slightly more than half of the patients were really enthusiastic about the result of their operation. In our study we asked the patients: "Would you undergo intertrochanteric osteotomy again?" The result of 219 replies was 134 "yes" and 79 "no", with six undecided.

What is the reason for this change in the patients' subjective assessment? There is no doubt that today patients compare their results with those of patients with total hip arthroplasty: Today the criteria for a hip operation are set by the exciting early results of primary total hip arthroplasty, not by those with a fusion, or a Girdlestone procedure. In the subjective assessment, the disadvantages of the intertrochanteric osteotomy become apparent. These disadvantages consist, as already mentioned, of a less than satisfactory primary result and a much harder and more difficult postoperative rehabilitation than after total hip replacement. Only 15 to 20 years ago, a patient with osteoarthritis of the hip was happy to get relief of pain from an operation, but today, it is often difficult to persuade even younger patients of the advantages of an intertrochanteric osteotomy and to dissuade them from an artificial hip joint for patients expect a normal joint following surgery and do not wish to settle for less.

In assessing the results of intertrochanteric osteotomy, we have to consider that the appearance of poor results as late as 5 years or more after the intervention means that the osteotomy was at least worthwhile, and cannot therefore be designated a complete failure. Figure 7 shows the "failures" of intertrochanteric osteotomy correlated with the time after operation when they appeared. One-third of the SMS failures and 14% of our own failures are failures right from the beginning, but the number of failures appearing each year decreases with time. A result which is still good after some years therefore has a better chance of remaining good for several years longer.

Our own results correspond with those of other authors. Collert and Gillström [4] found in a recent prospective study of 94 hips at the 5-year follow-up that only 45.5% have an acceptable result (pain absent or only slight). In a rather rough estimation, we can declare that intertrochanteric osteotomy gives a long-lasting excellent result in one-third of cases, in one-third the result has to be judged more or less satisfactory, and in one-third a total hip arthroplasty has to be done later on. In the last group the success or failure depended clearly on at

Varus		*Valgus*
Lateral	sclerosis	medial
In abduction	congruency	in adduction
Lateral	narrowing of the joint space	medial
Minor deformity	head	pronounced deformity

Fig. 8. Indications for varus and valgus osteotomy

what point between osteotomy and arthroplasty the evaluation was carried out. In cases where the total hip was done more than 5 years following the osteotomy, the intertrochanteric osteotomy was probably worthwile.

Let us now come to the question of whether intertrochanteric osteotomy still represents an alternative to total hip arthroplasty in osteoarthritis of the hip joint. The answer to this question is without doubt "yes", but unfortunately only in a minority of cases. The statistics from Switzerland (Fig. 1) show that today total hip replacement is performed in about 90% of cases and intertrochanteric osteotomy in only 10%. This is a fact we cannot overlook.

Summarizing our experience in osteotomy over more than 20 years it should be possible to describe in a computer-like way the ideal patient for osteotomy. This patient should have the following characteristics: age below 50 years; no marked obesity; secondary, mechanically caused arthritis; white-collar profession; good congruency in functional X-rays; X-ray signs of overload, such as sclerosis, cyst formation and localized narrowing of the joint space. In such a patient, a favorable result can be expected – provided that there has been good preoperative planning, good operative technique, and good rehabilitation with an extended period of non-weight-bearing. The choice between valgus or varus osteotomy depends mainly on the localization of the sclerosis, better congruency in abduction or in adduction, the localization of the narrowing of the joint space and the deformity of the femoral head, as outlined in Fig. 8.

The supreme advantage of an intertrochanteric osteotomy over total hip arthroplasty is that one does not burn one's bridges and that a hip replacement can always be done later on. A "second line of defense" is preserved, and this should always be one of the important principles in orthopedic surgery!

References

1. Arnoldi CC (1971) Immediate effects of osteotomy on the intramedullary pressure of femoral head and neck in patients with degenerative osteoarthritis. Acta Orthop Scand 42:453–455
2. Arnoldi CC (1972) Venous engorgement and intraosseous hypertension in osteoarthritis of the hip. J Bone Jt Surg 54B:409–421
3. Bombelli R (1983) Osteoarthritis of the hip. Pathogenesis and consequent therapy. 2nd edn. Springer, Berlin Heidelberg New York
4. Collert S, Gillström P (1979) Osteotomy in osteoarthritis of the hip. Acta Orthop Scand 50:555–561
5. Langlais F, Roure JL, Maquet P (1979) Valgus osteotomy in severe osteoarthritis of the hip. J Bone Jt Surg 61B:424–431
6. McMurray TP (1935) Osteoarthritis of the hip-joint. Br J Surg 22:916
7. Morscher E (1971) Die intertrochantere Osteotomie bei Coxarthrose. Huber, Bern
8. Müller ME (1969) Die Varisationsosteotomie bei der Behandlung der Koxarthrose. In Rütt (ed) Die Therapie der Koxarthrose. Thieme, Stuttgart, pp 49–63
9. Müller ME (1971) Die hüftnahen Femurosteotomien. Thieme, Stuttgart
10. Müller ME (1975) Intertrochanteric osteotomies in adults: planning and operating technique. In: Cruess, Mitchell (eds) Surgical management of degenerative arthritis of the lower limb. Lea & Febiger, Philadelphia
11. Pauwels F (1963) The importance of biomechanics in orthopedics. Postgraduate course. IXème Congrès de la Société Internationale de Chirurgie Orthopédique et de Traumatologie, Wien
12. Pauwels F (1965) Atlas zur Biomechanik der gesunden und kranken Hüfte. Springer, Berlin Heidelberg New York
13. Phillips RS (1966) Phlebography in osteoarthritis of the hip. J Bone Jt Surg 48B:280–288
14. Phillips RS (1967) Venous drainage in osteoarthritis of the hip. J Bone Jt Surg 49B:301–309

Treatment of Osteoarthritis of the Hip by Corrective Osteotomy of the Greater Trochanter

H. WAGNER and J. HOLDER

The spacial relationship of the greater trochanter to the center of rotation of the hip, or the center of the femoral head, has a profound influence on the forces acting about the hip joint. Under normal anatomic and functional conditions the tip of the greater trochanter is level with the center of the femoral head. The length of the femoral neck, which acts as a lever arm to transmit forces about the hip, varies with body size and habitus. As a general rule, however, the distance from the tip of the trochanter to the center of rotation of the hip, which corresponds roughly to the length of the lever arm of the pelvitrochanteric muscles, is equal to the diameter of the femoral head (Fig. 1). In the horizontal plane, because of the physiological anteversion of the neck, the greater trochanter is 15° posterior to the center of the femoral head. On X-rays the tip of the greater trochanter appears to lie about 20° posterior to the midline of the femoral neck. Because the center of insertion of the pelvitrochanteric muscle mass on the greater trochanter is approximately in line with the femoral neck axis, in biomechanical terms the line of action of these muscles in the horizontal plane corresponds roughly to the anteversion of the femoral neck.

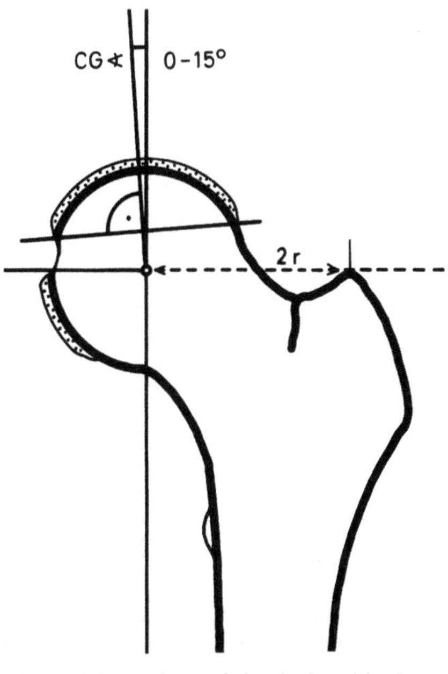

Fig. 1. Normal spacial relationship between the greater trochanter and the center of the femoral head

The loads on the hip joint are determined not only by the length of the femoral neck (the "effort arm"), but also by the distance between the center of hip rotation and the center of body gravity (the "load arm"). The distance from the center of rotation to the median plate is approximately twice the distance from the center of the femoral head to the tip of the greater trochanter. The center of body gravity is not fixed in its location. Only in the two-legged stance, with weight borne equally on both legs, does the center of gravity lie on the median plane of the body. In the one-legged stance, the weight of the unsupported leg is added to that of the trunk, which causes the center of gravity to be shifted toward the unsupported side. This lengthens the lever arm of the body weight (the "load arm") and increases the load on the hip. By bending the upper trunk toward the side of the supporting leg, it is possible to shift the center of gravity back toward the weight-bearing hip, thereby shortening the "load arm" and reducing stresses on the hip. This load-alleviating mechanism is characteristic of the Duchenne gait (Fig. 2).

In the one-legged stance the pelvis can be kept in balance only if the femoral neck is of adequate length, because this enables the pelvitrochanteric muscles to exert their action on the hip joint efficiently. A shortening of the femoral neck will decrease the lever arm of the pelvitrochanteric muscles, which then must develop more tension in order to keep the pelvis balanced. Since this increased muscle tension adds

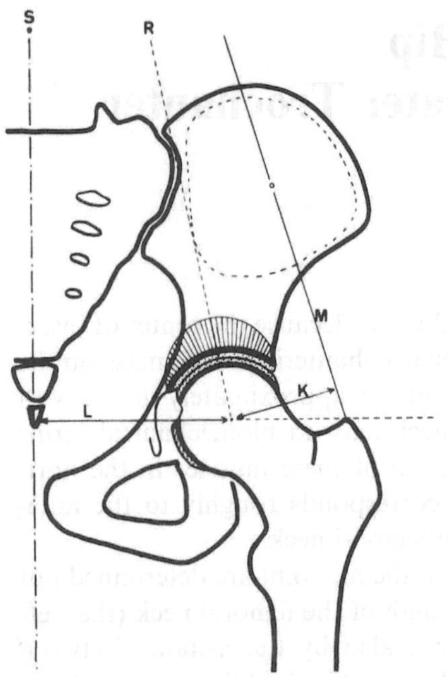

Fig. 2. Schematic diagram of the lever arms about the normal hip. *S*, center of body gravity; *M*, direction of pull of pelvitrochanteric muscles; *R*, resultant pressure force acting on the hip; *L*, load arm of body weight; *K*, effort arm of pelvitrochanteric muscles

to the loads on the joint, a short femoral neck tends to increase the pressure per unit area of the articular surfaces. This explains why the position of the greater trochanter has such a profound effect on hip loading and on the functional performance and stability of the hip.

A pathologic position of the greater trochanter can be the result of various causes. The most frequent cause is shortening of the femoral neck, with consequent elevation of the greater trochanter relative to the femoral head. This is usually the result of growth disturbances of the proximal femur in early childhood, which may be the result of damage to the epiphysis or growth plate of the femoral neck due to traumatizing surgical or conservative treatment of a congenitally dislocated hip. Similar deformities may develop secondarily to Perthes' disease or generalized skeletal dysplasias. Infantile osteomyelitis of the femoral neck and childhood fractures of the femoral neck are relatively infrequent causes of growth disturbances of this type.

All these growth deformities are ultimately based upon the same mechanism: an arrest of longitudinal femoral neck growth, combined with a continuation of growth of the greater trochanter (Fig. 3).

Intertrochanteric osteotomies can also alter the position of the greater trochanter in an unfavorable manner. An elevated trochanter is a typical and common consequence of a varus intertrochanteric osteotomy.

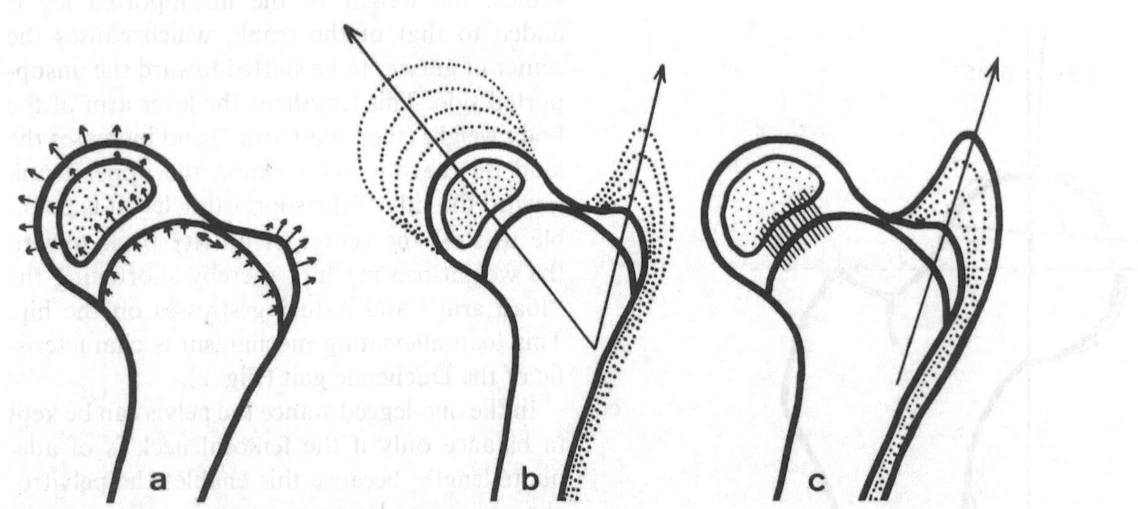

Fig. 3a–c. Growth of the proximal femur. **a, b** The arrows indicate the site and direction of growth. Growth takes place in the superficial germinative layer of the articular and epiphyseal cartilage. Bone tissue grows into the cartilaginous substance from the core of the epiphysis and from the metaphysis. **c** If the growth potential of the femoral neck (or head) is impaired, there will be an arrest of longitudinal growth at that location, with continued growth of the greater trochanter. The consequent shortening of the femoral neck leads to a relative elevation of the greater trochanter

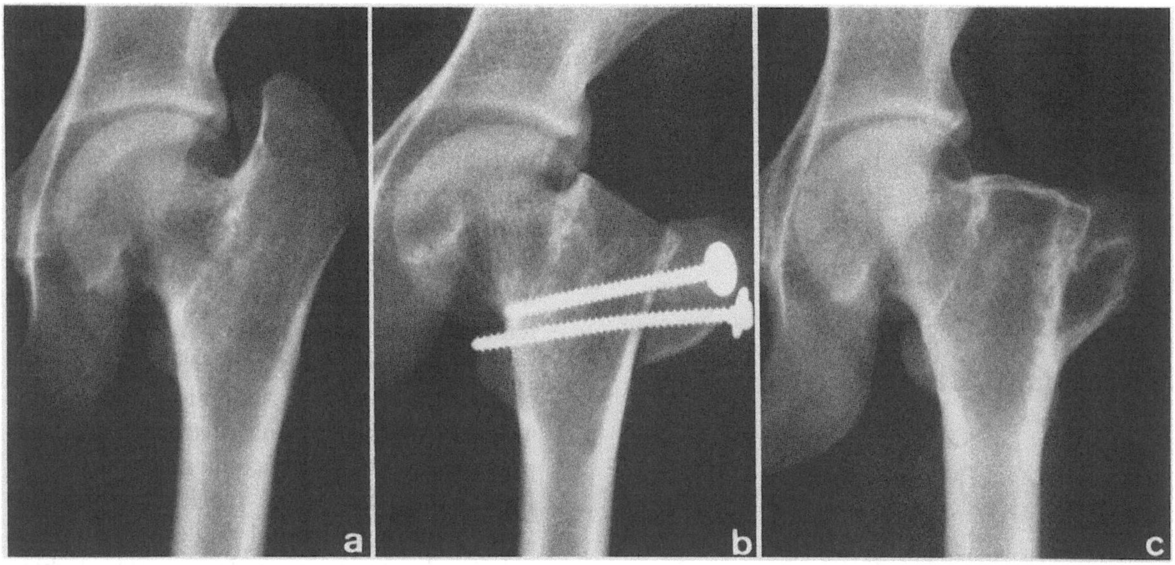

Fig. 4a–c. Compensation of the deformity of the proximal femur by corrective osteotomy of the greater trochanter. **a** The marked shortening of the femoral neck with trochanteric elevation in this 17-year-old girl resulted from growth impairment of the proximal femur in early childhood secondary to the conservative treatment of a congenitally dislocated hip. **b** Corrective osteotomy of the greater trochanter produced a *relative* lengthening of the femoral neck and an *absolute* lengthening of the lever arm of the pelvitrochanteric muscles. **c** Two years later there is a definite remodeling of trabecular bone in the femoral neck, femoral head, and acetabular roof

Finally, elevation of the trochanter can be the result of surgical intervention, as for example a femoral head resection for extensive necrosis or cysts, or following the removal of a cup prosthesis that has loosened because of reactive bone resorption with bone loss from the proximal femur.

Regardless of the mechanism responsible for malposition of the trochanter, the functional consequences are always the same (Fig. 4):

1. Elevation of the trochanter decreases the tension and mechanical efficiency of the pelvitrochanteric muscles, thereby compromising the muscular stability of the hip.
2. Shortening of the femoral neck moves the greater trochanter closer to the center of rotation of the hip, thereby decreasing the lever arm of the muscles. This impairs muscular stabilization of the hip, and leads to a greater degree of muscular contraction required in order to keep the pelvis balanced in the one-legged stance. As noted earlier, the increased muscular tension increases the pressure load on the joint.
3. Shortening of the femoral neck also moves the greater trochanter medially in relation to the ilium, and the line of action of the pelvitrochanteric muscles assumes a more vertical orientation (Fig. 5). As a result, the pressure forces acting on the hip also become more vertical, which moves the resultant pressure force closer to the superior rim of the acetabulum. This is particularly damaging in patients with acetabular dysplasia, because in them it increases the pressure forces concentrated over an area of joint surface that is already diminished (Fig. 6).
4. With extreme shortening of the femoral neck, the medialization of the greater trochanter may be such that it impinges on the rim of the acetabular roof when the leg is abducted, thereby limiting the range of hip motion.

Surgical repositioning of the greater trochanter strives to eliminate all these unfavorable anatomic and functional factors and aims at restoring normal conditions to the greatest extent possible. This may require that the greater trochanter be transferred distally, laterally, or even

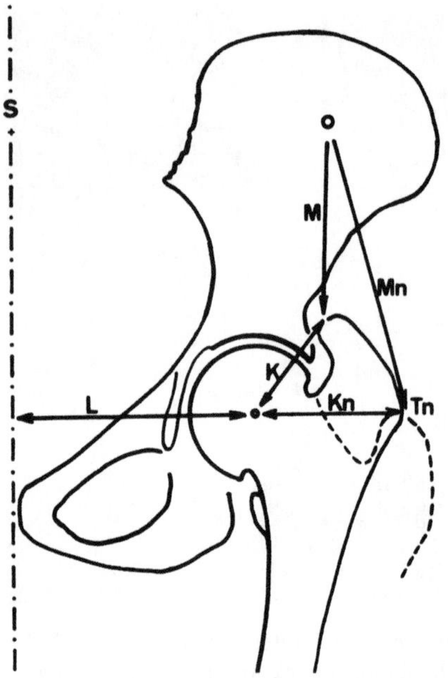

Fig. 5. Malposition of the greater trochanter alters the lever arms about the hip and changes lines of muscular action (drawn from the clinical example in Fig. 4)

anteriorly, depending on the nature of the deformity:

1. Transferring the greater trochanter distally, so that it is level with the center of the femoral head, restores normal tension to the pelvitrochanteric muscles and improves their mechanical efficiency.
2. Lateral transfer of the greater trochanter increases the distance between the tip of the trochanter and the center of hip rotation. This not only lengthens the lever arm of the muscles, thereby improving muscular stability and diminishing pressure on the joint, but it also increases the distance between the femoral head and trochanter, which effectively lengthens the femoral neck. This increases the range of abduction and creates a space for the eventual insertion of a cup prosthesis, should it become necessary.
3. Lateral transfer of the trochanter also imparts a more horizontal angle to the line of pelvitrochanteric muscular action, which shifts the resultant pressure force on the hip farther medially. This has three advantages:
   a) Pressure from the femoral head is directed more toward the center of the acetabulum.
   b) Loads are therefore distributed over a greater area of the acetabular roof, which reduces the pressure per unit area.
   c) By redirecting the forces acting on the hip, bone remodeling is stimulated throughout the hip region. This is particularly advan-

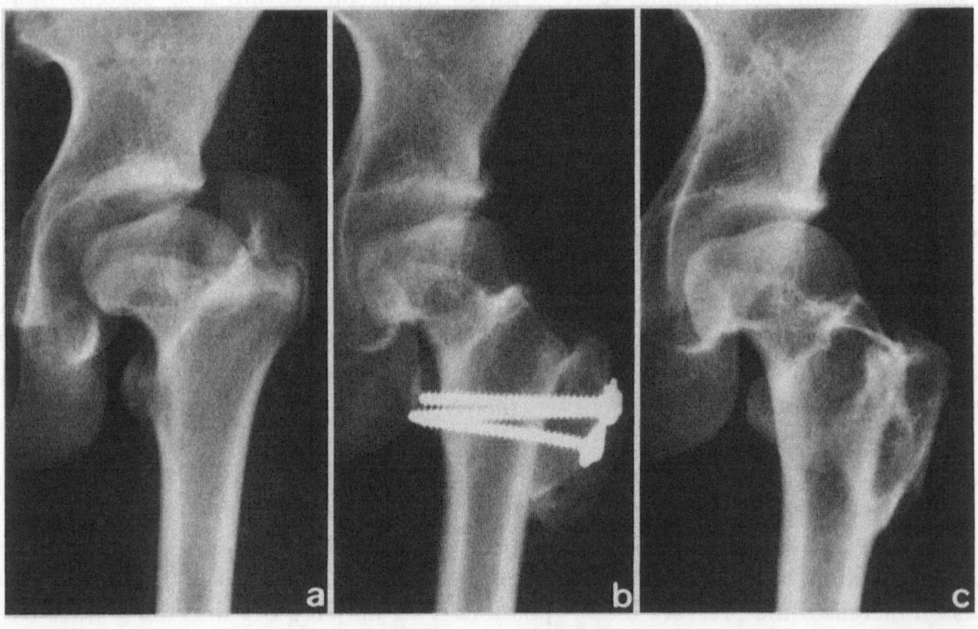

Fig. 6. a, b Corrective osteotomy of the greater trochanter in a 15-year-old girl. **c** Four years after surgery

tageous for the healing of osteoarthritic cysts.

4. In patients with excessive anteversion of the femoral neck, anterior transfer of the greater trochanter will functionally compensate for the excessive anteversion.

A corrective osteotomy of the greater trochanter is useful only if one of the foregoing deformities of the proximal femur is present. It is not indicated if the femoral neck length is normal and the greater trochanter is in a normal anatomic position.

Surgical Technique

The patient is placed in the supine position, preferably on a radiolucent operating table, and the operation is done through a lateral approach. The fascia lata is incised longitudinally, and the vastus lateralis is released from its origin on the greater trochanter. The anterior border of the gluteus minimus is exposed, and a narrow, blunt, curved elevator is passed carefully along its medial surface toward the trochanteric fossa. To improve orientation for the osteotomy, a Kirschner wire is inserted toward the fossa from that point on the greater trochanter from which the tendon of origin of the vastus lateralis was previously detached. Generally this Kirschner wire should be in line with the upper border of the femoral neck. Its tip should point to the trochanteric fossa but should not emerge from the bone. The use of an image intensifier at this stage greatly facilitates orientation. It should be noted that excessive anteversion of the femoral neck is frequently present, which will cause the shadows of the greater trochanter and femoral head to overlap somewhat in the intensifier image. The procedure is therefore much simpler if the leg is internally rotated to whatever degree necessary to provide full coverage of the greater trochanter. This will also give a clear view of the trochanteric fossa. The configuration of the proximal femur may make it difficult or impossible to osteotomize the greater trochanter in line with the upper border of the femoral neck. In such cases a more vertical osteotomy may have to be performed. The Kirschner guide wire will then have to be inserted at a correspondingly greater angle. The tip of the wire, however, must always point toward the trochanteric fossa. This will reduce the risk of vascular injury with consequent partial necrosis of the femoral head.

Once the guide wire is in position, a flat, blunt retractor is placed along the posterior edge of the greater trochanter to retract and protect the soft tissues. The osteotomy is carried out along the distal edge of the Kirschner wire, preferably with a low-speed oscillating saw. To avoid vascular damage, the saw is stopped a few millimeters before it reaches the medial cortex of the trochanter (Fig. 7). This cortex is initially left intact. Once the cut is made, a flat osteotome is inserted into the osteotomy, which is then pried open until the medial cortex fractures. Then, with a slow, prying motion of the chisel, but in the opposite direction, the osteotomy gap is also opened on the medial side, whereupon the greater trochanter is mobilized and gently pushed in a cranial direction. It is then pulled laterally and cranially with a fine-toothed forceps, and the tough connective tissue adhesions between the trochanter and joint capsule are divided with dissecting scissors flush with the medial surface of the trochanter. Frequently the greater trochanter and joint capsule will be in close apposition as a result of femoral neck shortening, even if X-rays show a space between the trochanter and femoral head. In such cases the trochanter must be detached from the joint capsule with extreme care. In all cases it is imperative that the blood vessels in the trochanteric fossa be spared when one separates the scar adhesions, and that the cutting instrument be directed toward the trochanter or the muscle insertions on the greater trochanter, and not toward the hip joint itself.

If traction on the greater trochanter meets with elastic resistance from the attached muscles, it may be assumed that adequate mobilization has been attained. If firm resistance is felt when the trochanter is pulled laterally or distally, additional adhesions have to be located and freed.

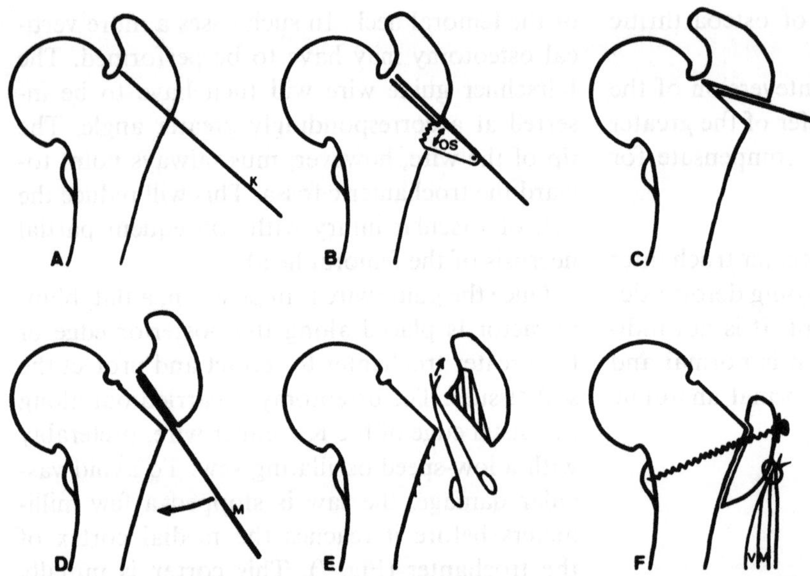

Fig. 7 A–F. Schematic representation of the surgical technique for corrective osteotomy of the greater trochanter. **A** A Kirschner wire marks the direction and level of the osteotomy. **B** The bone is cut distal to the Kirschner wire with an oscillating saw. The medial surface of the trochanter is left intact to avoid vascular injury. **C** The osteotomy is slowly wedged open with a flat chisel, in order to break the medial cortex. **D** The greater trochanter is carefully displaced with a slow, opposite prying movement of the chisel. **E** Scar adhesions between the trochanter and joint capsule are divided. The scissors are directed toward the trochanter to avoid damage to the vessels in the trochanteric fossa. **F** The trochanter is attached to the lateral aspect of the femur with two or three screws. A tension-band suture is placed between the reapproximated vastus lateralis and the gluteus medius tendon to absorb potentially damaging stresses and protect the internal fixation

The next step is to transfer the greater trochanter distally and laterally. It is also transferred anteriorly if excessive anteversion of the femoral neck is noted. The area on the lateral femoral cortex to which the trochanter is to be attached should be freshened superficially with an osteotome in order to encourage rapid consolidation following the transfer.

The trochanter is tentatively attached to the femur with Kirschner wires, and its position is carefully checked. When an image intensifier is used, it is helpful to place the legs together and lay a long Kirschner wire across the groin over the center of the femoral head and parallel to a line connecting the iliac spines. This will mark the horizontal plane on the monitor screen. The tip of the greater trochanter should be level with the center of the femoral head, and the distance between them should be 2–2.5 times the femoral head radius.

Fixation of the greater trochanter is best done with two screws inserted in a craniolateral-to-caudomedial direction. These screws should be fitted with washers and should compress the area of bony contact between the trochanter and femur. By their orientation, the screws will also neutralize tensile forces from the pelvitrochanteric muscles, thus providing an effective safeguard against trochanteric displacement. At the site where the screws enter the greater trochanter, the insertion of the gluteus medius should be incised in line with its fibers so that the screw heads and washers will have direct bony contact and will not cause soft tissue necrosis. Burying the screw heads in this way will also prevent local mechanical irritation postoperatively.

To ensure stable attachment of the trochanter, the metal fixation is supplemented by weaving a strong tension-band suture between the reapproximated origin of the vastus lateralis and the insertion of the gluteus medius. This suture will help to absorb tensile forces from the pelvitrochanteric muscles and prevent tro-

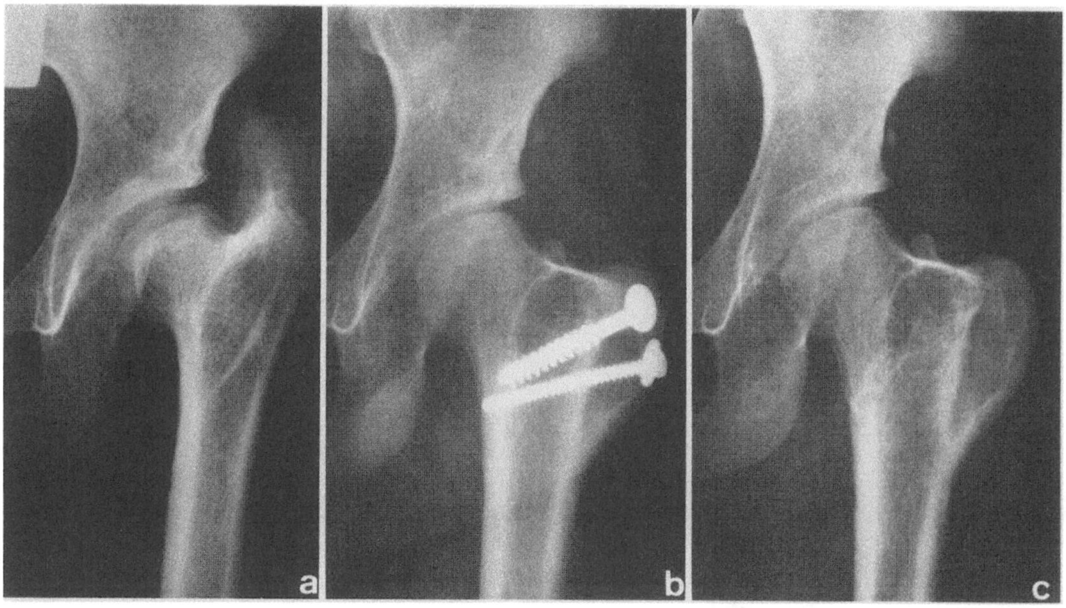

Fig. 8. a Shortening of the femoral neck and elevation of the greater trochanter in a 12-year-old girl who underwent conservative treatment in early childhood of a congenitally dislocated hip. **b** Two years after corrective osteotomy of the greater trochanter. **c** Five years postoperatively

chanteric avulsion. This mode of fixation is so secure that the patient should be able to stand with the aid of crutches on the first postoperative day. Active exercises of the pelvitrochanteric muscles are, however, not permitted until three weeks following surgery. For the first three weeks the patient should also avoid sitting in an upright posture, as this causes the gluteus medius to impart a strong rotational moment on the trochanter which may be sufficient to cause dislodgement (Fig. 8).

In cases where shortening of the femoral neck is not associated with elevation of the trochanter, but has simply decreased the distance between the tip of the trochanter and the femoral head center, the lever arm of the pelvitrochanteric muscles can be increased by lateralizing the greater trochanter (Fig. 9). The initial stages of this operation are as described above. After the trochanter has been mobilized, it is transferred laterally (and anteriorly in cases with excessive antetorsion), but not distally. This leaves a wide gap between the greater trochanter and the lateral femoral surface. The position of the trochanter is maintained by two long, fully-threaded cancellous bone screws that are inserted horizontally as "positioning

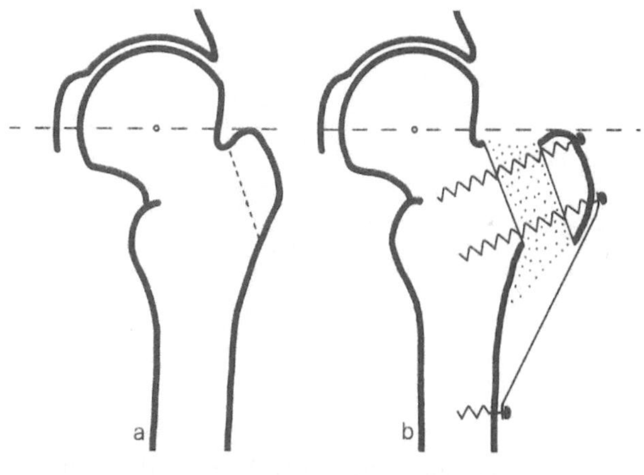

Fig. 9. Lengthening the greater trochanter by lateralization. A tension band protects the positioning screws from bending stresses. The gap between the trochanter and lateral femoral aspect is packed with cancellous bone

screws", meaning that the screw threads engage both the trochanter and the femur and maintain a constant distance between them (Fig. 10). To secure the fixation, a wire tension band is stretched tightly between the necks of the fixation screws and an anchoring screw inserted farther down the femoral shaft. The gaping defect between the trochanter and femur is packed

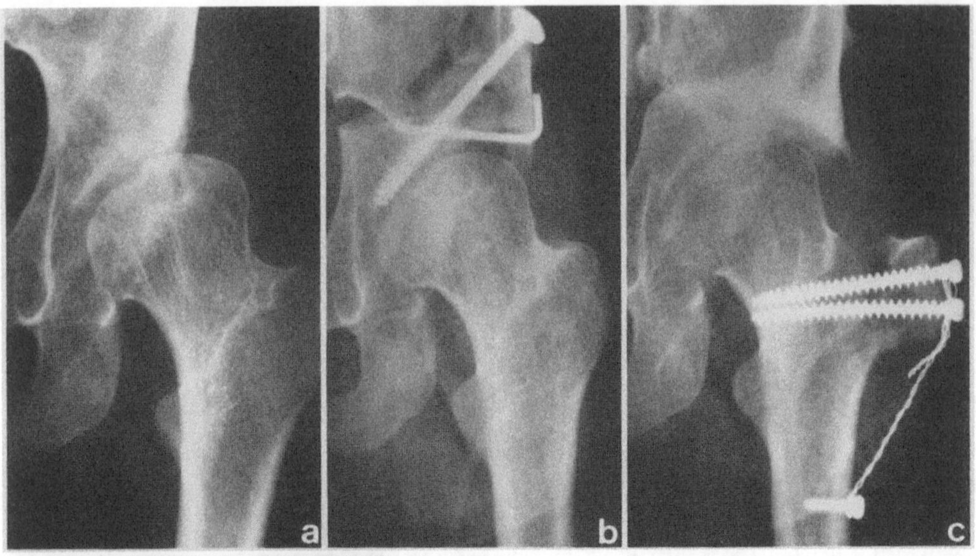

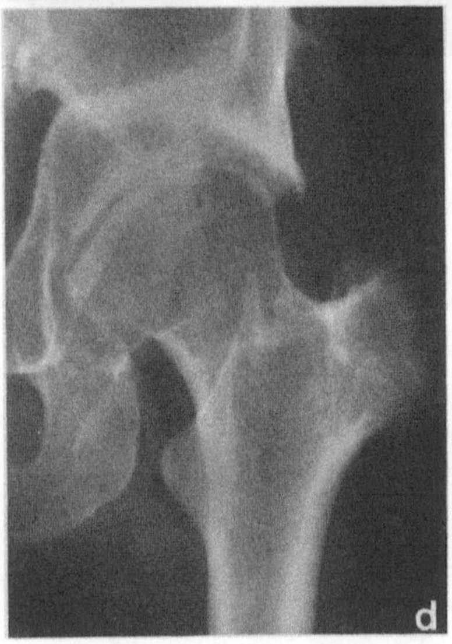

Fig. 10. a Example of lateral transfer of the greater trochanter in a 34-year-old woman with painful osteoarthritis secondary to dysplasia. **b** Initially a Chiari pelvic osteotomy was performed. **c** Due to muscular deficiency with a positive Trendelenburg sign, lateral transfer of the greater trochanter was undertaken. **d** Six years after the pelvic osteotomy and 4 years after the trochanteric transfer there is good bone remodeling with healing of osteoarthritic cysts

with cancellous bone chips. Even with a simple lateral trochanteric transfer, it is recommended that a tension-band suture be placed between the vastus lateralis and the gluteus medius.

Indications for Trochanteric Transfer

An abnormal pathologic position of the greater trochanter is the only indication for a trochanteric transfer. The aim of such surgery is always to normalize the anatomy and the biomechanics of the proximal femur to the greatest extent possible. A number of other problems may be considered as indications for transfer.

A. Trochanteric Transfer as a Reconstruction Procedure

A trochanteric transfer may be used as a reconstructive procedure to improve the prognosis and load-bearing capacity of the hip. This type of procedure is done only in patients under the age of 25 who have not yet developed degenerative hip disease. The goal of surgery in this group is to delay the onset of degenerative arthritis for as long as possible. A great many of these patients are mildly symptomatic or asymptomatic, and frequently their only complaint is a slight proneness to fatigue during long walks. Frequently a positive Trendelenburg sign is also present. Radiographs at this stage show a wide joint space, smooth articular surfaces, and a strong, regular bony structure. Many of those asymptomatic patients are seen only because they had a dislocated hip and present for radiographic examination only as part of their routine follow-up. The selection of these patients for trochanteric surgery is a difficult matter, firstly because their anatomic deformity implies a poor prognosis, and secondly because they are free of complaints and so are not particularly anxious to have surgery. A sound decision requires a careful consideration and experience from the orthopedic surgeon as well as intelligence and understanding on the part of the patient or his parents, who must appreciate the long-term benefits of an operation done prophylactically for a patient who is either asymptomatic or whose symptoms are only minimal.

The best time for a reconstructive trochanteric transfer is between the ages of 13 and 18. Surgery is rarely indicated prior to the closure of the growth apophysis of the greater trochanter. The operation may be considered if the deformity of the proximal femur is so severe that the position of the greater trochanter may cause lateralization of the femoral head, predisposing the patient to further secondary damage.

If a trochanteric transfer is necessary before closure of the apophyseal plate, the osteotomy should be performed distal to the plate, leaving a thin metaphyseal bone disc adherent to the growth cartilage. This will improve chances for bony consolidation of the trochanter on the lateral aspect of the femur. As a general rule, however, transfer of the greater trochanter should be deferred until the growth plate has fused. Surgery prior to that time has two disadvantages:

1. Because the femoral head and greater trochanter share a common epiphyseal plate, a premature trochanteric osteotomy can retard future growth of the femoral head and neck.
2. A premature trochanteric osteotomy can arrest the growth of the trochanter, resulting in a deficiency of bone stock in the proximal femur. This is unfavorable from a reconstructive standpoint, because the small size of the trochanter necessarily shortens the lever arm of the pelvitrochanteric muscles.

The trochanteric transfer may be done as a sole operation in the treatment of a CDH, or it may serve as one component of a comprehensive operation in which the femoral neck and acetabulum are also reconstructed.

B. Trochanteric Transfer as a Curative Procedure

Transfer of the greater trochanter may be done as a curative procedure. This has proved useful in patients with a short femoral neck and elevated trochanter who develop degenerative arthritis requiring surgical intervention. The value of the transfer in such cases is that a marked degree of improvement can be effected with a relatively minor operation.

As stated previously, the trochanteric transfer lengthens the lever arm of the pelvitrochanteric muscles, which in turn relieves pressure on the osteoarthritic hip. But the redirection of the pressure forces acting on the hip also carries an important benefit: by redirecting the resultant pressure force in a more medial direction, the load is distributed over a greater area of the articular surface, and so the pressure per unit area is decreased. This redirection of forces also stimulates structural changes in the bony tissue, leading to a rapid bone remodeling that is conducive to the healing of osteoarthritic cysts (Fig. 11).

Recurrent pain at the insertions of the pelvitrochanteric muscles due to overexertion is a relatively rare indication for a trochanteric transfer in adults.

Osteoarthritis of the hip is an excellent indication for a trochanteric transfer, because the effect of the procedure in such cases is two-fold: First, the improvement in the loads imposed on the hip will in all likelihood lead to clinical, radiologic, and subjective improvement of the osteoarthritic condition, provided sufficient hip mobility still exists. Second, the procedure im-

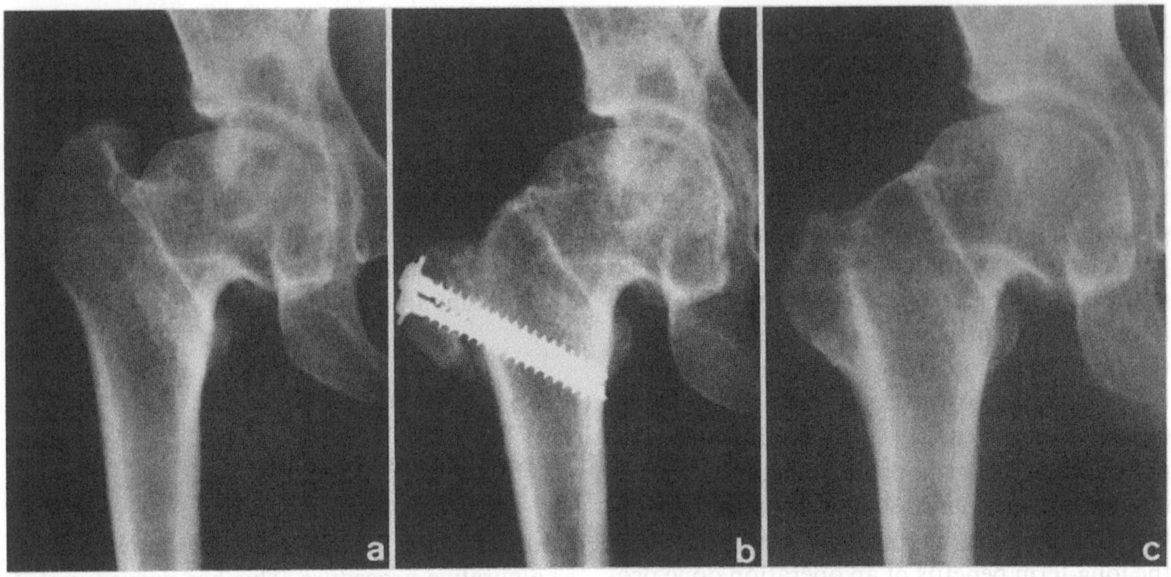

Fig. 11. a, b Transfer of the greater trochanter for painful dysplasia-associated osteoarthritis with cyst formation in a 41-year-old woman. **c** Six years after surgery the bone structure about the joint line is normal and the patient ambulates without pain

proves the anatomy of the proximal femur, the most important benefit being an effective "Lengthening" of the femoral neck. Without this anatomic revision it would be considerably more difficult, if not impossible, to undertake future operations in that region. These include pelvic osteotomy (Chiari type), intertrochanteric osteotomy, surface-replacement arthroplasty, and total hip arthroplasty. Thus, even if the trochanteric transfer does not afford the expected degree of improvement in osteoarthritic complaints, it still broadens the range of surgical options that are available at a later date.

C. Trochanteric Transfer for Mechanical Reasons

Transfer of the greater trochanter for mechanical reasons is indicated only in a relatively small group of patients for whom true reconstructive surgery is not feasible and the only goal of surgery is to improve stability of the hip. This group includes hips in which degenerative arthritis is so advanced that surface-replacement arthroplasty is indicated but has little prospect of restoring adequate stability because of marked shortening of the femoral neck. In such cases we perform the trochanteric transfer in a separate operation session, either before or after the arthroplasty (Fig. 12).

Trochanteric transfer in this group is also useful after failure of a cup prosthesis. As already noted in an earlier publication (Wagner 1978), the simple removal of a loose cup prosthesis followed by the insertion of the femoral neck stump directly into the acetabulum coupled with a trochanteric transfer can be an acceptable salvage procedure in cases where deficient bone quality precludes the insertion of a new prosthesis. Transfer of the greater trochanter should always be a part of this procedure. This seats the femoral neck stump more deeply in the acetabular fossa, and gives the pelvitrochanteric muscles a longer lever arm and better tension. Both factors greatly enhance the stability of the "resection arthroplasty" and give a decidedly better functional result than a "resection osteotomy" following the removal of a conventional total hip prosthesis (Figs. 13 and 14).

Finally, the trochanteric transfer can perform a similar function when there has been a pathological dislocation of the hip as seen following infantile osteomyelitis, where a rudimentary

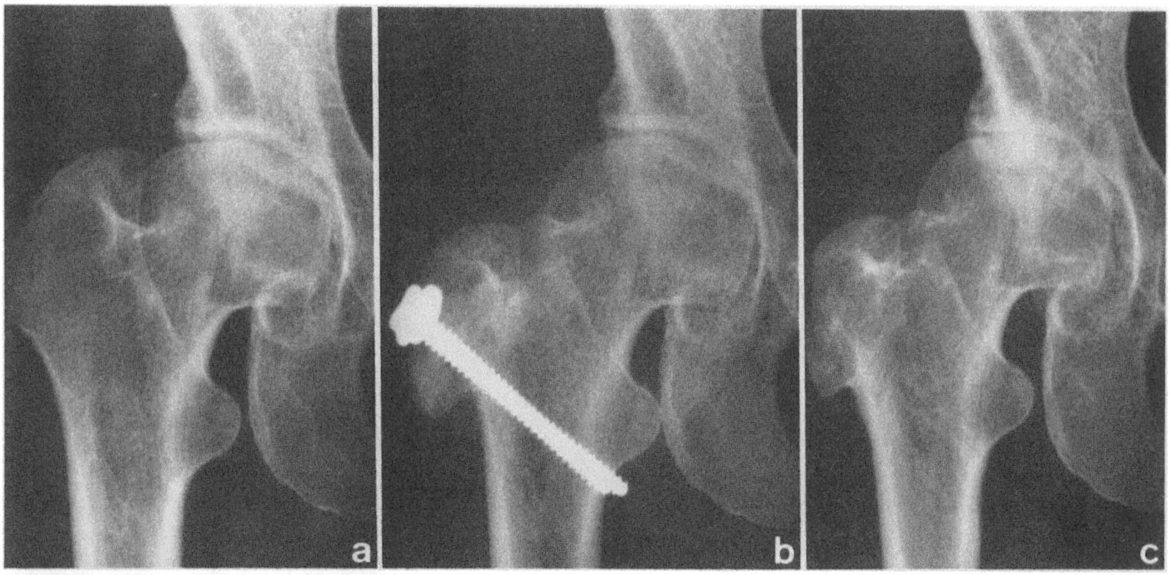

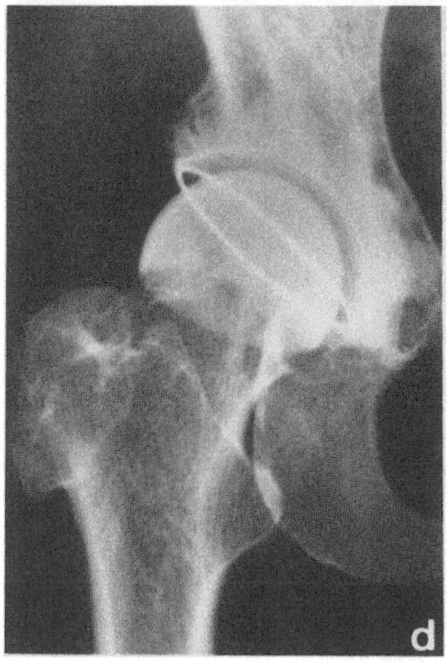

Fig. 12a–d. Transfer of the greater trochanter to lengthen the femoral neck, done here as a preliminary to surface replacement arthroplasty in a 52-year-old woman with osteoarthritis secondary to dysplasia

femoral neck stump covered with scar tissue abuts against the acetabulum. Here, too, the transfer of the greater trochanter can significantly improve the muscular stability of the hip.

Results

During the period from 1967 to 1980 we performed 609 trochanteric osteotomies. This review will be confined only to the transfer done for patients with congenital dysplasia of the hip or for patients with degenerative arthritis secondary to dysplasia. Other indications, such as post-traumatic femoral head necrosis, arthroplasty, or reconstruction of the proximal femur made necessary by post-traumatic deformity or destructive dislocation, are omitted.

Our review is further limited to operations performed during the period 1967–1978 (300 hips) so that at least 3 years' follow-up could be presented (Table 1). In all of these cases the operation was performed for the sequelae of congenital hip dysplasia. This accounts for the predominance of women (86%).

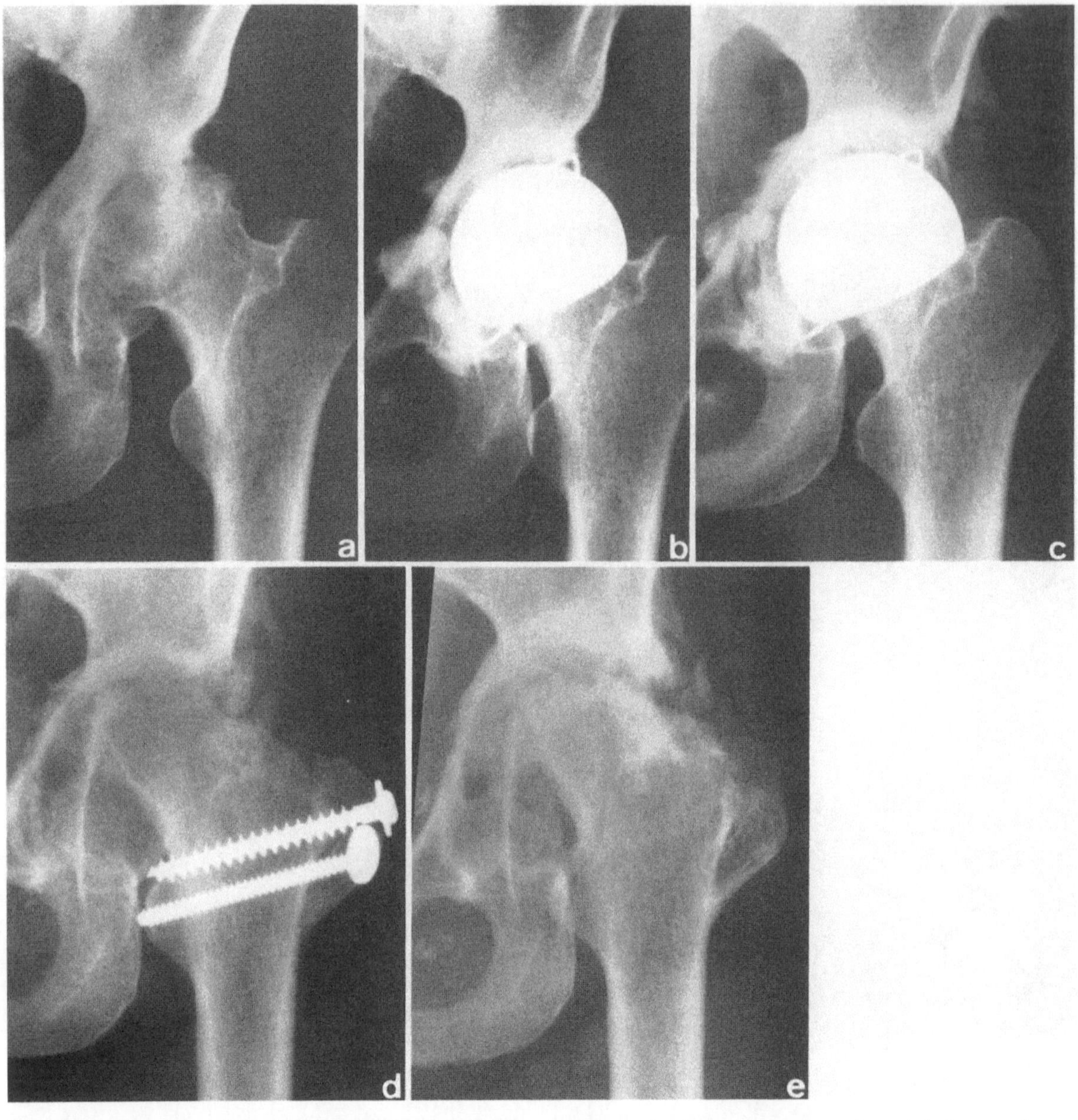

Fig. 13. a–d Transfer of the greater trochanter to stabilize the hip following the removal of a loose cup prosthesis in a 38-year-old woman. Special care was taken to preserve the caudal joint capsule so that direct contact between the femoral head and acetabular roof was avoided. **e** Two years after surgery there is good evidence of bone remodeling about the joint line

The average age was 25.5 years (range 8–72 years). We assessed our results on the basis of simple clinical and radiologic criteria that could be easily evaluated.

We also attempted to measure the improvement of abductor power after the trochanteric transfer. We developed a device which permitted an objective measurement of this parameter (Fig. 15). The laterally recumbent patient, by abducting the leg, compressed a pneumatic cylinder by means of a sling attached about the ankle. The pneumatic pressure was read directly from a manometer. This device provided a simple and accurate means of measuring abductor power. We did not take these results into account in the present review, however, because

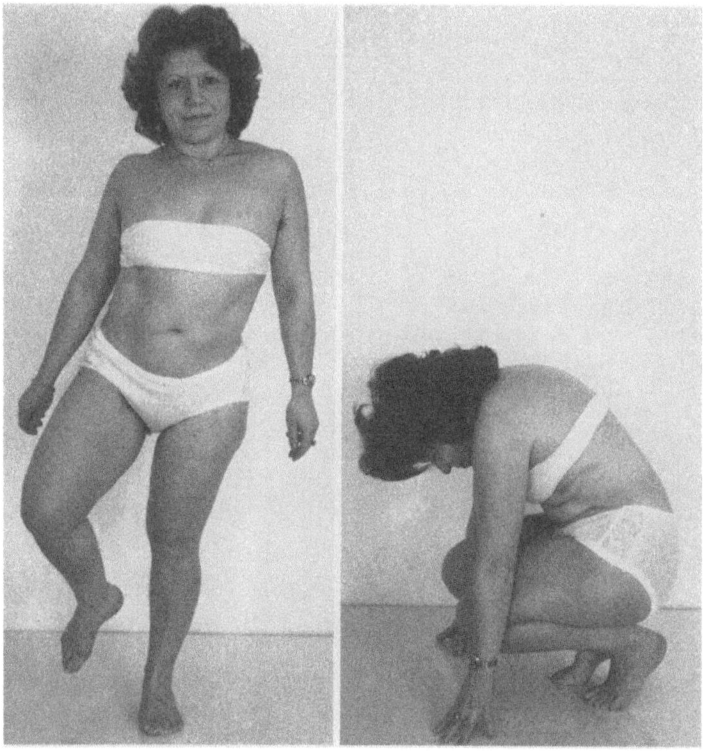

Fig. 14. Hip in which the greater trochanter was transferred following the removal of a loose cup prosthesis (same case as in Fig. 13). There is good mobility and a negative Trendelenburg sign

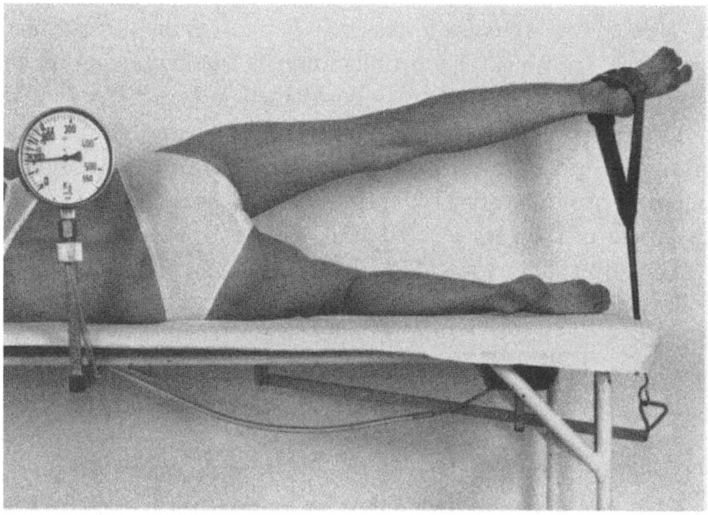

Fig. 15. Apparatus for measuring the abduction power of the pelvitrochanteric muscles

Table 1. Trochanter osteotomy in congenital hip dysplasia in 300 hips (1967–1978)

	Operated	Evaluated
Group I	180	159
Group II	50	48
Group III	70	68
Total	300	275

it is not yet possible to distinguish the effects of surgery from the effects of muscle training. This became apparent when we found that even preoperative isometric exercises markedly increased the power of the pelvitrochanteric muscles. After surgery the patients were again placed on a program of regular muscle training. Thus, the dramatic improvement in abductor power that was often measured after the tro-

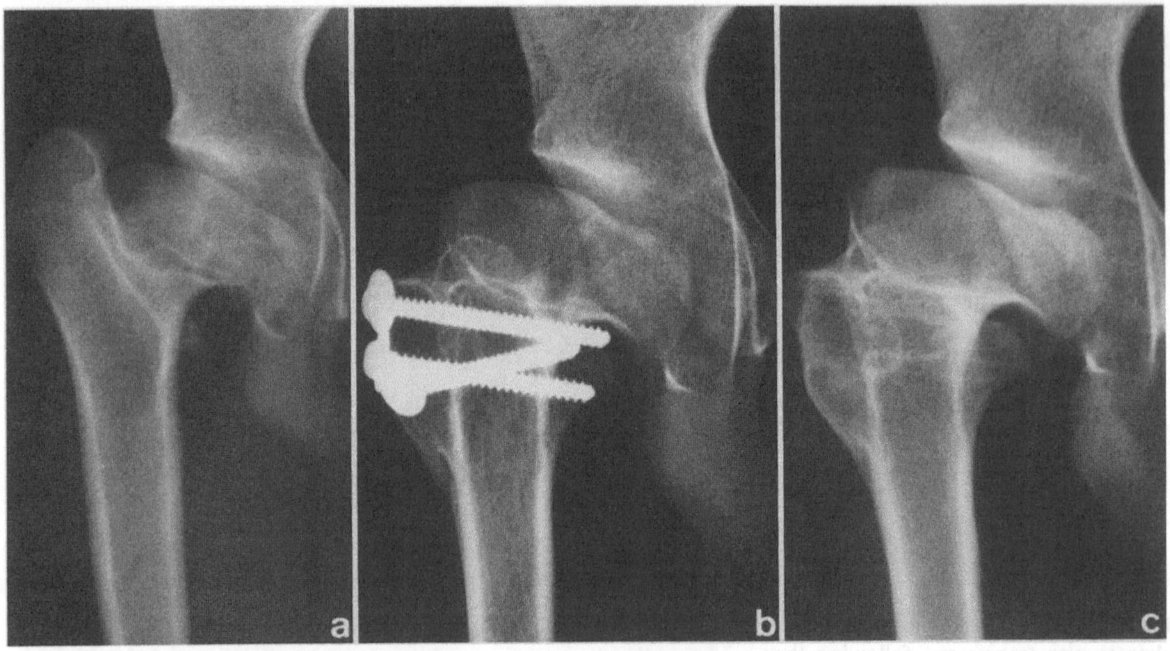

Fig. 16a–c. Partial correction of the greater trochanter in anticipation of a subsequent valgus osteotomy due to a cylindrical deformity of the femoral head

chanteric transfer could not be attributed to the surgery alone, because it was partly the result of muscle training. This problem merits further study. It is hoped that tests performed before preoperative exercises are initiated, and again after postoperative exercises are concluded, will one day provide more accurate information on the effect of the surgery alone.

The subjective, clinical, and radiologic signs following the trochanteric transfer showed a high degree of correlation in most patients, i.e., subjective improvement was accompanied by a favorable objective clinical and radiologic change.

Ideally, the aim of the trochanteric transfer is to place the greater trochanter in an anatomically normal position relative to the center of rotation of the hip. This means that the tip of the greater trochanter should be level with the center of the femoral head, with the distance between them equal to the diameter of the femoral head.

An ideal correction cannot always be achieved, and, an "ideal" correction is not always the most expeditious. Thus, for example, scar adhesions can reduce the elasticity of the pelvitrochanteric muscles and offer such great resistance to displacement of the greater trochanter that a partial correction is the only prudent alternative. Under no circumstances should the surgeon "force" a transfer against muscular resistance, as this will create pressure that is damaging to the joint.

A partical correction of the greater trochanter may also be advantageous in cases where deformity of the femoral head strongly suggests that an intertrochanteric valgus extension osteotomy will eventually be required. In such cases the greater trochanter is transferred laterally to correct for femoral neck shortening, but the tip of the greater trochanter is left above the center of the femoral head in anticipation of the time when a subsequent valgus osteotomy will move the trochanter to the ideal level without placing undue tension on the muscles (Fig. 16).

Occasionally, an overcorrection of the greater trochanter may be indicated if the pelvitrochanteric muscles show a marked degree of laxity and satisfactory tension cannot be obtained in the "ideal" position (Fig. 17).

Patients were selected for the trochanteric surgery for a variety of anatomic, biomechani-

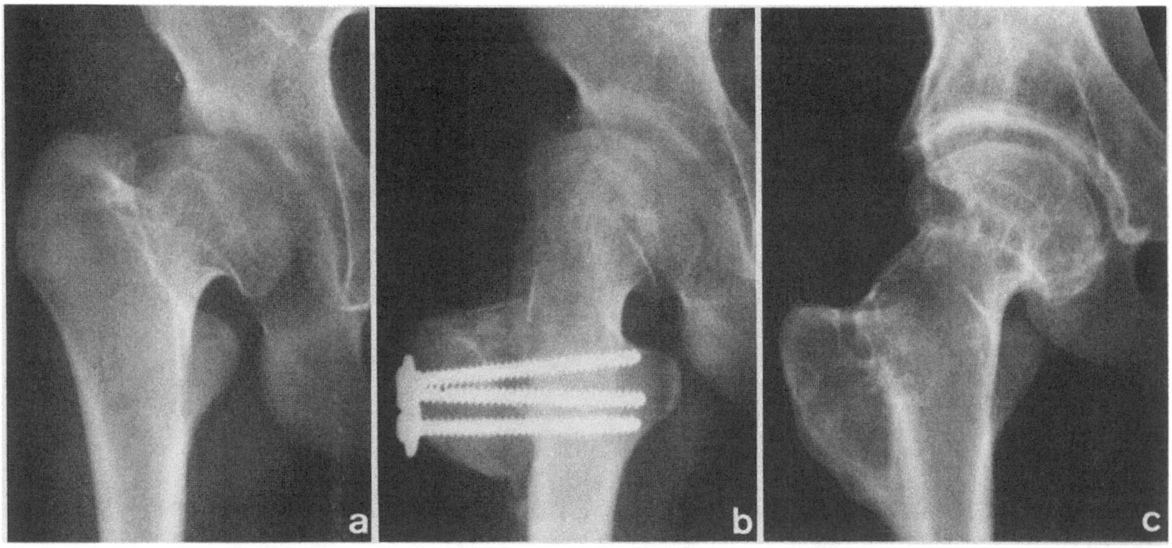

Fig. 17a–c. Overcorrection of the greater trochanter for laxity of the pelvitrochanteric muscles. The patient, a 13-year-old girl, initially underwent a trochanteric transfer (**b**) and 3 months later a spherical acetabular osteotomy was performed. **c** Ten years postoperatively there is normal hip function with good radiographic evidence of remodeling

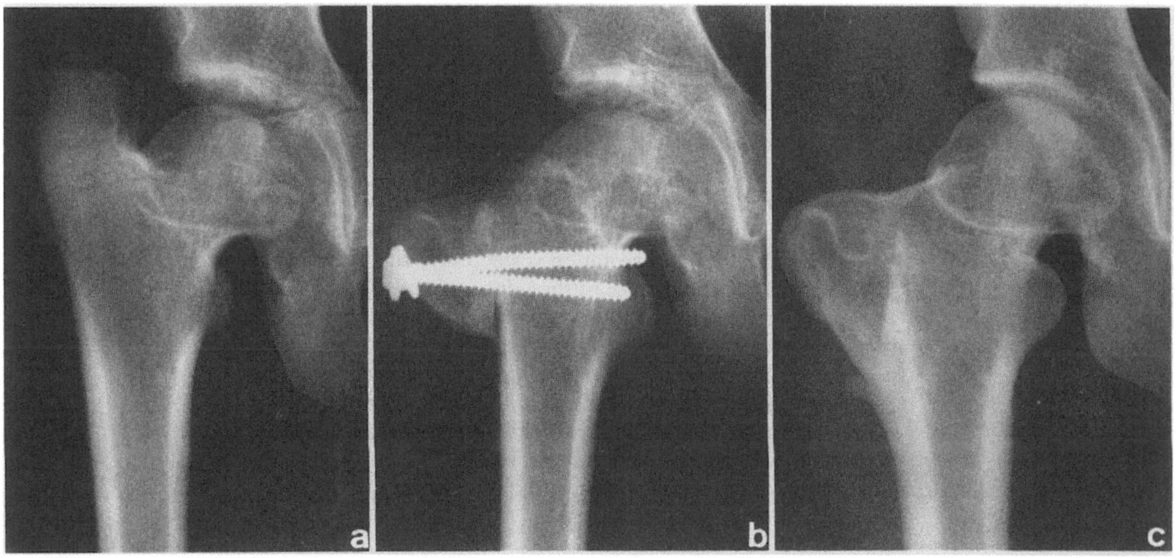

Fig. 18. a, b Transfer of the greater trochanter in a 13-year-old girl with shortening of the femoral neck secondary to conservative treatment of a congenitally dislocated hip. **c** Six years postoperatively there is normal hip function with good bone structure

cal, and clinical reasons. Thus, the results of the operation varied somewhat from one patient to the next. To present our results more meaningfully we have arranged the patients into three groups.

Group I

In group I the main concern was to improve the function and weight-bearing ability of the hip. Indications for the transfer were femoral

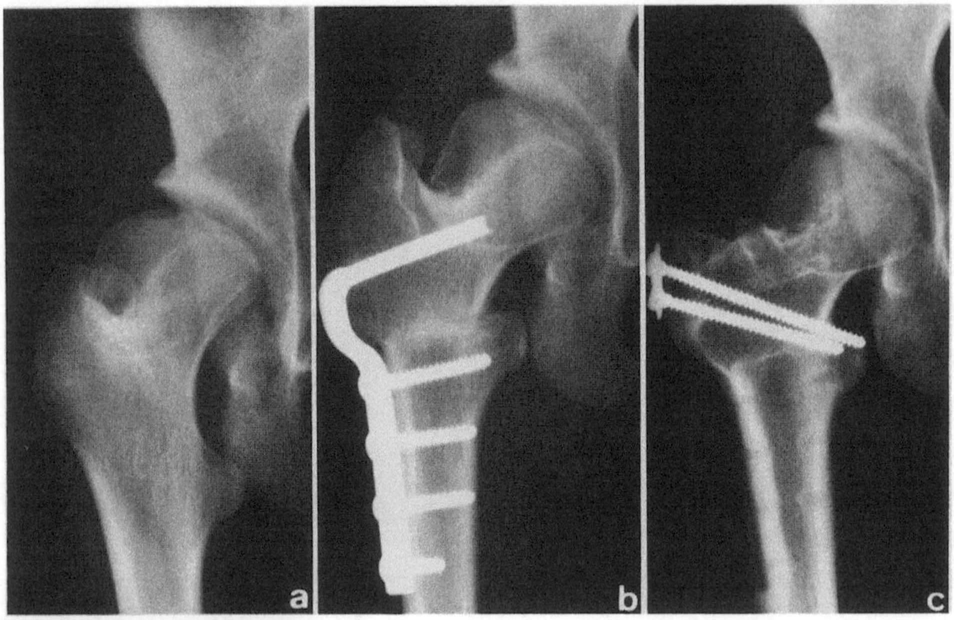

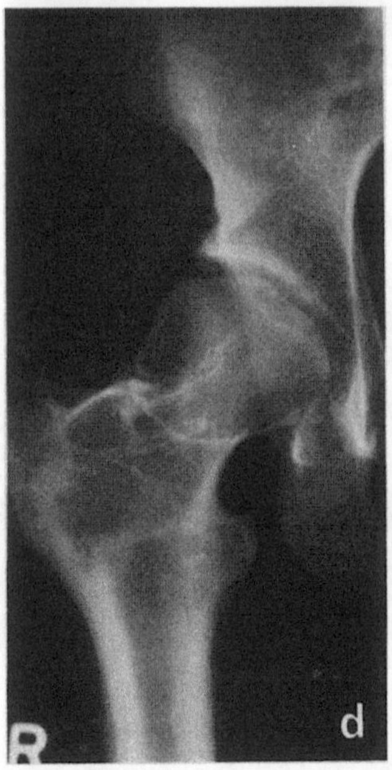

Fig. 19. a Deformity of the proximal femur with eversion of the articular surface of the femoral head. **b** An intertrochanteric varus derotation osteotomy significantly improved the congruence of the joint surfaces, but moved the greater trochanter to an unfavorable position. **c** When the patient returned for removal of the internal fixation material, a corrective osteotomy of the greater trochanter was performed. **d** Six years after the the intertrochanteric osteotomy and 5 years after the trochanteric osteotomy, hip function was normal and the trabecular pattern of the bone closely approximates that of the normal hip

neck shortening with elevation of the trochanter and muscular insufficiency of the hip, a positive Trendelenburg sign, a limp due to hip insufficiency, and inability to walk long distances (Fig. 18). Another major indication in this group was muscular insufficiency due to elevation of the trochanter following an intertrochanteric varus osteotomy (Fig. 19).

A total of 180 hips were operated upon in this group. Twenty-one patients who had a unilateral trochanteric transfer were lost to follow-up, leaving a total of 159 hips available for evaluation. Women predominated (138:21; =87%). The average age was 18.2 years. In 28 patients the transfer was bilateral. The longest follow-up after surgery was 148 months, with an average of 58 months. In 43 cases a Chiari pelvic osteotomy had to be done to stabilize the hip, and a Wagner spherical acetabular osteotomy was required in 20 cases.

Subjective Complaints. In this series of 159 hips, 99 were free of complaints both before and after surgery. The transfer in these cases was done to correct muscular insufficiency. In 53 hips in which the transfer was done for complaints associated with fatiguability with sustained walking, significant improvement was effected by the trochanteric surgery. In five hips, complaints were not relieved by surgery. In two hips, initial improvement after surgery was followed by a gradual recurrence of complaints, beginning 4 years postoperatively in a 33-year-old man and 7 years postoperatively in a 15-year-old girl (Table 2).

Ambulatory Status. Forty-one hips showed no evidence of a limp either before or after surgery. In 81 hips, a limp due to hip insufficiency was corrected by the trochanteric transfer. In 36 hips a limp was present both before and after the operation, but only five of these hips showed a positive Trendelenburg sign. In one hip the limp became worse within 5 years after the trochanteric transfer (Table 2).

Trendelenburg Sign. In 41 hips the Trendelenburg sign was negative before and after surgery. In 113 hips a positive Trendelenburg sign preoperatively became negative following the transfer. In three hips the surgery did not improve an initially positive Trendelenburg sign, and in two severely deformed hips the sign became more pronounced after surgery (Table 2).

Table 2. Clinical data for group I

	Preoperative	Postoperative
Pain		
No pain	99	99+53
Pain	60	5
Worse		2
Gait		
No limp	41	41+81
Limp	118	36
Worse		1
Trendelenburg		
Negative	41	41+113
Positive	118	3
Worse		2

In our radiographic evaluation, we took into account both the extent of the surgical correction and the structural changes that were present in proximity to the joint line:

Position of Greater Trochanter. In 68 out of 159 hips, the tip of the greater trochanter was higher than the joint line preoperatively. In 42 of these hips the greater trochanter was transferred to the ideal position of correction, with its tip level with the center of the femoral head. In nine hips only a partial correction was undertaken, because the elliptical deformation of the femoral head made it likely that an intertrochanteric valgus osteotomy would eventually be required, at which time the greater trochanter would be moved to its ideal position. In 17 other hips, laxness of the pelvitrochanteric muscles made it necessary to overcorrect the trochanter slightly, bringing its tip below the center of the femoral head.

In 63 hips the tip of the greater trochanter was level with the joint line preoperatively. A partial correction was performed in five of these hips, an ideal correction in 45, and, for the reasons stated, a slight overcorrection in the remaining 13.

In 28 hips the tip of the greater trochanter was already lower than the joint line preoperatively. The main problem in these cases was that the greater trochanter was situated too far medially as a result of femoral neck shortening, thereby decreasing the lever arm of the pelvitrochanteric muscles. The main goal of surgery, therefore, was to move the greater trochanter farther laterally. In 14 hips the tip of the trochanter was moved level with the femoral head center, and in another 14 a slight overcorrection was made distally (Table 3).

Joint Space. The radiographic joint space showed postoperative improvement in 50 out of 159 hips. This was evidenced by a greater regularity of the joint margins and a widening

Table 3. Radiologic data for group I

	Preoperative	Postoperative
Tip of trochanter		
Above joint space	68	
Level with joint space	63	
Below joint space	28	14
Level with head center		101
Below head center		44
Joint space		
No change		107
Widening		50
Narrowing		2
Bone structure		
No change		98
Improvement		58
Worsening		3

of the space. In 107 cases, no radiographic changes were noted during the follow-up period. In two cases there was a gradual loss of regularity in the joint margins and a narrowing of the radiographic joint space (Table 3).

Bone Structure. The bone structure in proximity to the joint line was improved in 58 out of 159 cases. Areas of increased density and atrophic rarefaction were replaced by a stronger and more uniform osseous structure. This homogenization of bone structure was most apparent in areas where stresses that had been highly concentrated preoperatively were afterward distributed over a larger area of joint surface as a result of the trochanteric transfer. In 98 cases no change of bone structure was evident, and in three cases a deterioration of bone structure, with marked density variations, developed over a period of years (Table 3).

Group II

Patients in group II had severe, complex deformities of the hip for which the trochanteric transfer did not represent a definitive correction, but served only to facilitate reconstructive surgery at a later date. These joints were characterized by severe dysplastic changes of the acetabulum in which a Chiari pelvic osteotomy or Wagner spherical acetabular osteotomy was required to improve the coverage of the femoral head, but could not be done immediately due to femoral neck shortening or trochanteric elevation. Transfer of the greater trochanter was a necessary preliminary to these operations.

A total of 50 hip joints were operated upon in this group. Two patients were lost to follow-up, leaving 48 hips available for review. Women predominated (45:3; 94%). The average age was 19.4 years. In 16 patients the transfer was bilateral. The longest duration of postoperative follow-up was 116 months, with an average of 57 months. In 30 hips the trochanteric transfer was supplemented by correction of the acetabulum – Chiari pelvic osteotomy in 19 and Wagner spherical acetabular osteotomy in 11.

Originally, correction of the acetabulum was intended for all 48 hips in this group. It was carried out in only 30 hips because in the other 18, the trochanteric transfer improved hip biomechanics to such a degree that corrective surgery of the acetabulum could be deferred.

Subjective Complaints. Thirty of the 48 hips were free of complaints before and after surgery. In the remaining 18 patients, the complaints were significantly improved following the transfer (Table 4).

Ambulatory Status. Thirty hips showed no evidence of a limp either before or after surgery. In 13 hips, a limp due to hip insufficiency was corrected by the trochanteric transfer. In three hips a limp was present both before and after surgery, and in two hips the limp became worse within 5 years after the transfer (Table 4).

Trendelenburg Sign. In 35 hips the Trendelenburg sign was negative before and after surgery. In 10 hips a positive Trendelenburg sign preoperatively became negative after the transfer. In two hips the surgery did not improve an initially positive Trendelenburg sign, and one hip even experienced an exacerbation of muscular insufficiency with passage of time (Table 4).

Table 4. Clinical data for group II

	Preoperative	Postoperative
Pain		
No pain	30	30+18
Pain	18	
Worse		0
Gait		
No limp	30	30+13
Limp	18	3
Worse		2
Trendelenburg		
Negative	35	35+10
Positive	13	2
Worse		1

Table 5. Radiologic data for group II

	Preoperative	Postoperative
Tip of trochanter		
Above joint space	15	
Level with joint space	23	
Below joint space	10	4
Level with head center		29
Below head center		15
Joint space		
No change		35
Widening		12
Narrowing		1
Bone structure		
No change		34
Improvement		13
Worsening		1

Position of Greater Trochanter. In 29 of the 48 hips, the greater trochanter was placed in the ideal position of correction. In four hips the correction was partial, and in 15 hips an overcorrection was done due to laxity of the pelvitrochanteric muscles (Table 5).

Joint Space. In 34 hips the width of the radiographic joint space was unchanged after surgery. In 13 hips a widening of the space was seen during postoperative follow-up, and in one hip the space narrowed over a 5-year period (Table 5).

Bone Structure. The bone structure adjacent to the radiographic joint line is an important index of the functional status of the hip. Bony atrophy, circumscribed sclerosis, and the presence of subchondral cysts give important information on pressure distribution and degenerative changes in the joint. In 34 of the 48 hips in this group, no change in bone structure was observed postoperatively. In 13 hips the bone structure gradually became more homogeneous after the transfer, and a gradual deterioration of bone structure was seen in only one hip (Table 5).

Group III

The patients in group III had already developed marked osteoarthritis secondary to their dysplasia, and transfer of the greater trochanter was done as a curative measure. All these hips showed shortening of the femoral neck with elevation of the greater trochanter. The aim of the transfer was to ameliorate biomechanical deficiencies about the hip (reduce intra-articular pressure and stimulate remodeling by the redirection of forces) for the purpose of relieving symptoms, improving the weight-bearing ability of the hip, and retarding the progression of degenerative changes.

A total of 70 hips were operated on in this group. Two patients were lost to follow-up, and so 68 hips were available for review. Women predominated (54:14; 79%), and average age was 42.3 years. In two patients the transfer was bilateral. The longest duration of postoperative follow-up was 137 months, with an average of 56 months. In 54 hips, treatment of the degenerative arthritis required adjunctive operative measures: Chiari pelvic osteotomy in 31 hips, intertrochanteric osteotomy in 21 hips, and total arthroplasty in two hips. Fourteen hips were treated by transfer of the trochanter alone.

Subjective Complaints. In 13 of the 68 hips, complaints were mild or absent both before and

Table 6. Clinical data for group III

	Preoperative	Postoperative
Pain		
No pain	13	13+50
Pain	55	2
Worse		3
Gait		
No limp	13	13+29
Limp	55	26
Worse		0
Trendelenburg		
Negative	32	32+30
Positive	36	6
Worse		0

Table 7. Radiologic data for group III

	Preoperative	Postoperative
Tip of trochanter		
Above joint space	19	
Level with joint space	25	
Below joint space	20	10
Level with head center	4	40
Below head center		18
Joint space		
No change		28
Widening		36
Narrowing		4
Bone structure		
No change		28
Improvement		38
Worsening		1

after surgery. In 50 hips complaints were significantly improved by the transfer. In two hips, complaints associated with sustained walking persisted after the operation. In three hips load-dependent complaints recurred 6–8 years after the transfer: In a 37-year-old women with severe osteoarthritis and dysplasia, a trochanteric transfer and subsequent pelvic osteotomy were followed by an initial symptom-free interval. Six years later the patient reported a recurrence of complaints, whereupon an intertrochanteric valgus osteotomy was performed. In two hips the complaints gradually returned and intensified despite the trochanteric transfer (Table 6).

Ambulatory Status. Thirteen hips showed no evidence of a limp before or after surgery. In 29 hips a limp due to hip insufficiency was corrected by the trochanteric transfer. In 26 hips a limp was still present after the transfer (despite a negative Trendelenburg sign in four cases) (Table 6).

Trendelenburg Sign. In 32 hips the Trendelenburg sign was negative before and after surgery. In 30 hips a positive Trendelenburg sign preoperatively became negative after surgery. In six hips the surgery did not improve an initially positive Trendelenburg sign (Table 6).

Position of Greater Trochanter. In 40 hips the greater trochanter was placed in the ideal position of correction, with its tip level with the center of the femoral head. In 10 hips only a partial correction was performed, placing the tip of the greater trochanter between the level of the joint line and the center of the femoral head, because the elliptical deformity of the femoral head made it likely that an intertrochanteric valgus osteotomy would eventually be required, at which time the greater trochanter would be moved to the ideal position. In 18 hips, laxity of the pelvitrochanteric muscles made it necessary to overcorrect the trochanter slightly, bringing its tip below the center of the femoral head (Table 7).

Joint Space. In 36 of the 68 hips, transfer of the greater trochanter was followed by structural improvement and widening of the radiographic joint line, which coincided with an improvement in clinical findings. No change was observed in 28 hips, and in four hips an initially narrow joint space showed further narrowing after surgery (Table 7).

Bone Structure. Despite the poor initial bone status, 38 of the 68 hips showed an improvement of bone structure about the articular surfaces after the transfer. In 29 hips no change was observed, and one hip showed a further deterioration of bone structure postoperatively (Table 7).

Complications

Corrective osteotomy of the greater trochanter is seldom associated with complications, and when they occur, they tend to be minor.

The most frequent and serious complication was avulsion of the greater trochanter in the postoperative period, with resulting loss of correction. The risk of trochanteric displacement depends largely on the quality of the mechanical fixation. When there is severe atrophy of the bone, as commonly associated with osteoarthritis and considerable hip stiffness or in patients with failed operations on the proximal femur, the screw heads and washers may sink into the soft bony surface and lose their stabilizing effect. Moreover, the all-important tension-band suture that is woven between the reattached vastus lateralis and the tendon of the gluteus medius may be unable to prevent trochanteric dislodgement if the suturing technique is poor or the muscles atrophied. Avulsion of the greater trochanter may also result from excessive mechanical stresses during the postoperative period. Overactivity on the part of the patient during the first days after surgery, excessive weight-bearing on the operated limb, and accidental falls are frequent causes. Occasionally the displacement occurred gradually and was unnoticed by the patient.

Another important cause of loosening is premature sitting in an upright posture. This is because the tension-band wire between the vastus lateralis and gluteus medius exerts its tension-absorbing action when the hip is in full extension. When the patient sits upright, the origin of the gluteus medius on the wing of the ilium is moved anterior to the thigh, and the lines of action of the gluteus medius and vastus lateralis are at right angles to each other. This exerts a rotational moment on the greater trochanter, with a corresponding risk of displacement.

Table 8. Complications in 275 hips

Secondary dislocation of greater trochanter	5
Fatigue fracture of screws	5
Revision of hematoma	4
Delayed bone healing	3
Ectopic ossification	6
Infection	0

Displacements occurred in five of 275 hips (Table 8). Three were caused by a fall in the 2nd postoperative week, and open refixation was required. Healing was uneventful. In two other cases a gradual, unrecognized displacement occurred, causing approximately 50% loss of the original correction. The clinical result was, however, satisfactory.

Fatigue fractures of the metal screws are another potential complication of this procedure. It must be realized that even when properly placed, the screws that anchor the greater trochanter are subject to bending stresses. This can lead to fatigue fracture of the screws, particularly if the muscle suture is deficient or if the bony consolidation is delayed. Even if full consolidation has occurred, the elasticity of the bone can eventually lead to implant fracture. The screws should therefore be removed as soon as possible.

We observed screw fractures in five of the 275 hips. In four cases this had no effect on the position of the greater trochanter or bony consolidation. In one case, however, fatigue fracture of the screws led to the development of painful pseudarthrosis. While this was not associated with significant trochanteric displacement, the resultant pain and disability required that an open refixation be performed. Uneventful healing ensued in all.

In four of the 275 hips, a hematoma had to be operatively evacuated. This was done on postoperative day 7 in two cases, day 10 in one case, and day 20 in one further case. All four cases went on to heal uneventfully. No wound infections occurred.

We observed a significant delay of bony consolidation in only three cases. All three healed without complications, although two of the patients had to walk with a crutch for 3 months. In a 32-year-old alcoholic, who cooperated poorly with the treatment program, bony consolidation was delayed for $1^1/_2$ years.

Finally, in six of the 275 hips we observed heterotopic ossifications in proximity of the trochanteric osteotomy, but this did not affect the operative result.

Discussion

Growth abnormalities of the proximal femur as a complication of treatment of a congenitally dislocated hip can lead to marked deformities about the hip. Shortening of the femoral neck with elevation of the greater trochanter is a typical example. This deformity has two major effects on the hip joint:

1. The greater trochanter becomes elevated and medialized relative to the center of rotation of the hip. The elevation of the greater trochanter removes tension from the pelvitrochanteric muscles and decreases their efficiency. The medialization of the greater trochanter places it closer to the center of the femoral head, and thus to the center of hip rotation. This shortens the lever arm of the muscles, and causes them, in stabilizing the hip, to develop more tension than would be the case if the femoral neck length were normal. This increased muscle tension adds to the loads imposed on the hip. Hence, a shortening of the femoral neck has the effect of increasing pressure on the joint. The increased muscle tension needed for joint stability, combined with the loss of muscular efficiency due to elevation of the trochanter, results in a higher degree of muscular exertion, which leads to rapid fatiguability even with normal gait. The short femoral neck also places the greater trochanter closer to the acetabular roof, thereby restricting the range of hip motion, especially abduction. Moreover, the line of action of the pelvitrochanteric muscles acquires a more vertical orientation, which causes the pressure forces to become concentrated in the lateral part of the joint. This is particularly damaging since most of these hips have a shallow acetabulum with poor femoral head coverage. Thus, the lateralization of the pressure forces concentrates them over an already relatively small area of the articular surfaces.
2. The anatomic alterations, particularly the shortening of the femoral neck, tend to hamper or prevent important operative measures such as intertrochanteric osteotomy, pelvic osteotomy, and surface replacement arthroplasty (Wagner).

Corrective osteotomy of the greater trochanter can improve or eliminate all these functional and morphologic deficiencies. By increasing the relative length of the femoral neck and normalizing the lever arms about the hip, this operation is beneficial in three respects:

1. The increase in the lever arm of the muscles improves hip performance. This is particularly apparent in the Trendelenburg test.
2. The normalization of the lever arms about the hip reduces the pressure loads on the joint. The redirection of the lines of muscle action leads to a distribution of the pressure over a larger joint area. This explains the value of the trochanteric osteotomy in preventing late degenerative disease. The redirection of forces has the added advantage of stimulating bone remodeling and promoting the healing of osteoarthritic cysts.
3. The relative lengthening of the femoral neck by the trochanteric transfer creates morphologic conditions that are favorable for subsequent operations on the proximal femur and acetabulum.

Dysplastic hips in which the femoral neck is shortened and the greater trochanter is elevated have a strong tendency to develop degenerative arthritis with passage of time. If treatment is deferred until degenerative changes appear, surgical correction of the greater trochanter will still be required. This provides a sound rationale for the early selection of a trochanteric osteotomy before degenerative disease appears, so that the valuable prognostic effect of the procedure can be fully utilized.

Weighing the minor nature of the operation against its highly beneficial effect on hip joint mechanics, one might characterize corrective osteotomy of the greater trochanter as the most efficient joint-saving operation that may be performed about the hip.

Problems and complications are infrequent and minor, but the operation does require careful technique. Three points in particular must be reemphasized:

1. During the osteotomy, care must be taken not to injure the blood vessels in the trochanteric fossa, or femoral head necrosis could result.
2. When mobilizing the greater trochanter, one must carefully free all adhesions between the medial aspect of the trochanter and the joint capsule so that the trochanter can be mobilized, without force, against the *elastic* resistance of the attached muscles.
3. When the greater trochanter is fixed to the lateral aspect of the femur, good bony contact must be established to ensure rapid consolidation. In addition, a strong tension-band suture must be placed between the vastus lateralis and the insertion of the gluteus medius. This suture will absorb much of the tension from the pelvitrochanteric muscles, and protect the fixation screws from excessive bending loads, which makes early physiotherapy possible.

It should be emphasized that corrective osteotomy of the greater trochanter is indicated only if the position of the trochanter is pathologic. It has no role in the treatment of osteoarthritic conditions in which the proximal femur has a normal anatomy.

Summary

Corrective osteotomy of the greater trochanter was performed in a series of 300 hips which showed shortening of the femoral neck and elevation of the greater trochanter as a result of congenital dislocation. Late follow-up was possible in 275 hips.

The patients were selected according to three general criteria:

Group I: Muscular insufficiency of the hip, chiefly in young patients

Group II: As part of surgical reconstruction of complex deformities about the hip

Group III: Osteoarthritis of the hip secondary to dysplasia

In all three groups, trochanteric osteotomy was found to be a highly effective mode of treatment. In patients with muscular hip insufficiency, the major effect of the surgery was to improve the Trendelenburg sign. In patients with significant osteoarthritis secondary to dysplasia, pain relief and improved bone structure were the principal benefits. Complications and problems were minor and infrequent. The operation is not indicated for osteoarthritis of the hip in which the anatomy of the proximal femur is normal.

References

Chiari K (1955) Ergebnisse mit der Beckenosteotomie als Pfannendachplastik. Z Orthop 87:14–26

Wagner H (1978) Femoral osteotomies for congenital hip dislocation. Progr Orthop Surg 2:85–105

Wagner H (1978) Experiences with spherical acetabular osteotomy for the correction of the dysplastic acetabulum. Progr Orthop Surg 2:131–145

Wagner H (1978) Surface replacement arthroplasty of the hip. Clin Orthop 134:102–130

Subject Index

R. Bombelli

Osteoarthritis of the Hip

Classification and Pathogenesis
The Role of Osteotomy as a Consequent Therapy

With a Foreword by M. E. Müller
2nd, revised and enlarged edition. 1983. 374 figures (partly in colour).
XVIII, 386 pages. ISBN 3-540-11422-X

Renato Bombelli, Professor of Orthopedics at the University of Milan, has treated more than 1500 cases of primary and secondary osteoarthritis of the hip in the last 20 years. This book is the result of his clinical, radiological and surgical observations in the course of this distinguished career. In it, Prof. Bombelli details the biomechanics of the normal and diseased hip and shows that the natural healing process can be accelerated through changes induced by surgery on the forces acting on the hip. Bombelli's intertrochanteric osteotomy subjects the superior capsule of the hip to tension to induce osteophyte formation along the superior lip of the acetabulum, forming a physiological "shelf" and thereby increasing the weight bearing area of the hip. His procedure is shown to produce excellent results, particularly in young adults. For this second, revised and enlarged edition, Prof. Bombelli has further refined his classification of osteoarthritis of the hip, his theory of hip biomechanics, and the indications for osteotomy. He has also included updated clinical statistics which lend credence to his conclusion that, whereas the best hip replacement is of unknown but certainly finite duration, a hip healed after osteotomy will often last a lifetime.

The Cementless Fixation of Hip Endoprostheses

Edited by **E. Morscher**

1984. 230 figures. XV, 284 pages. ISBN 3-540-12254-0

This book examines the problems associated with hip endoprostheses, emphasizing the possibilities and limitations of cementless fixation.
It surveys the biomechanics of prosthetic loosening, the biochemistry of implants, and the choice of implant material. Special consideration is also given to the design of acetabular prostheses, the character of the prosthetic surface, and the elastic and mechanical properties of the implant.
The volume comprises the papers presented at a symposium on cementless hip endoprostheses, held in Basle in June, 1982. This was the first symposium ever held which dealt exclusively with this topic. There were presentations on various methods of hip endoprosthetic attachment used at present, as well as those still being tested and assessed. This is the first comprehensive account of cementless hip prostheses and provides an overview of the special problems in this field. It summarizes the current state of knowledge and indicates the direction of future developments.

Springer-Verlag
Berlin
Heidelberg
New York
Tokyo

P. G. J. Maquet

Biomechanics of the Hip

As Applied to Osteoarthritis and Related Conditions

1984. Approx. 285 figures. Approx. 56 tables. Approx. 300 pages

ISBN 3-540-13257-0

Surgery of the Hip Joint

Volume 1

Editor: R. G. Tronzo

2nd edition. 1984. Approx. 500 figures. Approx. 548 pages

ISBN 3-540-90922-2

E. W. Somerville

Displacement of the Hip in Childhood

Aetiology, Management and Sequelae

1982. 262 figures. XIII, 200 pages. ISBN 3-540-10936-6

E. Letournel, R. Judet

Fractures of the Acetabulum

Translated from the French and Edited by R. A. Elson

1981. 289 figures in 980 separate illustrations. XXI, 428 pages

ISBN 3-540-09875-5

J. Charnley

Low Friction Arthroplasty of the Hip

Theory and Practice

1979. 440 figures, 205 in colour, 22 tables. X, 376 pages

ISBN 3-540-08893-8

R. Liechti

Hip Arthrodesis and Associated Problems

Foreword by M. E. Müller, B. G. Weber

Translated from the German edition by P. A. Casey

1978. 266 figures, 35 tables. XII, 269 pages. ISBN 3-540-08614-5

F. Pauwels

Biomechanics of the Normal and Diseased Hip

Theoretical Foundation, Technique and Results of Treatment

An Atlas

Translated from the German by R. J. Furlong, P. Maquet

1976. 305 figures, in 853 separate illustrations. VII, 276 pages

ISBN 3-540-07428-7

Springer-Verlag
Berlin
Heidelberg
New York
Tokyo

MIX
Papier aus verantwortungsvollen Quellen
Paper from responsible sources
FSC® C105338

If you have any concerns about our products,
you can contact us on
ProductSafety@springernature.com

In case Publisher is established outside the EU,
the EU authorized representative is:
Springer Nature Customer Service Center GmbH
Europaplatz 3, 69115 Heidelberg, Germany

Printed by Libri Plureos GmbH
in Hamburg, Germany